The Social Context of Birth

The Social Context of Birth

SECOND EDITION

Edited by

CAROLINE SQUIRE

Senior Lecturer
Faculty of Health and Human Sciences
Thames Valley University

Radcliffe Publishing
Oxford • New York

Radcliffe Publishing Ltd
18 Marcham Road
Abingdon
Oxon OX14 1AA
United Kingdom

www.radcliffe-oxford.com
Electronic catalogue and worldwide online ordering facility.

Reprinted 2009, 2010

First Edition 2003

Caroline Squire has asserted her right under the Copyright, Designs and Patents Act 1998 to be identified as the author of this work.

British Library Cataloguing in Publication Data

A catalogue record for this book is available from the British Library.

ISBN-13: 978 184619 253 1

The paper used for the text pages of this book is FSC certified. FSC (The Forest Stewardship Council) is an international network to promote responsible management of the world's forests.

Printed on totally chlorine-free paper.

Typeset by Pindar NZ, Auckland, New Zealand
Printed and bound by TJI Digital, Padstow, Cornwall, UK

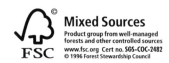
Mixed Sources
Product group from well-managed forests and other controlled sources
www.fsc.org Cert no. SGS-COC-2482
© 1996 Forest Stewardship Council

Contents

Preface to the second edition

This book seeks to engage with the social context in which women give birth in the UK. To me and like-minded midwives, childbirth is much more than a biological event or a set of case notes with a number. No one has an 'uneventful' pregnancy and there are always stories through which women can explain and try to make sense of what has happened to them, why it happened and how they feel about it now. Giving birth *always* occurs within a social context, and an understanding of that context enriches the understanding a midwife must have if she is to work *alongside* a woman and her family throughout their pregnancy and birth in an insightful, intelligent and informed manner.

The UK is an industrialised, capitalist, technological society, and that is the context in which women give birth and the culture in which we, as midwives, work. In this sociocultural milieu, a business culture prevails where non-clinical managers must balance the books and make decisions that profoundly affect the resources available to midwives and obstetricians. Here, also, the biosciences have achieved dominance. 'A' must equal 'B', the rituals of childbirth must be followed 'just in case', particularly in an era of (perceived) risk management, women should *be delivered* in hospital and 'authoritative knowledge' is scientific. In this positivist environment, the importance of the social aspects of birth is denied; women are muted and learn to mistrust their bodies. Often, midwives feel muted and find it hard to act as advocates where thinking is in absolutes and care is often fragmented. Currently, midwives feel stretched and tired in a role that can be so rewarding and enriching – but can also be so draining emotionally and physically when resources become scarce and it becomes impossible to do one's best for women. Possessing knowledge of the culture of midwifery as well as the social context in which women birth their children must be beneficial to midwives as we struggle to create a more woman-centred environment and make our own work practices more enabling not only for birthing women but also for ourselves.

The first few chapters set the scene. Chapter 1 considers not only women who give birth in the UK but also the lives of midwives because we are, in the main, female. The midwifery profession is considered alongside the progression of women over the last hundred years or so. It seems reasonable to think that how we, as midwives, view ourselves as women affects how we interact with pregnant women and how we perform as advocates. Are we with women, with maternity unit policies, with institutions, with obstetricians? Is it still a man's world? Are mothers valued? Are midwives valued? Do midwives value themselves? Does UK society value technological midwives more than midwives with the great skills of patience, intelligent observation and skills of listening to women, and who possess great belief in women's ability to birth children naturally? So many questions and many more to answer. To be a midwife and a woman is challenging enough, but we also have to possess knowledge and understanding of how other women feel and behave and the differences and similarities that exist between us in order to be 'with woman' and practise in a so-called 'woman-centred' manner.

Sandy Nelson considers the fundamental issue of sex in Chapter 2, in order to inform the reader of the sexual lives of other women including pregnancy and sexuality and cultural differences. Strands of this chapter interweave with Cathryn Britton's chapter on breastfeeding (Chapter 18). The UK still has a poor record on breastfeeding, but it is not surprising when one considers the social context in which women feed their babies.

Chapter 3 considers the problems that women specifically encounter when they are poor. These include lone parenthood and the gender issues pertaining to paid work, for example, part-time work and low pay. These issues are also touched upon in Val Dunn-Toroosian's chapter about the family (Chapter 4). In this chapter, the many diversities of what is considered a family are critically analysed. During these discussions, the lone-parent family is key in any critical exploration of poverty and social exclusion and most lone parents are women struggling to keep children and participate, if they can, in the arena of paid work. The issues of poverty and social exclusion are further explored in Dave Sookhoo's chapter on 'race' and ethnicity (Chapter 5), where the vexed problems of racist attitudes are addressed, which are uncomfortable for some midwives but important to approach.

Chapter 6 looks at the social lives of refugee women, while Chapter 8, by Comfort Momoh, considers women who have experienced genital mutilation. These chapters inform us of how women experience their lives in very different social contexts and how important it is for midwives to have knowledge of their specific needs. In Chapter 7, Sally Cottrell discusses domestic violence and pregnancy, a problem that is pandemic, occurring in every kind of domestic arena throughout the world. An important consideration is the issue of midwives in the UK experiencing domestic violence and how this might affect their practice. This idea, of ourselves as midwives experiencing social problems such as those of the pregnant women we work alongside, is very important to tackle as it occurs again and again. An example is in Chapter 15, which explores childhood sexual abuse and childbirth. It may have occurred to any pregnant woman, and to any midwife.

Fortunately, most women love their children but some experience difficulties in relating to their babies and in making the transition to being a mother. In Chapter 9, Nicola Winson discusses the many transitions women make when becoming mothers, particularly for the first time, and in Chapter 10, Cathy Rowan considers maternal–infant attachment and, importantly, describes how scientific technologies have affected this attachment for better or worse. Key questions are asked as to whether we, as society, value mothers and their role of raising families. Tim Blackshaw considers fathers and childbirth in Chapter 13, in terms of how industrialisation and hospitalisation of childbirth contributed to both the absence and subsequent attendance of fathers at the births of their children. This is an area that has altered greatly over the years with unprecedented numbers of fathers being present at the births of their children. In the last few years, the question of how midwives can support husbands and partners has gained interest.

In Chapter 12, Chris McCourt considers the importance of social support in childbirth in all of its complexities and in a society where families may well be physically separated by long distances. The concept of social support is often not well understood, but it can be argued that a sophisticated understanding is fundamental to being an insightful midwife. It is also crucial to the experiences of becoming a mother and this is explored by Christine Grabowska in Chapter 14 concerning unhappiness after childbirth. This chapter delineates clearly the difficulties many women face after they give birth in a society where their psychological needs may not be taken seriously, particularly if they have birthed a healthy child and they seem to be healthy themselves.

Chapters 11, 16 and 17 concerning the medicalisation of childbirth (Alyson Henly-Einion), assisted conception (Marilyn Crawshaw), and fetal surveillance (Christine Grabowska) engage with the rise and dominance of a scientific culture. Clearly, there have been many benefits to childbirth from technology, but there have also been drawbacks. Many women have felt that they were objectified in hospital and lost much of their control over themselves and their ability to give birth. There are many questions to ask. For example, does society control the lives of fetuses through screening? Does the fetus have human rights? What are the ethical considerations that surround the field of medically assisted conceptions?

The complexities of screening and ethics bring us to the concept of disability and the inclusion in this second edition of a fresh chapter on this subject. In Chapter 19, Harriet Clarke has contributed an important discussion focusing on the attitudes of society to disability, and to disability and parenthood. As midwives, we need to be aware of the social context of the disabled and those embarking on the journey to becoming parents so that we can practise insightfully and be sensitive to their special needs.

This book does not attempt to approach all the key issues relating to women, women as midwives and women giving birth. It will, however, help the reader to understand the similarities and differences between women so that the concept of being midwife – 'with woman' – becomes a little clearer and easier to grasp.

Caroline Squire
March 2009

About the editor

Caroline Squire is a senior lecturer at Thames Valley University. She qualified as a midwife in 1981, and practised in a variety of inner and outer London hospitals before qualifying as a lecturer in 1988.

She has a key interest in women's studies, particularly in cross–cultural contexts, and has a degree in Medical Anthropology. At the university where she works her areas of specialisation include women who have experienced domestic abuse, female genital cutting and those who are giving birth following sexual abuse when they were children.

Caroline is also an acupuncturist and oriental herbal medical practitioner. She runs a clinic at the university for members of staff and students, which has been running since 1999.

List of contributors

Kate H Beverley MSc, MA, Cert Ed, RN, RM, RCNT
Senior Lecturer (retired)
Faculty of Health and Human Sciences
Thames Valley University

Tim Blackshaw MSc, BSc (Hons), CSCT (Cert), RCNT, RN
Senior Lecturer
Faculty of Health and Human Sciences, Thames Valley University

Cathryn Britton RN, RM, ADM, PGCEA, MSc, PhD
Lecturer
Department of Health Sciences, University of York

Harriet Clarke BA, PhD
Lecturer
Institute of Applied Social Studies, University of Birmingham

Sally Cottrell BSc, RM, MCGI, NNEB
Consultant Midwife
North Bristol NHS Trust

Marilyn Crawshaw MA, CQSW
Senior Lecturer
Department of Social Policy and Social Work, University of York
Adviser to UK Donorlink

Val Dunn-Toroosian RN, RNT, BA, MSc
Senior Lecturer
Faculty of Health and Human Sciences, Thames Valley University

Christine Grabowska MSc, BSc (Hons), RN, RM, ADM, PGCEA, LicAc, LicOHM, DipCST, Postgraduate Diploma (Research Methods)
Senior Lecturer
Faculty of Health and Human Sciences, Thames Valley University

Alyson Henley-Einion RN, RM, DipHE (Nursing), BSc (Hons), PGCEA, MA, MAPD
Senior Lecturer
Faculty of Health and Life Sciences, University of the West of England, Bristol

Jo James MSc, RGN
Clinical Redesigner, BECaD Project
Central Middlesex Hospital

Christine McCourt BA, PhD
Professor of Anthropology and Health
Centre for Research in Midwifery and Childbirth, Thames Valley University

Comfort Momoh MBE, PhD, RN, RM, FPN, BSc
Female Genital Mutilation/Public Health Specialist Midwife
Guy's and St Thomas' Hospital Trust

Sandy Nelson BEd, MA
Senior Lecturer
Faculty of Health and Human Sciences, Thames Valley University

Cathy Rowan MA, RM, RN, ADM, PGCEA, Postgraduate Diploma (Research Methods)
Senior Lecturer
Faculty of Health and Human Sciences, Thames Valley University

Dave Sookhoo PhD, MEd, BA, RN, RMN, DipN
Principal Lecturer (Research)
Faculty of Health and Human Sciences, Thames Valley University

Caroline Squire MSc, RM, RN, ADM, PGCEA, LicAc, LicOHM Postgraduate Diploma (Research Methods)
Senior Lecturer
Faculty of Health and Human Sciences, Thames Valley University

Nicola Winson MA, RN, RM, ADM, PCGEA
Senior Lecturer
Faculty of Health and Human Sciences, Thames Valley University

Acknowledgements

I would like to acknowledge the invaluable help of Julia Magill-Cuerden with the first edition of this book. I would also like to thank Marc Forster, Subject Librarian at the Learning Resource Centre at Thames Valley University for his constant patience and support. Finally, I give my thanks to my midwifery friends and colleagues for their friendship and support over many years.

This edition is dedicated to my godson Tom, Fleur and Louise, my late cousin Sue, Nigel, Jonathon, Peter, June, my godson Roger, Becky, Christopher, Kate, my goddaughter Stephanie, Suzanne and Michael, Richard, Isobel, Tom, Sue, David, Pat, Nikki, Nicky, Neil, Eva, Anna, and the many other members of my family.

CHAPTER 1

Women and society

Caroline Squire

Pregnancy and childbirth are unique events in the lives of women. Midwives and health professionals need to have knowledge and understanding of the social and cultural context that influences women and their lives, and in which they give birth. Midwives and health professionals also need to understand the culture of maternity services in which they work and how it supports or impedes so-called 'woman-centred' midwifery. Women's subjective and collective experiences of life will depend upon such factors as age, ethnicity, social and economic background and how these factors interrelate, contradict and intersect with each other. The study of women's lives is complex but necessary for midwives and health professionals in order to be able to practise in a so-called 'woman-centred' manner. This chapter discusses the key feminist theories that have contributed to explanations about the experiences of being women as well as consideration of the sex/gender debate. The concept of 'woman-centred practice' is also addressed with particular reference to postmodernist feminist theory.

INTRODUCTION

'She is defined and differentiated with reference to Man and not he with reference to her; she is the incidental, the inessential as opposed to the essential. . . . He is the Subject, he is the Absolute – she is the Other' (de Beauvoir 1953: xiv). This is from the translation of de Beauvoir's seminal [sic] text, published in 1949. There is a popular view that times have changed for the better, that women have achieved equality. Is this true or an illusion? Certainly, in this country, individual women seem freer and more powerful than before. They drive fast cars, appear on television interviewing politicians (as opposed to being 'weather girls'), become Members of Parliament (MPs), become Prime Minister, down pints of beer in the pub, live alone, pay the bills, marry men but do not promise to obey their husbands, have children or decide not to have children, and so the list continues.

However, a brief look at the major systems and structures that underpin our society reveals a very different story. Religion remains a major influence in every society

1

whether one attends church or not. There are no female Roman Catholic priests, very few female Anglican priests (*see* Table 1.1), and no Islamic, Hindu or Buddhist female clerics.

TABLE 1.1 Proportion of ordinations by gender: 1994–2006 – www.cofe.anglican.org

	1994	1995	1996	1997	1998	1999	2000	2001	2002	2003	2004	2005	2006
Stipendiary men	244	245	201	186	174	199	223	190	199	181	143	155	128
Stipendiary women	72	65	67	57	67	78	90	105	112	120	92	99	95
Non-stipendiary men	55	30	46	69	73	61	81	65	67	55	63	81	82
Non-stipendiary women	34	42	59	67	87	76	107	89	104	77	93	108	118

(Archbishops' Council 2008)

The path before and since the ordination of women to the priesthood in 1992 has not been smooth and heated debate continues over the decision taken in July 2008 by the General Synod of the Church of England to allow for the consecration of women bishops. The following are press releases to illustrate what has been reported in some of the media. The first two are from before the decision was taken and the last was published afterwards:

1,300 CLERGY THREATEN TO DEFECT IN THE WOMEN BISHOPS ROW –
DAILY MAIL

More than 1,300 clergy have written to the Archbishop of Canterbury saying they will defect from the Church of England if women are consecrated as bishops.

Members of the group, which includes 11 serving bishops, say they will take decisive action if two votes are passed this weekend to allow female bishops.

By *Caroline Grant*
Last updated at 1:54 a.m. on 1st July 2008

CHURCH OF ENGLAND MUST GO AHEAD WITH PLANS TO CREATE WOMEN BISHOPS, SAYS SENIOR CLERGYMAN – ***DAILY MAIL***

A senior bishop urged the Church of England yesterday to ignore warnings that allowing women to become bishops would 'shatter the unity of the Church' – and to plough ahead with the historic reform.

The Bishop of Manchester, the Rt Rev Nigel McCulloch, told the General Synod in York that there were 'hard choices' to be made.

But he warned it would be a 'sad day' and 'dangerous' if members delayed establishing equality in the top ranks.

By *Mail-on-Sunday* reporter
Last updated at 10:38 p.m. on 5th July 2008

CHURCH IS NOT WOUNDED AND BLEEDING, SAYS WILLIAMS – *GUARDIAN*

Archbishop acknowledges 'unfinished business'
  Pledge to engage with bishops in boycott
  The archbishop of Canterbury yesterday acknowledged the alienation and grievance felt by traditionalists following a decision to allow women bishops, but insisted the church was not 'a bleeding, hunted animal with arrows in its side'.

By *Riazat Butt*, religious affairs correspondent
Guardian, 22nd July 2008

There are many more comments such as the above from the media. Attention has been paid to this topic because of the, at times, vitriolic backlash against the consecration of female bishops. It appears anachronistic in this postmodern age but Judeo–Christianity underpins UK Society in terms of the laws of the land and, arguably, moral codes of conduct and opinion and it is an important marker to illustrate the status of women in UK society.

MPs rule the country politically. There has been but one female Prime Minister (Margaret Thatcher), one female Speaker of the House of Commons (Bettie Boothroyd), and only a handful of female Secretaries of State (no Chancellors of the Exchequer). Table 1.2 shows the slow progression of women members of parliament (MPs) in the UK.

The number of women MPs in the UK doubled in 1997 and this was under the Blair Labour Government of that time. These female MPs were then referred to as 'Blair's babes' – a derogatory and infantilising term. Currently, in 2008, the UK has 7 female cabinet ministers of 24 cabinet members. The situation is different in other countries within the European Union. Spain has 9 women ministers out of 17 in its Cabinet, Finland 12 out of 20 and France 7 out of 15 (Owen 2008). The UK does not seem to welcome women at senior level. In any event, this woeful under-representation of women within conventional politics in the UK is crucial in thinking about democracy and gender (Abbot, Wallace and Tyler 2005).

The legal system within a society may be said to prevent anarchy and, thus, is absolutely fundamental to social cohesion and function of any civilised society. The legal profession may profess that more than half of all newly qualified lawyers are women but where do they go? Table 1.3 records a depressingly static state of affairs in terms of the numbers of women in the higher echelons of the judiciary in England and Wales from 2003–07 (Lord Chancellor's Department 2008).

TABLE 1.2 Women in the House of Commons: House of Commons Information Office Factsheet M4 (2008)

Women members elected at General Elections: 1918–2005

Date of election	Total	% of all MPs
14 Dec 1918	1	0.1
15 Dec 1922	2	0.3
6 Dec 1923	8	1.3
29 Oct 1924	4	0.7
30 May 1929	14	2.3
27 Oct 1931	15	2.4
14 Nov 1935	9	1.5
5 Jul 1945	24	3.8
23 Feb 1950	21	3.4
25 Oct 1951	17	2.7
26 May 1955	24	3.8
8 Oct 1959	25	4.0
15 Oct 1964	29	4.6
31 Mar 1966	26	4.1
18 Jun 1970	26	4.1
28 Feb 1974	23	3.6
10 Oct 1974	27	4.3
3 May 1979	19	3.0
9 Jun 1983	23	3.5
11 Jun 1987	41	6.3
9 Apr 1992	60	9.2
1 May 1997	120	18.2
7 Jun 2001	118	17.9
5 May 2005	128	19.8

There has been very little change over the last five years in terms of women in the higher echelons of the judiciary, which means that, broadly speaking, women still remain judged by men.

In October 1999, the Equal Opportunities Commission (EOC) launched 'Valuing Women', a major three-year campaign for equal pay (Equal Opportunities Commission 2002). Ahead of the campaign launch, the EOC commissioned three studies to assess current attitudes towards, and awareness of, equal pay. Some of the overall key findings were as follows:

- There is a low level of awareness of the gender pay gap.
- Half of all women and men think the gender pay gap is unfair.

TABLE 1.3 Annual diversity statistics: Lord Chancellor's Department 2008

Post	Year	Total	Female No.	Female %
Lords of Appeal in ordinary	2007	12	1	8.3
	2006	12	1	8.3
	2005	12	1	8.3
	2004	12	1	8.3
	2003	11	0	0
Lord Justices of Appeal	2007	37	3	8.1
	2006	37	3	8.1
	2005	37	2	5.4
	2004	37	2	5.4
	2003	35	3	8.6
High Court Judges	2007	108	10	9.3
	2006	107	11	10.2
	2005	107	10	9.3
	2004	105	8	7.6
	2003	106	6	5.7

- Most people do not know what their colleagues earn and only a minority have ever asked.
- Almost half of all students state that equal pay would influence their choice of job; women are much more likely to state this than men.

Interestingly, in research with line managers, both male and female line managers regarded men as the main breadwinners, whose key role is to provide for their families. Male line managers generally regarded women as secondary earners, a view which some (but not all) women shared. Looking at these comments, it is not difficult to see how men may be reluctant to promote women and to give them equal pay. This campaign was followed up with a report monitoring its progress in 2003 (Neathey, Dench and Thomson) and, of course, the Equality Act of 2006. The latest publication is the Framework for a Fairer Future – The Equality Bill (Government Equalities Office 2008) presented to Parliament in June 2008. One of its clauses (p. 23) states:

> The Equality Bill will outlaw pay secrecy clauses and make it unlawful to stop employees discussing their pay.

It also recommends the further use of equal pay job evaluation audits, which ascertain how women and men are rewarded as employees in an organisation and will expose any gender pay gap. It will be interesting to see how this develops in the future.

Many women are, of course, perfectly at ease with never having paid employment during their marriages/partnerships, or with interrupted careers. This situation is not problematic unless the partnership breaks up and/or divorce occurs, with children often involved. Then, many women find themselves experiencing poverty. Furthermore, women who never experience paid employment are often in the position whereby the household does not rely financially on two wages. Arguably, women in lower socio–economic groups are rarely able to experience 'career breaks' or not having to work for financial gain.

At the top end of the labour market, the situation remains iniquitous with the so–called 'glass–ceiling' remaining evident. Almost half of the top one hundred companies have no women on the board. Only eight of them employ female executive directors and the number is falling, not rising (Connon 2001). There have also been several high profile law suits taken out, against leading banks and insurance companies in particular, for sexual harassment and discrimination – see Gammell (2008) as an example. However, on the plus side, the first female chairman of a FTSE 100 company commenced that role in January 2002. Whether this will have any effect on the employment of women in higher or lower paid work is seriously doubtful but remains to be seen.

The picture remains poor in the fields of obstetrics and gynaecology, surely an area where a preponderance of female practitioners might be expected. In the year 2000, there were 1246 consultants, of whom 274 (24%) were women (RCOG 2001). Table 1.4 illustrates some improvement since 2000.

TABLE 1.4 Number of consultants in obstetric and gynaecology posts in England and Wales, 2003–07: (RCOG 2008)

	2003	2004	2005	2006	2007
Total	1384	1466	1544	1600	1629
Male	1020	1063	1094	1141	1114
Female	364 (36%)	403 (38%)	450 (41%)	459 (40%)	515 (46%)

These figures seem particularly ironic and contradictory considering they relate to a field of medicine that is directly pertinent to women and can have dramatic effects on the lives of women for better or for worse. There has been some improvement and many, though not all, hope that women will soon constitute over 50% of consultant posts. Higham and Steer (2004) on the other hand are concerned about the so–called anti–male environment for medical students in maternity services and state:

> Excluding men from important aspects of reproduction is fundamentally unwise; the lack of adequate male role models is already widely cited as a problem afflicting society as a whole. (Higham and Steer 2004: 143)

This seems an extraordinary example of self importance. However, whether having more female than male consultants will contribute to maternity services being more 'woman–centred' is debatable since the role of consultant is traditionally a male gendered role and it remains to be seen what happens in the future.

It would be possible to continue giving examples of women's absence from key positions of power and influence within the social system. Does this matter one might think? This chapter will argue that this is a matter of real concern and will address key feminist theories that have informed women's thinking. Radical feminism and postmodernist feminism will be focused upon and comparisons made with the history of midwifery and childbirth in the 20th century. The sex/gender debate will also be discussed; it will conclude that women and men are different and analyses of similarities and differences between women may be fruitful in the future. The chapter concludes with a discussion about postmodern feminist theory and how it helps to explain the differences and similarities in women's experiences of the complexities and contradictions in their lives.

FEMINIST THEORIES

There are a number of feminist theoretical approaches to the explanation of gender inequalities. As these theories differ markedly from one another, it is not possible to consider the socialisation of women from a single feminist perspective. The diverse range of theories mirrors the complexity and variation to be found within women's lives across society and across different societies.

The word 'feminism' engenders many different, but profound, feelings amongst women and men alike. Stereotypes of feminists such as butch and man-haters abound. The following description from a health and beauty magazine in contemporary media provides an illustration:

> For too long women have had to choose the hard or soft option – you were either feminist or feminine, careerist or carer, pinstripes or pincurls, hard-nosed or high-heeled. Thankfully, most of us no longer feel the need to take sides. Our mothers might have had to burn their bras to make a point, but now – with due credit to them and the Battle of the Sexes they fought on our behalf – we can wear an Agent Provocateur push-up balconette to work, without feeling like an extra in a Carry On movie. (Allen 2001: 37–8)

So, feminists are the 'hard option': careerist, pinstriped and hard-nosed. These words may seem amusing to some but, in truth, are sexist pejorative labels meant to discredit and humiliate women, who are perceived by some men and women to be a threat to the patriarchal status quo. Incidentally, the infamous photograph taken in the 1970s of women burning their bras was fallacious. Women were seen to be throwing their bras into a waste bin, but the image of the flames was superimposed.

This section of the chapter seeks to relate the development of feminist theories from the modernist period (1960s and 1970s) to the contemporary postmodern period. These perspectives are, themselves, manifestations of the struggle to enable women in academia to have their voices articulated within mainstream (male-stream) sociological discourse. Sociology, as an academic discipline, only acknowledged the 'validity' of feminist theory in the 1970s. Such theories offer particular analyses and explanations of how and why women have less power than men and how this imbalance can be challenged and transformed. Knowledge such as this is of clear, fundamental importance to midwives and healthcare professionals who work with women; indeed the word 'midwife' means 'with woman'. Midwives are encouraged to practise in a 'woman-centred' manner and, thus, an understanding of how other women live their lives is imperative. Furthermore, the vast majority of midwives and nurses are women themselves and it is important that such practitioners have insight and self-awareness as to how they view themselves as women in order to assist other women in childbirth in a sensitive, empathetic and, so-called, woman-centred manner. Also, feminist perspectives may enable midwives to reappraise the constraints and limitations to which midwifery practice has been/is subjected in a maternity culture that is largely technological, positivist and hierarchical, with more men by far occupying the powerful roles of Chief Executive and Consultant Obstetrician.

Definitions

Feminism has been referred to as a philosophy, a worldview, a theory and method of analysis (McCool and McCool 1989). There is no single definition because there are multiple perspectives, but it may be useful to consider the following definition as a possible base-line:

> At the very least a feminist is someone who holds that women suffer discrimination because of their sex, that they have specific needs which remain negated and unsatisfied, and that satisfaction of these needs would require a radical change (some would say a revolution even) in the social, economic and political order. (Delmar 1986: 8)

Thus, a feminist is someone who recognises that there is discrimination against women, that their specific needs are unsatisfied and that there is necessity for radical change in order to meet these needs. However, when seeking the reasons and solutions to these problems, there are differing views or perspectives. The main feminist perspectives will now be considered briefly. It can be seen that they are broadly social constructionist in that the role of society is fundamental, the exception being radical feminism.

RADICAL FEMINISM: ITS CONTRIBUTION TO CHILDBIRTH AND PATRIARCHY

Of all the 'feminisms', radical feminism has been the one most misunderstood and most threatening to men (and to many women). The word 'radical' here means 'the root of'; it has a direct relationship with radical midwifery (Klima 2001). In terms of chronology, it can be seen that the development of women's position in society relates clearly to the recent history of midwifery and women's services, as shown in Table 1.5.

Radical feminism developed during the 1960s and 1970s as a theory to explain oppression of women. It coincided with the surge of the use of science and technology in childbirth, which many women were beginning to regale against due to their experience of loss of control and invisibility (Donnison 1977, Stanworth 1994, Tew 1998). Radical feminist theorists contend that the oppression of women is based centrally on patriarchy, the domination of women by men. The family is seen as a key instrument of the oppression of women through male control of women and children (with marriage, patrilineal heritage and the taking of the man's name as central to this control). Men, it is argued, systematically dominate women in every sphere of life, and all relationships between men and women are institutionalised relationships of power and therefore an appropriate subject for political analysis. Thus, radical feminists are concerned to reveal how male power is exercised and reinforced in all spheres of life. Included in the thrall of patriarchy are personal relationships, child rearing, housework and marriage

TABLE 1.5 History of women's position in society related to history of midwifery/women's services

Woman's Movement		History of Midwifery/women's services	
1897	The National Union of Women's Suffrage Societies formed: President: Millicent Fawcett	1902	The Midwives Act
1903	The Women's Social and Political Union, formed by the Pankhursts	1918	Second Midwives Act
1928	The Equal Franchise Act gave the vote to all women over 21 years	1929	British College of Obstetricians and Gynaecologists formed
1937	The Matrimonial Causes Act extended grounds for divorce to cruelty, desertion and insanity	1936	Third Midwives Act
1964	The Married Women's Property Act enabled a divorced wife to keep half of anything she had saved from any allowance given by her husband	1956	Natural Childbirth Association (NCA) formed in response to the medicalisation of childbirth, which developed rapidly during the 1950s and 1960s
1960	The beginnings of 'second-wave' 1970s radical feminism	1961	National Childbirth Trust formed (name changed from NCA)
1970	The Equal Pay Act		
1975	The Sex Discrimination Act		
	The Employment Protection Act		
1976	The Domestic Violence Act	1981	First women's march on an NHS maternity hospital due to its over-medicalised policies
		1986	Foundation of the Association of Radical Midwives
1990s	The development of postmodernist feminist theory	1992	House of Commons Select Committee, Second Report
		1993	Department of Health, Changing Childbirth, Part 1: Report of the Expert Maternity Group
2006	The Equality Act	2007	Department of Health: Maternity Matters: Choice, Access and Continuity of care in a safe service

and the range of sexual practices including rape, prostitution, sexual harassment and sexual intercourse.

An analogy of the patriarchal nuclear family and the relationships between doctors, nurses and patients has been made by Littlewood (1991). It can be adapted to midwifery as follows – *see* Figure 1.1.

Here, obstetrics is seen as a male gendered profession – scientific, technological, active and patriarchal in its belief system. There is no room for women's individual

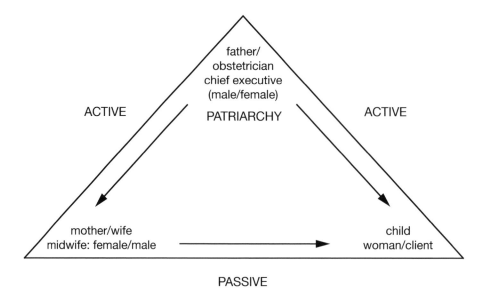

FIGURE 1.1 Representation of an analogy between the patriarchal nuclear family and relationships between obstetricians, midwives and women

emotional needs here. The midwife is seen as analogous to the 'wife' – necessary and useful, but inferior and, therefore, passive, in the hierarchy. She is there to be kind and caring and to support the obstetrician. And what of the woman? She is portrayed as passive and at the bottom of the hierarchy. If she is 'good', she will book early, make use of all the technology offered to her and will give birth in the hospital. The analogy is that of the child in the nuclear family. The Chief Executive has been added here in order to illustrate the shift in power relations in the NHS today. In this Capitalist system, it seems those with control of finances have the power to give or to take. Birth centres are being opened and yet closed depending on the location. Choices are being given and yet denied, depending on the location and the decisions of non-clinical managers.

Male science has been used to legitimise the ideologies that define women as inferior, and women's role as domestic labourers (Abbott, Wallace and Tyler 2005, Stanworth 1994). In the field of childbirth, the new reproductive technologies are now very fundamental to maternity services and becoming increasingly widespread. Crozier (2001), however, questions whether technology should be viewed as a purely masculine domain of knowledge which oppresses women since many women feel the technology to be empowering and beneficial in making choices. To think otherwise renders women as passive and subordinate. Are women, who profess to be in control when they use technology in childbirth, really in control or have they been frightened into believing the rhetoric of those whose interests lie in the use of technology – obstetricians and pharmaceutical companies for example? This is a vexed question that will tax midwives and healthcare professionals increasingly in the future.

Patriarchy

To return to the wider field of radical feminism, Mitchell (1974) is a key radical feminist theorist who has made a significant contribution to the understanding of the concept of patriarchy. She sees patriarchy as a universal feature of human societies, but argues that its origins are cultural rather than biological and that its maintenance is primarily through ideology. The ideas and beliefs through which women make sense of their lived experience are accomplished through socialisation and education. Arguably, it is men who write the gender socialisation scripts and thus ensure the continual reproduction of dominant masculinity and dominated femininity. An example of this would be domestic ideology, which identifies women particularly with the home, and the complementary 'bread-winner' ideology, by which men are supposed to provide financially for their families (Walby 1994, Connell 1994). These ideologies are obviously linked and co-contribute to making sense of the world, usually by supporting the status quo and reinforcing power relations so that they seem inevitable and the way it should be (Crowley and Himmelweit 1992). Mitchell (1974) suggests that what is needed is a specific struggle against patriarchy involving a cultural revolution to counter ideological notions of the feminine as being subordinate within society.

However, the concept of patriarchy has not been used within feminist theory in any simple or unified way. Its use varies from attempts to trace the origins of women's subordination, to the seeking of explanations as to how patriarchy works in terms of the different activities of women and men in society (Stacey 1993, Connell 1994).

Delphy (1984) has also made an important contribution to the debate concerning patriarchy. She considers there are two modes of production: the industrial mode of production, which is the arena of capitalist exploitation, and the family mode of production, in which men exploit women's labour. Men, she says, benefit from women's provision of domestic services and unpaid child rearing within the family and, therefore, women's reproductive and productive activities in the household are the main form of women's oppression.

Patriarchy also exerts influence over women in that 'motherhood' is set out as the superordinate role for all women. The depths of women's identification with this are revealed in the agonies that infertility brings. It is threatening the very essence of woman–identity. Furthermore, women who do not 'fit the mould' are disparaged and stigmatised. It may be considered tragic if a woman is unable to bear children, but she is abnormal if she has chosen not to be a mother.

Walby (1990, 1994) is another feminist writer who has made a major contribution to the debate surrounding patriarchy. She sees patriarchy and capitalism as two distinct systems, and notes that capitalism may benefit from patriarchy in that female domestic labour is unpaid and sustains male labour (an historical basis). However, she does not view women as victims and sees it as mainly due to women's own efforts that (in Britain) they have partly broken out of private patriarchy and achieved a stronger position on paid work.

Walby (1990) presents six main structures within which patriarchy occurs:
- paid employment ('glass ceiling', low pay, low status, part-time)
- household production (child rearing, housework, production of food)
- culture (including religion, media, education)
- sexuality (including definitions of sex as male orientated)
- male violence (domestic violence including marital rape, rape, pornography, childhood sexual abuse)
- the State.

Walby (1990) then considers that these six main structures of patriarchy are linked to private and public patriarchy. In private patriarchy, male domination occurs directly within the household structure and also by the exclusion of women from public life. In public patriarchy, women play roles within paid employment and in other structures, but their subordination is implemented by segregating them from the main areas of wealth, power and status (e.g. clerical work, low numbers of female consultant obstetricians). This analysis can be applied to midwifery in terms of historical social construction and devaluation of what is perceived as women's work (Brennan 2005). Importantly, Walby also considers that women have moved from being excluded from the main areas of wealth, power and status to being segregated within these areas. For example, more women work outside the home for money, so they are not excluded from paid work but they tend to take low-paid, part-time work and may fail to achieve the higher positions.

For midwives and healthcare professionals, patriarchy can be a useful tool for analysis in that it takes the male body as the 'standard, prototype', with the female body seen as 'defective, inferior'. This is particularly relevant to women, reproduction and the negative aspects of the medicalisation of childbirth whereby birth is only seen as normal in retrospect. Also, it can be argued that much of women's experience of ill health stems from their relationships with men and male dominated institutions (Doyal 1995). These experiences of ill health may include the sequelae of domestic violence, stress and poverty, which have profound effects on women and/or fetuses/children (Lewis 2007, Gary, Sigsby and Campbell 1998).

Liberal feminism

Historically, liberal feminism has concerned itself with equal opportunities for women and men and is considered reformist in nature. The Equal Pay Act (1970), the Sex Discrimination Act (1975) and the Equality Act (2006) could be said to be the results of a widely supported effort to achieve liberal equality between the sexes. Liberal feminists consider a woman's sex as irrelevant to her rights. They propose that, in Western industrial societies, women are discriminated against on the basis of sex in so far as certain restrictions are placed on women as a group without regard to their own individual wishes, interests, abilities and needs (Abbott, Wallace and Tyler 2005). Once discrimination is removed, it will be possible for women and men to be treated as individuals and women will be given the chance to show that they are as capable as men in all the key positions in society currently denied to them (Crowley and Himmelweit 1992). This was clearly demonstrated in Britain in the Second World War when women performed men's work (but not political leadership).

Liberal feminism is a useful theoretical approach in that equal opportunities, for example, are important to women. However, it does not address the underlying oppressive ideologies of the status of women in society (Crowley and Himmelweit 1992). It seeks to reform women's position to that of equality with men without a deconstruction of pervading masculinist ideologies and replacement with structures representing the views and needs of women.

Marxist feminism

In the 1970s, a number of feminist theorists began to draw on the writings of Marx in order to explain the oppression of women. In doing so, they had to extend his theories in order to make women 'visible' because Marxist analysis is essentialist in nature in that it presumes the biological basis of gender (power) relations. Here, women's oppression is seen to be tied to forms of capitalist exploitation of labour, and thus women's paid and unpaid work is analysed in relation to its function within the capitalist economy (Stacey 1993). Capitalism compounds women's oppression by systematically excluding them from the Labour Market, denying them the chance to sell their labour power. Marxist feminists have critiqued the state as not acting in women's interests and reinforcing relations of power. They have attempted to analyse the part played by the state in establishing and maintaining women's dependence within the family household and wage labour as interrelated systems (Watson 1999). Figure 1.2 below sets out the sexual division of labour in diagrammatic form.

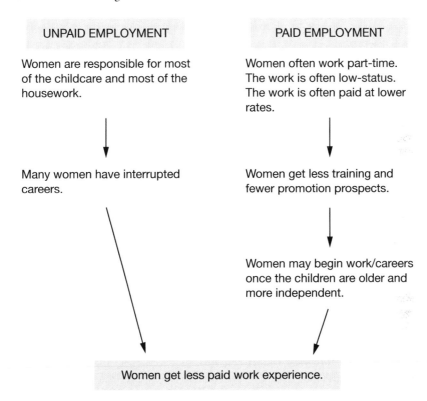

UNPAID EMPLOYMENT	PAID EMPLOYMENT
Women are responsible for most of the childcare and most of the housework.	Women often work part-time. The work is often low-status. The work is often paid at lower rates.
Many women have interrupted careers.	Women get less training and fewer promotion prospects.
	Women may begin work/careers once the children are older and more independent.

Women get less paid work experience.

FIGURE 1.2 The Sexual Division of Labour

In conversations with many women, midwives and healthcare professionals, it would seem the above holds true. Letvak (2001) considers that in Great Britain, traditional images of motherhood are enduring, pervasive and incompatible with paid employment. However, in a society with radically reconstructed structures favouring connection and respect between women and men, an alternative model of paid/unpaid work may be represented as shown in Figure 1.3.

Clearly, such a model needs a radical, ideological change to the structures and systems that make up society. Patriarchy has no place here. The ethos is of mutual respect, sharing and connection. In recent years, some maternity units have become much more flexible with midwives who need career breaks or wish to work part-time, but the change

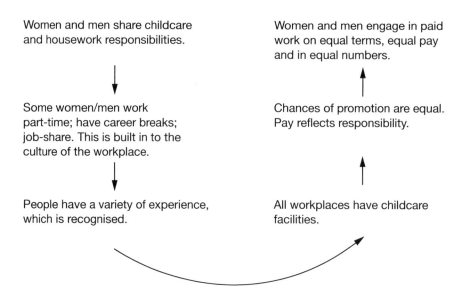

Women and men share childcare and housework responsibilities.

↓

Some women/men work part-time; have career breaks; job-share. This is built in to the culture of the workplace.

↓

People have a variety of experience, which is recognised.

Women and men engage in paid work on equal terms, equal pay and in equal numbers.

↑

Chances of promotion are equal. Pay reflects responsibility.

↑

All workplaces have childcare facilities.

FIGURE 1.3 An alternative model of paid/unpaid work for women and men

is largely because of the shortage of midwives rather than a radical change in the culture of the workplace.

Black feminism

Black feminists have been critical of the lack of centrality given to issues of ethnic difference, racialisation and racism in feminist theory and research (Abbott, Wallace and Tyler 2005). Anthias and Yuval-Davis (1992) go further by saying that black, minority and migrant women have been, on the whole, invisible within the feminist movement in Britain and they describe the feminist movement as white, middle-class and racist. Whilst class and gender may be seen as central to women's subordination, race is another form of social exclusion. The ways in which class, race and gender interact with one another may be different for black, minority and migrant women. Women who are oppressed and exploited by racism, and/or by imperialism, have powerful interests in common with their men, and these stand in opposition to those of white Western men and women. Therefore, the issues here are complex, revealing solidarities, contradictions and struggles with which women globally have to interact in their lives (Aziz 1992).

Stereotypes abound in healthcare literature concerning 'different' women, whether different by skin colour, religion, language or between themselves. Asian women are represented as passive and as being controlled within patriarchal family systems. Afro-Caribbean women are seen as dominating and running matriarchal family structures. Both stereotypes are devoid of analysis of class or gender despite the fact that many black women occupy low-paid, low-status jobs, experience poverty, and are particularly vulnerable to oppression (Abbott, Wallace and Tyler 2005). Again, despite the fact that there has been development of black and Asian middle classes, they will, nevertheless, suffer discrimination and prejudice. Bowler (1993), in her study of Asian women who had given birth, found clear evidence of stereotyping and prejudice among the midwives she interviewed including lack of maternal instinct, overuse of the service and non-use of contraception. Similarly, Katbamna (2000) found that periods of rest after childbirth can be interpreted as being indolent by some midwives. Further examples may be found in Dave Sookhoo's analysis of 'race', ethnicity, culture and childbirth (*see* Chapter 5).

This consideration of black feminism has been brief. However, it is important for midwives and health professionals to have a real understanding of the complex lives and experiences of black, migrant and minority women in order to practise in insightful ways.

POSTMODERN FEMINISM

Postmodernism constitutes a critique of traditional theorising and proposes that there can no longer be a claim that scientific theories actually 'capture' reality. Instead, theories are to be understood as partial representations or approximations of a reality that is more complex and multifaceted. Central to postmodern theory is the recognition of difference – race, sex, age – and deconstruction – a multiply divided subject in a multiply divided society (Abbott, Wallace and Tyler 2005). Women have similarities and differences and, therefore, so do midwives and healthcare professionals. It may be that a postmodern approach is best suited in terms of contributing to sensitive midwifery practice and trying to understand what it really means to work in partnership with women. 'Realities' in childbirth are always too complex for objective understanding, and recognition of this may lead to more sophisticated approaches in the attempt to understand what women want/need. The differing views of women and their relationship with technology and control, as mentioned earlier, is perhaps an example.

Postmodern feminists reject biological determinism and the notion of sex differences. Furthermore, they reject the idea of substituting feminist theories for male-stream ones because they argue that there is no possibility of true knowledge, only a multiplicity of truths. Instead, it is suggested that there is a need to deconstruct truth claims, to seek knowledge, but to recognise that knowledge is a part of power (Abbott, Wallace and Tyler 2005). Flax (1990) summarises the focus of postmodernism as how to understand and reconstitute the self, gender, knowledge, social relations, and culture without resorting to linear, holistic or binary ways of thinking and being.

However, postmodernism is problematic. It can be argued that difference is a way of not having to think about oppression and subordination and this makes it possible to ignore the centrality and reality of male power that has been fundamental to other feminisms. A politics of difference also assists in the rejection of the notion that there is a hierarchy of oppressions, that some oppressions are more salient than others or that oppressions are additive. Thus, the focus shifts to the ways in which each of these relations interact, reinforce and contradict each other in specific contexts (McDowell and Pringle 1992). Patriarchy, as 'reality', is denied and oppression ignored.

Postmodernism, therefore, is the antithesis of the biomedical system in which midwives work which encourages binary, linear models of thought. It may be that this form of theorising leads to a more sophisticated understanding of the complexities of different women's lives and may be of use to midwives and healthcare professionals in their interactions with different women and their families and with each other. The challenges are enormous. Midwives work in hierarchical institutions dominated by men, where both the ethos and structures are generally highly masculinised (Pringle 1995), and where binary ways of thinking abound. Roles, such as those of Chief Executive and Consultant Obstetrician, are male gendered even if occupied by females. It would be incredibly difficult to think in terms of a multiplicity of truths in a culture where scientific rigour is supposed to underpin practice. It is not suggested here that patriarchy, as a theory, should be abandoned but that postmodernism may contribute to a better understanding of difference. Nor is it suggested that any notion of women having beliefs, values or interests in common should be denied. Indeed, Zadoroznyj (1999), for example, found that social class had a strong effect in the shaping of identity in her study of birthing narratives. Information such as this is useful in trying to understand the experiences of different women. In summary, it is a question of balancing the different approaches of patriarchy and postmodernism in the quest for insightful practice.

Until now, this chapter has focused on the structural issues concerning women and society and on the contribution of primarily radical and postmodernist feminist practice to midwifery. It now addresses the nature/nurture debate and its contribution to the differences between women and men.

SEX AND GENDER

In the study of women and socialisation, the differences between the concepts of sex and gender have been problematic. The term 'sex' relates to nature and biology and since the 1970s, feminist theory has attempted to explain differences between being female and male as being socially constructed. Thus, the biologically orientated and deterministic theories, considered patriarchal, have been supplanted by more socio-culturally orientated models (Sebrant 1999). However, whilst acknowledging the importance of social construction in attempting to understand the experiences of being a woman, it would appear reasonable to state that women and men are different but that attention should focus on the unequal power relations resulting from these differences.

Sex

In general, the term 'sex' is used to refer to the chromosomal differences that underlie male and female bodies. Biologically determinist theories define what women are, or can and cannot do because of their sex (Crowley and Himmelweit 1992). Therefore, women have been represented as 'naturally' more caring, nurturing, less aggressive with smaller brains and ruled by hormones, which is why women tend to look after the home and family while men are more likely to be engaged in activities that need more logical brain activity (Giddens with Griffiths 2006). Such ideology pervades much of the media in contemporary society where women are viewed as passive and beautiful and men as strong, active and muscular. This serves to reinforce the heterosexist notions of femininity and masculinity and a binary divide which, in turn, supports heterosexual relations and a patriarchal society (Kent 2000). It is interesting to note that, historically, female genitalia were regarded as the same as the male except that they were located inside the body:

> The spermatick vessels (fallopian tubes) in women, called preparing because they
> prepare and convey to the testicles (ovaries) the blood, of which seed is engendered,

differ not from those in men, either in number, or use, but only in their insertion and manner of their distribution. (Mauriceau 1697: 22)

Biological determinism can be applied also to men, but it could be argued that the symmetry ends there because such a theory ultimately valourises existing relations of power. Male dominance and aggression, and female passivity and domesticity are portrayed as biological and, therefore, 'natural' and 'normal' (Birke 1992). There have even been media reports that men are naturally more intelligent than women. The example below from the *Daily Mail* (Clerkin and Macrae 2006) is but one.

MEN ARE MORE INTELLIGENT THAN WOMEN, CLAIMS NEW STUDY –
DAILY MAIL

Battle of the sexes: Are men more intelligent than women?

It is research that is guaranteed to delight men – and infuriate the women in their lives. A controversial new study has claimed that men really are more intelligent than women.

The study – carried out by a man – concluded that men's IQs are almost four points higher than women's.

British-born researcher John Philippe Rushton, who previously created a furore by suggesting intelligence is influenced by race, says the finding could explain why so few women make it to the top in the workplace.

He claims the 'glass ceiling' phenomenon is probably due to inferior intelligence, rather than discrimination or lack of opportunity.

The University of Western Ontario psychologist reached his conclusion after scrutinising the results of university aptitude tests taken by 100 000 students aged 17 and 18, of both sexes.

By *Ben Clerkin and Fiona Macrae*
Last updated at 13:38 14 September 2006.

There is no evidence that this is true of course.

Some modernist feminist writers, however, do not refute the biological differences and celebrate the capacity of women's bodies to nurture and reproduce. Assister (1996) argues that there is value in the distinction made between gender and sex. Concerning biology and sex, she considers there is a minimally necessary set of bodily or biological features present in every female (chromosomes, hormones, genitalia and secondary sex characteristics) which form 'the real essence' of what it is to be a woman and are significant in influencing social and psychological identity. She argues for a universalist basis for feminism such that refocusing on nature and on the importance of the minimal biological body should provide a basis for a shared identity among women.

However, Annandale and Clark (1996) critique what they call the negative consequences that can arise from feminist thinking premised upon a binary division between women and men, male and female, and sex and gender. In their paper concerning sociology and human reproduction, they consider these consequences to include:

- the universalising and valourising of gender differences
- a preoccupation with the abnormalities of women's reproductive health
- a focus on women to the neglect of gender (and men's health), which, it is argued, inhibits the ability truly to understand the experience of being a woman.

Birke (1992) also is not comfortable to reject the biological, but suggests incorporation of gene theories into postmodernist feminist discourse. She argues that female and male bodies are different; it is the usage of biological determinism to reinforce inequalities of status and power between women and men that is the problem. She advocates a dynamic interaction between sex and gender as follows:

> What this line of thought emphasizes is that what you are now – your biological body, your experiences – is a product of complex transformations between biology and experiences in your past. And those transformations happening now will affect any such transformations in the future. Biology, in this view, does have a role: but it is neither a base to build on, nor determining. (1992: 75)

This theory, which is termed the concept of 'transformative change', would appear to look at women's lives in a more holistic way. It suggests that a woman is affected by the society she lives in, her particular social and economic background, and by the fact that she carries the XX (female) chromosomes. This theory also incorporates the changes that may occur in the future as a result of the complex relationship between experiences of the social and of being biologically female. Thus, the sense of being female may change through life with the various experiences that may occur. The following list contains examples of such possible experiences:

- poverty or acquiring disposable income
- marriage or deciding not to be married in a relationship
- altered sexual identity
- being homosexual
- the joy of having children – or the unhappiness
- making the decision not to have children
- finding oneself being unable to have children due to not having a relationship with a man
- finding oneself being unable physically to conceive a child
- miscarriage
- termination of pregnancy
- getting divorced or separating from a partner
- bereavement of a loved adult, stillborn/miscarried baby, child
- having been sexually abused as a child – the effects that has on survivors
- having experienced domestic violence
- relating to and being influenced by the experiences of peers and family.

Many women will experience some of the above and so will midwives and other health-care professionals.

Gender

Gender, in contrast, refers to socially constructed notions of femininity and masculinity. Gender theory, especially in the 1970s and 1980s, highlighted the social construction of gender difference and was important for underpinning feminist struggles for equality and liberation. Social constructions of femininity and the role of women differ, however, according to whether a woman is born in the United Kingdom or, for example, Nepal. All countries are stratified whether it be by social class, economic class or, for example, the caste system. How women are viewed depends very much on the nature of the system of stratification they are born into. Furthermore, each individual woman within a given society will experience life in unique ways making generalisation difficult and invalid. Patterns of behaviour and attitudes can be distinguished, usually referred to as 'social norms'. These include norms governing gender identities and are transmitted/learned in the course of socialisation. When a midwife assists a woman to give birth to female children, the babies may not look significantly different at birth. However, the midwife will know from her knowledge of social sciences that their lives will vary considerably depending upon factors such as social or economic class and attitudes to women held by their parents and social group with whom they will grow up.

Socially constructed notions of femininity and masculinity in any society are difficult, if not impossible, to circumvent when bringing up and, therefore, socialising children. They are there in everyday social interactions, in the media, and even begin at birth when considering the differences in how female and male babies are cared for. It may be that male babies are picked up and cuddled less (Nicholson 1984) and, certainly, different language is adopted when referring to male or female children such as 'what a big, strong boy you are' as opposed to 'she's so sweet and pretty'. A recent visit to a department store (18 January 2009) to look for toys revealed the following stereotypes:

Toys for boys	Toys for girls
Military walkie talkie	Doll like a real baby:
	• feed her from her bottle
	• cries real tears
	• change her nappy
Battle bashers	Honeymoon nails and rings (age 3+)
Battleline robots	Wedding tiara
Action man	Fashion doll:
	• goes shopping
	• goes to the beauty centre
Paratrooper	Nails and jewellery kit
Fireman Sam	
Cowboy	

Obviously, British Society has clear views on what are appropriate toys for male and female children to play with (Wajcman 1994).

The proposition that gender is more fundamental than other social divisions has been critiqued in terms of its representation of all women as homogenous (universalist), belonging to the same oppressed group. Doyal (1995) rejects what she calls crude universalism. She points to the fact that women from diverse social contexts/life-styles, such as lesbians, black women, women with disabilities and women from non-industrialised countries, have challenged the white, Western, middle-class domination of feminist theory and practice.

Postmodernist feminism has highlighted the limitations of generalisations, stressing instead the importance of understanding and acknowledging the diversity of the lived experiences of being a woman. A more sophisticated understanding and emphasis of the relationships between race, class and gender, and of the differences between women can be developed from such a perspective. Needless to say, there are problems inherent here. For example, is it appropriate to consider that cultural practices should *always* be respected, because to do otherwise would denigrate customs and practices that are different from our own? This could lead to a refusal to take action, for fear of being considered racist, when a female child has been genitally mutilated, or a refusal to condemn male violence in cultures where it is widely condoned (Doyal 1995).

Doyal (1995), however, does not believe that the focus should rest solely on difference. She feels that the possibility of shared beliefs, values or interests should not be denied. For example, many women share the reality of occupying subordinate positions in most social and cultural contexts. There is much commonality in the psychological struggle to make sense of themselves, as women, against strong cultural messages that define women as inferior.

With regard to women's employment, much of which is part-time in order to care for children, the State and employers do little to facilitate women in these dual roles. Letters to the Royal College of Midwives' journal, *Midwives*, reveal that some returning midwives are employed at a more junior level than they were when they were employed full-time, surely a state of affairs not likely to induce experienced midwives to return to work after giving birth. Such inequity is replicated throughout the labour market. The clear message is that such workers are perceived to be of less value than their full-time colleagues. Thus, there is a material dimension to women's experiences of subordination since many women are obliged to deal with the consequences of poverty and economic inequality between the sexes (Abbott, Wallace and Tyler 2005).

CONCLUSION

This chapter has explored a number of different theories that attempt to explain the basis of particular socialisation difficulties women face in their lives. Feminist perspectives have been examined in terms of their differing approaches to the explanation of gender inequalities. Radical feminism has been discussed in relation to its influence upon evolving approaches to midwifery practice. The various theories offer analyses and explanations of how and why women have less power than men and how this imbalance can be challenged and transformed. Many women are at ease being married, having children and being responsible for childcare, housework and the domestic infrastructure. However, it has been seen that ideologies of women as being only suited to domesticity have been harmful to many women, and their needs should be addressed. The debate concerning sex/gender or nature/nurture is complex and will no doubt continue, but such binary ways of thinking are not sophisticated enough to consider the complexities of interactions and power relations between men and women.

It is suggested that postmodernism offers a different understanding of women's lives and may be a useful theory for enhancing midwifery practice. Feminism as a 'lay' concept has been much maligned and misunderstood but can offer relevant insight and understanding to midwives and healthcare professionals who work with women and who profess to be 'woman-centred'. Midwives, as women, have close ties to the patriarchal medical and scientific world. This makes analysis of women's lives all the more pertinent, not just to women who give birth but also to the lives of female midwives and health professionals. As Elizabeth Davis asks 'What could be more feminist than the practice of midwifery?' (1987: 5). Midwives need to deal with oppression in the workplace and in their own lives in order to make an impact on what the concept of 'woman-centred' practice and being 'with woman' really could mean.

KEY POINTS

- ⊛ Feminist theories enable analysis of women's lives, how and why women have less power than men and how this can be addressed.
- ⊛ A feminist is not someone who hates men.
- ⊛ Analysis of the similarities and differences between women would lead to a deeper understanding of 'being woman'.
- ⊛ Such analysis is vital for midwives and healthcare professionals who are mainly women, who work with women, and sit juxtaposed to a patriarchal medical and scientific community within hierarchical, patriarchal institutions.

GLOSSARY

Social Constructionism: 'a sociological theory of knowledge that considers how social phenomena develop in particular social contexts' – society and social roles are constructed/shaped by interest groups/people in society.

Essentialism: 'a doctrine that certain traditional concepts, ideals, and skills are essential to society and should be taught methodically to all students, regardless of individual ability, need, etc.' – the traditional concept highlighted in this chapter being that gender and biological sex are synonymous.

Universalism: 'The condition of being universal; universality', e.g. women's oppression is common to all women.

REFERENCES

Abbott P, Wallace C, Tyler M. (2005) *An Introduction to Sociology: feminist perspectives.* 2nd ed. London: Routledge.

Allen C. (2001) Feel like a woman. *Health & Leave as is Beauty.* Winter; pp. 37–8.

Annandale E, Clark J. (1996) What is gender? Feminist theory and the sociology of human reproduction. *Sociol Health Illn.* 18: 17–44.

Anthias F, Yuval-Davis N. (1992) Contextualising feminism: gender, ethnic and class divisions. In:

McDowell L, Pringle R, editors. *Defining Women: social institutions and gender divisions*. Article 3.2. Cambridge: Polity Press in association with the Open University.

Archbishops' Council. (2008) *Church Statistics 2005/6*. Available at: www.cofe.anglican.org/info/ statistics/churchstats2005/statisticspg40.htm (accessed 8 Jan 2009).

Assister A. (1996) *Enlightened Women: modern feminism in a postmodern Age*. London: Routledge.

Aziz R. (1992) Feminism and the challenge of racism: deviance or difference? In: Crowley H, Himmelweit S, editors. *Knowing Women: feminism and knowledge*. Article 7.1. Cambridge: Polity Press in association with the Open University.

Birke L. (1992) Transforming biology. In: Crowley H, Himmelweit S, editors. *Knowing Women: feminism and knowledge*. Article 2.1. Cambridge: Polity Press in association with the Open University.

Bowler I. (1993) 'They're not the same as us': midwives' stereotypes of south Asian descent maternity patients. *Sociol Health Illn*. 15: 157–78.

Brennan D. (2005) The social construction of 'woman's work': nursing labour and status. *J Nurs Manag*. 13(4): 282–5.

Clerkin B, Macrae F. (2006) *Men are more intelligent than women claims new study*. London: Daily Mail; 14 September 2006.

Connell RW. (1994) Gender regimes and gender order. In: *The Polity Reader in Gender Studies*. Chapter 3. Cambridge: Polity Press.

Connon H. (2001) *Old girls' network takes on male bastion*. London: The Observer; 25 November 2001. p. 5.

Crowley H, Himmelweit S. (1992) *Knowing Women: feminism and knowledge*. Cambridge: Polity Press in conjunction with Blackwell Publishers and the Open University.

Crozier K. (2001) Technology: is it killing the art of midwifery? *RCM Midwives*. 4(12): 410–11.

Davis E. (1987) *Heart and Hands: a midwife's guide to pregnancy and birth*. 2nd ed. Berkeley, CA: Celestial Arts.

de Beauvoir S. (1953) *The Second Sex*. London: David Campbell Publishers Ltd.

Delmar R. (1986) What is feminism? In: Mitchell J, Oakley A, editors. *What is feminism?* Chapter 2. Oxford: Blackwell.

Delphy C. (1984) *Close to Home: a materialist analysis of women's oppression*. London: Hutchinson.

Donnison J. (1977) *Midwives and Medical Men: a history of interprofessional rivalries*. London: Schocken Books.

Doyal L. (1995) *What Makes Women Sick: gender and the political economy of health*. Basingstoke: Macmillan Press Ltd.

Equal Opportunities Commission. (2002) *Research Findings: attitudes to equal pay*. Available at: www. equalityhumanrights.com (accessed 23 Jan 2009).

Flax J. (1990) *Thinking Fragments: psychoanalysis, feminism and postmodernism in the contemporary west*. Oxford: University of California Press.

Gammell C. (2008) *Bank boys' club forced me out, claims City high-flier*. London: The Daily Telegraph; 22 April 2008. p. 5.

Gary F, Sigsby LM, Campbell D. (1998) Feminism: a perspective for the 21st century. *Issues Ment Health Nurs*. 19: 139–52.

Giddens A, with Griffiths S. (2006) *Sociology*. 5th ed. Cambridge: Polity.

Government Equalities Office. (2008) *Framework for a Fairer Future – The Equality Bill*. London: The Stationery Office. Available at: www.official-documents.gov.uk/document/cm74/7431/7431.asp (accessed 7 Jan 2009).

Higham J, Steer PJ. (2004) Gender gap in undergraduate experience and performance in obstetrics and gynaecology: analysis of clinical experience logs. *BMJ*. 328(7432): 142–3.

House of Commons Information Department. (2008) *Women in the House of Commons*. Factsheet M04. Available at: www.parliament.uk/parliamentary_publications_and_archives/factsheets/m04.cfm (accessed 6 Jan 2009).

House of Commons Select Committee. (1992) *Second Report: Maternity Services*. London: HMSO.

Katbamna S. (2000) *'Race' and Childbirth*. Buckingham: Open University Press.

Kent J. (2000) *Social Perspectives on Pregnancy and Childbirth for Midwives, Nurses and the Caring Professions.* Buckingham: Open University Press.

Klima CS. (2001) Women's health care: a new paradigm for the 21st century. *J Midwifery Womens Health.* **46**(5): 285–91.

Letvak S. (2001) Nurses as working women. *AORN J.* **73**(3): 675–82.

Lewis G, editor. (2007) *Saving Mothers' Lives: reviewing maternal deaths to make motherhood safer – 2004–2005.* The Seventh Report of the Confidential Enquiries into Maternal Deaths in the United Kingdom. Confidential Enquiry into Maternal and Child Health (CEMACH). London: CEMACH.

Littlewood R. (1991) Gender, role and sickness: the ritual psychopathologies of the nurse. In: Holden P, Littlewood J, editors. *Anthropology and Nursing.* London: Routledge.

Lord Chancellor's Department. (2008) *Annual Diversity Statistics.* Available at: www.judiciary.gov.uk/keyfacts (accessed 6 Jan 2009).

Mauriceau F. (1697) *The Diseases of Women with Child, and in Child-bed.* 3rd ed. Translated by Chamberlen H. London: Andrew Bell.

McCool WF, McCool SJ. (1989) Feminism and nurse-midwifery: historical overview and current issues. *J Nurse Midwifery.* **34**(6): 323–34.

McDowell L, Pringle R. (1992) *Defining Women: social institutions and gender divisions.* Cambridge: Polity Press in association with the Open University.

Mitchell J. (1974) *Psychoanalysis and Feminism.* Harmondsworth: Penguin.

Neathey F, Dench S, Thomson L. (2003) *Monitoring Progress Towards Pay Equality.* Manchester: Institute for Employment Studies for Equal Opportunities Commission.

Nicholson J. (1984) *Men and Women; how different are they?* Oxford: Oxford University Press.

Owen N. (2008) *He's back . . . the glamour team aiming to clean up the rubbish.* London: The Times; 16 April 2008.

Pringle K. (1995) *Men, Masculinities and Social Welfare.* London: University College London Press.

Royal College of Obstetricians and Gynaecologists. (2008) *Statistics Consultants in England and Wales.* Available at: www.rcog.org.uk (accessed 6 Jan 2009).

Sebrant U. (1998) Being female in a health care hierarchy. *Scand J Caring Sci.* **13**: 153–8.

Stacey J. (1993) Untangling feminist theory. In: Richardson D, Robinson V, editors. *Introducing Women's Studies,* Chapter 3. Basingstoke: Macmillan Press Ltd.

Stanworth M. (1994) Reproductive technologies and the deconstruction of motherhood. In: *The Polity Reader in Gender Studies,* Chapter 20. Cambridge: Polity Press.

Tew M. (1998) *Safer Childbirth? A critical history of maternity care.* 3rd ed. London: Chapman & Hall.

Wajcman J. (1994) Technology as masculine culture. In: *The Polity Reader in Gender Studies,* Chapter 19. Cambridge: Polity Press.

Walby S. (1990) *Theorising Patriarchy.* Oxford: Blackwell.

Walby S. (1994) Towards a theory of patriarchy. In: *The Polity Reader in Gender Studies,* Chapter 2. Cambridge: Polity Press.

Watson S. (1999) Introduction. In: Watson S, Doyal L, editors. *Engendering Social Policy.* Buckingham: Open University Press.

Zadoroznyj M. (1999) Social class, social selves and social control in childbirth. *Sociol Health Illn.* **21**(3): 267–89.

Women and sex

Sandy Nelson

The aim of this chapter is for readers to gain a critical understanding of the main theories of female sexuality. The relevance of the concepts of these theories to medicine, midwifery and nursing practice will be explored. The key themes that are considered are: scientific research on sexuality, ideological biases in the research, sexual health, the female body, Freudian theories, current images of female sexuality, heterosexuality and safer sex, pregnancy and sexuality, and cultural differences.

INTRODUCTION

Gender and sexuality pervade every aspect of our lives; from childhood onwards, we are curious about what it means to be female or male and what attracts us to certain people and not others. A vast amount of money is spent on research that sets out to explore the extent to which sexuality is based on our biological inheritance in the form of hormones, genes, or genitals, or whether childhood experience is more important. Other research examines the role of culture, and some looks at the extent to which power, social status and financial independence influence our ability to choose the sexual relationships we want.

The answers we give to these questions are not merely academic but have important consequences. For example, hormonal explanations of rape and sexual abuse have directly resulted in the use of 'chemical castration' to control sex offenders. Moreover, the law and medicine work hand in hand to judge whether sexual behaviour is natural or unnatural and, consequently, whether someone should be regarded as ill or criminal, or both. These norms change over time and reflect the cultural values of different periods. Masturbation, for instance, was believed to be harmful in Victorian England but today is regarded as a vital part of psychosexual therapy. Women are no longer 'routinely' given hysterectomies, and the National Health Service may provide gender reassignment for transsexuals.

It is ironic, therefore, that a subject of such importance, and one in which medicine plays a central part, is so little dealt with by healthcare workers. Despite the fact that sexuality is regarded as an important aspect of holistic care, sexual issues are rarely addressed with patients. When they are raised there is a tendency to reduce a person's sexuality to their marital status. This omission is more astonishing when we consider how ill health affects feelings of self-esteem and can create sexual difficulties in relationships. Imagine how people with stomas, scars, missing body parts, chronic tiredness or anxiety may feel about themselves as sexual beings. For many years within midwifery sexuality was barely mentioned and pregnancy was separated from conception as if all births were virgin births. The sexuality of the elderly was (and often still is) ignored. The specific needs of lesbian and gay patients, or the sexual concerns that people with psychiatric illnesses or learning difficulties may have, seldom appear in nursing care plans or in service provision. Antenatal HIV testing has placed sexuality on the agenda for midwives, but whether the test will be discussed within an infection control model or be raised as part of a more open discussion of any sexual concerns remains to be seen.

Maybe this omission is not so surprising. Many midwives and nurses do not feel confident in their ability to raise discussions about sexuality and fear they may hear disclosures of sexual abuse, sexual assault or homosexuality to which they would not know how to respond. It is difficult to find a language that feels comfortable and this reflects the conundrum that we live in a society with explicit images of sex everywhere but have little capacity in private to express sexual desires openly, or communicate and negotiate about sex verbally. Nevertheless, the medical profession is seen as an appropriate place to turn to for help with sexual difficulties; people hope that midwives and other healthcare workers will initiate discussions about sex, and show, by doing so, that they have permission to air their concerns. Moreover, sexual health is currently regarded as a fundamental component of general health (Baker 1992) with people believing they have a right to live sexually fulfilling lives. In order to be able to help people achieve this, and to feel more comfortable providing it, an understanding of the complexity of gender and sexuality is needed. Some awareness of the theories most commonly used, as well as a critical appreciation of their limitations should, hopefully, provide the basis for this.

SCIENTIFIC RESEARCH ON SEXUALITY

Since the late nineteenth century, science has been relied upon to describe, define and explain human sexuality. Most past research has been undertaken from the viewpoint that sex is a drive or instinct every individual is born with. The roots of sexuality are thought to reside in biological differences, though there are various theories about what these precise differences are. Researchers tend to fall into one of two groups: those who see sexuality as a good natural instinct corrupted by society (Masters and Johnson 1966, Kinsey, *et al.* 1953), and those who view it as a dangerous force that needs to be tamed for the benefit of civilisation (Freud 1905, Malinowski 1963). Biological differences, and the evolutionary drive to procreate are presented as sufficient explanations for all sexual behaviour.

The material body is at the centre of most of the research. The focus is on what can be measured and observed. The type and frequency of sexual activities, the prevalence of male and female homosexuality, and the physiological changes leading to orgasm have all been examined. The search is for facts and objective truth. Socio-biologists have amassed evidence based on animal behaviour to support their theory that women choose their partners on the basis of their superior genes to maximise the evolutionary potential of the human race (Dawkins 1978, Symons 1979). Homosexual men have been studied to see if they have smaller brains, different genes or lower levels of testosterone (Le Vay 1993, Hamer 1994). Biological abnormalities in gender characteristics (Money 1994), the impact of gender reassignment on sexual development (Money 1975), and the social impact of being raised in a biologically incorrect way (Luria, *et al.* 1987: 94–5) are studied by scientists to attempt to answer questions about how much of our sexuality is dependent on nature and how much on nurture.

IDEOLOGICAL BIASES IN THIS RESEARCH

This research is interesting and much may be useful in highlighting important aspects of sexuality; however, there is a problem in that it is presented as providing the unquestionable truth about our sexual nature. Biological explanations are given the force of moral authority. The assumptions that underpin the research are not seen as open to question, and, although many biologists are less deterministic than previously, the media continues to present reductionist and uncritical 'scientific' versions of sexuality as if they were the absolute truth. This is evident in press reports such as '*striking similarities between the brains of gay men and straight women . . . discovered by neuroscientists*' (Sample 2008) [my italics].

In fact, examination of scientific texts reveals an ideological bias in much of this research. Many of the supposedly neutral scientific descriptions are gender coded in ways that reflect stereotypical definitions of masculinity and femininity. For example, in the 1950s, John Money, an influential researcher, described a gene as the Sex Determining gene, also known as the Master Sex Determining gene (cited in Fausto-Sterling 1997). In its presence, the male is formed. The male embryo must *seize* its developmental pathway. The female, on the other hand is formed by the *absence* of the master gene. Recent research has suggested that the ovaries have an active role in conception. This contradicts previous descriptions of conception as a battle of fighting, active sperm gaining access to the passive, waiting ova. Although this may be seen to be merely a matter of semantics it is on a continuum with the credence given to biologists such as Randy Thornhill who has written a book arguing that rape is a normal mechanism for spreading genes (Thornhill and Palmer 2000). His theory is based on his observations of flies – evidence for various theories of human sexuality has been found by comparisons with monkeys, rats and sparrows, to name a few, as well as insects! He uses the word rape as a scientific term to describe his observations, with no apparent concern that this is a very subjective, human term with connotations of consent and conscious choice. This 'scientific' research is then, in a circular argument, cited as evidence that rape is 'natural' for men. The pernicious effect of this can be found in legal arguments, where this and similar theories are used, successfully, to justify and defend male sexual aggression (Ussher 1997b: 333–8).

The research reflects the political and ideological needs of the historical period. Research that highlights similarities between men and women gets little attention (Unger 1979, cited in Nicolson and Ussher 1992), whereas research that demonstrates differences commands widespread coverage in both scientific journals and the popular press. There is a close relationship between current social and political issues and the research undertaken and published. History provides very clear examples of this. For instance, in the late eighteenth century there was a sudden interest in differences between men and women, which previously had been seen as of little importance. This interest was not simply the result of advances in scientific knowledge, but seems to have become important because of the justification biological explanations could provide for political arguments (Laqueur 1997: 228). Both feminists and anti-feminists looked to biology to support debates about the role of women in society.

> New claims and counterclaims regarding the public and private roles of women were thus contested through questions about the nature of *their* bodies as distinguished from those of men. (Laqueur 1997: 239) [my italics]

Moreover, scientific research defines female sexuality in terms of male sexuality. Most of the renowned sex researchers have been male, but more than this, men have taken themselves as the norm for human sexuality, with women judged in relation to them as lacking, deficient or, at best, the mysterious 'other'. Men are seen as needing sex and women are regarded as the passive recipients of that sexual drive. This all-consuming male drive will find expression in 'deviations' or aggressive demands if denied legitimate outlets (Jackson 1987: 72). The penis is regarded as the essential sexual organ. The act of sex itself is defined as penetrative vaginal intercourse (Holland, *et al.* 1998), and anything else is not the real thing, mere foreplay. The fact that much research indicates that orgasm and sexual pleasure generally, for many women, has less to do with vaginal intercourse and more to do with 'foreplay' is ignored (Segal 1994: 95). It is only in imagination that we can think of sex as centred around the woman's experience of orgasm.

> The model not only reflects and legitimates the male supremacist myth that the male sexual urge *must* be satisfied; it defines the very nature of 'sex' in male terms . . . Male sexuality has been universalised and now serves as the model of human sexuality. (Jackson 1987: 73)

This has been reinforced by men's political, social and economic power, which has given them a great deal of control over female sexuality. A practical manifestation of this was the practice of stitching women extra tightly after episiotomies in order to increase the sexual pleasure of their 'male partners'.

It is not that women have just passively accepted male control of their sexuality. Many have actively struggled to define sexuality for themselves, and have found ways to resist and subvert the sexuality imposed upon them. Feminists, and lesbian and gay writers (Rich 1980, Butler 1990) have profoundly questioned the prevailing ideas about sexuality and, in recent history, women have claimed their own sexual desires and need for satisfaction. Theories of gender and sexuality have been radically transformed by the critical readings of scientific texts undertaken by contemporary writers (Connell and Dowsett 1992, Vance 1984, Weeks 1985) influenced by feminist and 'queer' perspectives.

Also, scientific research itself provides evidence of the actual complexity of the relationship between gender and sexuality, despite the reductionist versions presented by some scientists and the popular press. There is no straightforward relationship between biology, gender and sexual orientation. Many people born without clearly male or female sexual characteristics grow up with few problems related to their socially (rather than biologically) designated gender. Others, who feel they have been born in the wrong bodies and who seek gender reassignment have no biological abnormalities (Luria, *et al.* 1987: 445). The majority of transvestites have no desire to change from male to female (Blanchard 1990), and many homosexuals have no problems related to their gender (Luria, *et al.* 1987: 95). Transsexuals and transvestites may or may not remain heterosexual, still choosing partners opposite their original biological gender and the majority of us have some bisexuality (Kinsey, *et al.* 1948, 1953). Similarly, interest in sado-masochistic sex, paedophilia, fetishism or any other designated perversion defies biological explanations. The desire to have children can be strong for lesbians and gay men and absent for heterosexuals. Most attempts to categorise and explain human sexuality by reference to biology are undermined by the sheer variety of sexual behaviour.

SEXUAL HEALTH

Medicine is a dominant influence in defining sexuality and judging what is normal and abnormal, healthy and unhealthy, and midwifery and nursing practice are ways that those values are transmitted to individual women. As Frank Mort (cited in Weeks 2000: 138) convincingly argues, there is a substantial medico-moral tradition linking health and disease to moral and immoral sex. Public hygiene and cleanliness have been closely associated with 'dangerous sexualities'.

> 'Healthy' serves as the modern equivalent to 'normal' in terms of endorsing and recommending sexual scripts for what's done, why it's done, when, where, and with whom it's done . . . Health is morality nowadays. (Tiefer 1997: 105)

In the recent manifestation of this tradition, hygiene has been replaced by 'concerns about orgasmic efficiency and the management of erotic pleasures' (Hawkes 1996: 119). Sexual health is now, in practice, thought of as active engagement in a fulfilling sexual relationship, and there are concerns about people who are not interested in sex or who deviate from the norms prescribed by medical experts. Leonore Tiefer, an associate professor in a department of urology and psychiatry, gives an interesting example from a conference on aging and sexuality. A study had been done measuring erections during sleep of a group of older male volunteers with no sexual problems. One urologist looking at the results commented:

> So, these men did not have rigid nocturnal erections; they may actually have had disease. (Tiefer 1997: 108)

The 'epidemic' levels of erectile dysfunction (possibly 50% in men over 40 years old) and its treatment with Viagra also illuminates the medicalisation of sexual desire.

Medical authorities no longer discuss morality but talk instead of disease, as in the above example, or unhealthy behaviours; however, these descriptions are used in a pejorative way. The prescriptive nature of medical discourse is evident in the way that being unhealthy can be presented as if it is a personal failing. For example, the sexual activity of young women is no longer presented as morally wrong but as premature and potentially medically dangerous (Hawkes 1996: 84), yet the subtext is that it is a problem and ought to be stopped.

Generally, midwives and nurses are now more tolerant than in the past and express more awareness of the variety and complexity of sexuality. However, a more thorough examination soon reveals that sexuality remains bound by ideas of normal, good sexuality positioned above dubious, perverted or socially undesirable sexuality. The contentious and contradictory responses to sex education, for instance, reveal the actual hierarchical values, as well as the confusion, underlying overt acceptance. Homosexuality was not to be 'intentionally promoted' according to Section 28 of the Local Government (Amendment) Act, yet this prohibition was not meant to stop any health education necessary to prevent the spread of disease, such as, presumably, safer sex for gay teenagers at risk of contracting HIV. Section 28 was repealed in November 2003 but the memory of it still influences the uneasiness of many teachers about discussing homosexuality. Recent decisions, such as the vote to reject the amendment to the Fertilisation and Embryology Bill, which required fertility clinics to consider the need for a father prior to IVF treatment, demonstrate the changing attitudes to female sexuality and the recognition of the rights of lesbians and single mothers (Dobson 2008). Indeed the Human Fertilisation and Embryology Authority guidelines (2005, cited in Dobson 2008) specifically prohibit refusal of fertility treatment on the basis of sexual orientation. Nevertheless, political support for the family reinforces ideas of preferred sexual configurations and the political will behind attempts to make fathers take financial responsibility for their offspring has restrictive implications for women who choose to be single parents (Weeks 2000: 175). There was public outrage at the idea that lottery money could be used to support gay and lesbian organisations, prostitutes and drug users, despite the fact that the funds were to be used to work with individuals with HIV and AIDS. Awareness of the power of medical institutions to impose these values on individuals through the sexual healthcare offered will, hopefully, lead to better support for women receiving that care and greater appreciation of limitations they may perceive in the care offered.

THE FEMALE BODY

Women's healthcare needs continue to be assessed on the basis of common sense assumptions about female bodies and gender differences that are taken from scientific and medical research, with little awareness of the values that shape that knowledge and inform seemingly objective descriptions of human biology. Far from being described objectively, the female body is presented in medical texts as vulnerable, problematic and generally suspect. 'Raging hormones' take over in premenstrual tension and Nicolson and Ussher draw attention to the portrayal of women as:

> . . . erratic, unreliable and potentially dangerous. Their bodies make them so.
> (Nicolson and Ussher 1992: 43)

Menstruation, pregnancy and labour all require the expert attention of the medical profession. Postnatal depression is presented as a definite clinical diagnosis, despite the lack of evidence of a clear biological aetiology. Abortion is justified legally by presenting the woman or her fetus as vulnerable to medical or mental disorder if the pregnancy continued (Boyle 1992: 140). In some texts the menopause is described as an oestrogen–deficiency disease (Hunter and O'Dea 1997: 201). Breast milk has virtually been hijacked by the medical profession and is more and more being marketed as a health food. Questioning these explanations because of their negative and derogatory descriptions of women's bodies does not mean that women have no specific concerns related to their experiences of being in female bodies or that women do not themselves look to medical science to provide relief from debilitating experiences. The material reality of the body is important but needs to be understood in relation to the ideological shaping provided within purportedly neutral scientific texts, as these descriptions, explanations and theories about the female body profoundly influence women's own understanding of their bodily experiences.

Medical science conceives of the body in mechanistic ways. Consequently, sexual problems are responded to with penile pumps and Viagra. Female sexuality has always posed more problems because it is harder to reduce it to the specific functioning of one body part. Nevertheless, the quest to measure clitoral swelling, vaginal dryness and orgasmic strength continues. Sex therapists suggest masturbation exercises for women in 'laboratory' conditions to enable them to measure their physical responses to self-stimulation. This ignores the multiple means of achieving sexual satisfaction, and sees sexuality in individual rather than social or relational terms. Also, people are influenced by ideas that good sex involves penetration and leads to orgasm. It is difficult to define sexual satisfaction for oneself without taking on these stereotyped views about desirable outcomes. Yet we know that there are far more reasons for desiring sex than there are ways of being sexual (Whittier and Simon 2001: 161), and that simply describing sexual behaviour or counting the number of times intercourse occurs (Vance 1991: 880) tells us little that is useful about sex.

> Sexology's nomenclature of sexual disorders does not describe what makes women unhappy about sex in the real world, but narrows and limits the vision of sexual problems to failures of genital performance. (Tiefer 1992, cited in Heise 1995: 110)

Most of us recognise that we have sex for multiple purposes: to try to 'keep' a relationship, to bargain, because it is expected of us, for money, power, self-esteem, protection from violence, social acceptability, intimacy, to conceive, to prove something, as well as for physical pleasure. Research identified 237 reasons why people had sex 'ranging from the mundane . . . to the spiritual . . . from altruistic . . . to vengeful' (Meston and Buss 2007: 1). Satisfaction, in these terms, may come in many guises.

FREUDIAN THEORIES

When we consider how broad sexual satisfaction is, the role of the mind and fantasy can be seen to play at least as big a part as biology. The meanings we give to sexual acts are mediated by culture and personal history as much as by biology. Freud's contribution (Freud 1905) to our understanding of sexuality was his insight into the role of childhood experience and fantasy in shaping adult sexuality. In his theories, gender identity, heterosexuality and the desire to have children are all achieved through the child's struggle to make sense of its sensations, experiences of gender differences and parental sexuality; from this no single developmental path can be guaranteed. The sexual drive dominates the infant's unconscious fantasies, and if 'normal' development is thwarted then alternative outlets will be found. The child's experiences of sucking the breast or bottle, the way it is held and touched by both parents, the interactions with parents during toilet training, the responses of others to their pleasurable genital play all contribute to subsequent sexual preferences. For the child, gender is flexible. It is no more difficult to imagine growing up and turning into the opposite sex, than to imagine becoming like mother or father. Primary identification with the mother poses different problems for the boy and girl, but both have to find ways to separate from her and find their own adult selves. Initially, the child is interested in exploring its body with anyone and everything; there is no specific choice of male or female partners. It is only later that desire becomes related to particular genders, or age group or type of sexual activity. Even then it remains fluid for many, rigid and fixed for others. Finally, there will be fantasies around the capacity to reproduce. There will be fears and anxieties, hopes and dreams around producing babies. For the child these are focused on having babies with their mother or father, and it is through coming to terms with their exclusion from the parental couple that they are free to go on and find their own partners. All of these live on in adult fantasies where humans reveal a capacity to be aroused by a vast range of situations, people, objects and activities.

Freud's theories have been developed (Harding 2001), and contested by feminist psychoanalysts (Benjamin 1998, Chodorow 1994) since he wrote them. They continue to be of interest, however, because they offer a means to make sense of the varieties of sexual expression. Fetishism, transsexuality, sado-masochism, paedophilia and homo-sexuality, for example, can be understood using the framework he offered. Nevertheless, they contain major problems, particularly for women. Similarly to the biologists and sexologists, Freud's view of sexuality was phallocentric; women are viewed as castrated, defective versions of men, consumed with envy for the longed-for penis. Various female analysts (Horney 1932) questioned this and theorised male envy of the female capacity to bear children. Whilst this provides another useful piece of the pattern, it focuses attention on women as mothers rather than sexually desiring beings.

CURRENT IMAGES OF FEMALE SEXUALITY

Female sexuality continues, then, to pose problems for psychoanalysts, biologists, psy-chosexual therapists and, not least, for women themselves. Doubtless, Western women have more sexual choices and freedom than in most periods in our history. Yet many women put up with unhappy and frustrating relationships, forego their own sexual satisfaction, gain more pleasure from being an object of desire than from being the author of their own desires, and hope men will awaken and arouse them in a modern day version of the old romantic myths.

Language and culture do not present us with images of positive female sexuality. The cultural exaltation of the phallus as the sexual organ par excellence leaves women's sexuality mysterious and lacking to themselves, despite the distorted reflections they see everywhere, in the ubiquitous images of women's bodies. The language of active desire belongs to the penetrating male:

> . . . our culture presents all agency and power in phallic terms and there is no equiva-lent symbol to suggest female desire or potency. (Maguire 2001: 110)

Women's more diffuse experience of sexual pleasure is lost, absent or misunderstood in cultural representations. Sex scenes in films continue to be genitally driven and, although women initiate sex more readily, they more often remain objects of desire, frequently rewarded by successfully seducing the man pursued, than active subjects writing their own sexual scripts. There are more positive images of women's sexuality available currently, and a belief that women have as much right as men in satisfying their sexual needs and desires, but this is undermined by more traditional scripts that still have force. The voracious sexual predator counterposed to the respectable mother, wife and daughter remains alive in our culture and continues to prescribe female sexuality and rob women of their capacity to define sexual desire for themselves. Despite the rejection of these categories by most women, they continue to be used. Courts continue to take into account women's sexual histories in assessing rape charges, girls judge themselves and their peers on the basis of the number of boys 'slept' with and the term 'slag' is used to control and police teenage female sexuality (Holland, *et al.* 1990). The press presents women with HIV either as innocent victims or as predatory, promiscuous spreaders of the virus.

Although there may be awareness of the unfairness of the double standard, many parents understandably still feel the need to teach young women to protect themselves sexually. Girls are taught that their bodies will turn boys into lustful animals and that they must be the ones to take responsibility for controlling sexual interactions. Sex is presented as something dangerous to young women and desire is presented as coming from others, not from within. Women are vulnerable because of the power of the male sexual urge, although, if they are very attractive and cunning, they can use their physical attributes to gain sexual power over men. The contradictions within all these scripts leave girls with a confusing and difficult pathway to a strong sense of their own sexuality.

> Women must, on the one hand, allure, and, on the other hand, control and restrain; they must be sensuous, lovable and passionate, but on the other hand, scrupulously chaste. (Okin 1980, cited in Seidler 1987)

The constant threat of sexual violence or social disgrace, and the hierarchies of good and bad sex give women an idea of their sexuality as risky, disturbing and potentially troublesome. This is reinforced through legal judgements, such as the case of the window cleaner who was given a two-year sentence for raping a girl of 10 years old. Judge Hall stated that the girl had dressed provocatively and looked as though she was 16 (BBC News 2007). This is a very different story from the narratives of pleasure and passion. Moreover, even the more enlightened attitudes that also prevail can turn into injunctions that can be just as oppressive.

> In this brave new age of sex, the greatest sin is sexual boredom. (Hawkes 1996: 119)

As Hawkes goes on to argue, women's magazine articles leave people with what she calls an 'ignorance anxiety'. She contends that advertisers exploit women's sexual anxieties to sell their products. Their articles claim expertise about sex, and as a result women question their own desires and feel they ought to be having earth-shattering, adventurous, multi-orgasmic sex regularly. Readers are left insecure, and doubt their sexual capacity, as they measure their own experiences against the accounts to which they are exposed.

HETEROSEXUALITY AND SAFER SEX

In this climate, negotiating safer sex, and all kinds of sexual safety and pleasure remain difficult for women. Male-centred definitions of sex continue to dominate and are actively constructed by women as much as by men. Heterosexuality is rarely questioned or seen as the sexual category and organising principle that it is (Richardson 2000). Yet sexual desire is seen as distinctly heterosexual. Gay relationships are thought of as mimicking heterosexual ones and the anus is viewed as taking the place of the vagina in gay male relationships. This can stop us from identifying the anus as a source of pleasure for all human beings and allows us to forget that many heterosexuals also see the anus as a site for sex. The 'coital imperative' (Segal 1994) script is severely limiting. Heterosexual men are still regarded as exempt from the need to change and suggesting that heterosexual men give up penetrative vaginal sex is unthinkable, whereas gay men are expected to give up penetrative anal sex, as suggested in some safer sex campaigns (Richardson 2000: 135). The challenge of HIV for heterosexual women is to redefine heterosexual sex, expose male control of women's sexuality and produce a female-centred theory of sexuality from which women could insist on pleasurable and safe sex.

Women undermine themselves through ideas about romantic love and trust, which supersede any concerns they may have about infections. Trust is used in relationships as a reason why condom use cannot be discussed, either because they are seen as unnecessary or would jeopardise the relationship by suggesting disease or infidelity (Willig 1997). In the light of this it is ironic that:

> . . . most women now infected with HIV globally have been infected within a stable, long-term relationship or marriage. (Lewis 1997: 247)

Women knowingly put themselves at risk because of the idealisation of monogamous, heterosexual relationships, the kind of relationships thought to bring most status and esteem. The search for intimacy and the sense of being part of a loving relationship overrides sexual health issues (Sobo 1995). Greater love and intimacy are signified by non-use of a condom, which is why condom use is more likely to be found in casual than long-term relationships (Joffe 1997). I suggest that it is because of an implicit understanding of this that midwives feel unwilling to discuss HIV and, in particular, talk about safer sex and condom use during pregnancy.

PREGNANCY AND SEXUALITY

Pregnancy poses particular challenges related to the different constructions of masculinity, femininity and sexuality. At no other time are the differences between men and women so sharply delineated. Envy and resentment of one another's experiences can cause unexpected conflicts between men and women who were previously happy in their relationship. Having a child represents deeply felt hopes, fantasies, and fears for those involved. Old anxieties and powerful, primitive emotions are stirred as the expectant parents are reminded of their own early experiences. Childhood desires and ideas about sexuality and reproduction, long buried, rise to the surface in disturbing ways. Experiences as a child of dependency and vulnerability, closeness to and separation from mother get vividly recalled. How their own parents related to their sexual bodies, fertility and the quality of the sexual relationship established by the parents will affect the parents to be. The pregnancy can be seen as a demonstration of love, as evidence of femininity, potency and virility, as a solution to problems of identity or esteem, or as a route to adult status and social approval. Fertility is an important aspect of sexual identity and the ability to conceive is highly valued; consequently the pregnancy can be seen as a triumphant achievement. Women may feel fascinated and excited, and discontented and exhausted, in confusing mixtures. Men may feel envious and excluded, or relieved and guilt-ridden. These are often only semi-consciously experienced and can be difficult to talk about, emerging during sex and causing enormous anxiety. Of course, many couples manage these feelings and experience increased tenderness and closeness. Intimacy and sexual passion can be heightened and women may experience more intense orgasms. However, whether enhanced or inhibited, sexuality will be profoundly affected by pregnancy, and in particular by a first pregnancy.

> Pregnancy alters a woman's internal experience of her sexuality, as her spontaneous responses are shaped by unfamiliar bodily sensations and hormonal experiences, as well as by her psychic experience of the pregnancy. (Raphael-Leff 1993: 42)

The couple may feel that the baby in the womb represents a third presence in the bed, which must be protected from sex, with the penis seen as damaging and potentially causing miscarriage. The baby can be imagined as an audience to the sex, a voyeur or incestuous partner. Later in the pregnancy the liveliness of the baby can be inhibiting and lead to impotence. The woman may withdraw emotionally from her partner and feel her sexual energy is wrapped up in the baby. She may feel suddenly stripped of her adult independence or that her swelling body is sexually unattractive. Others may feel proud and strong, affirmed in their own identity and confirmed as a sexual woman.

Some women feel invaded, exploited and taken over and this may culminate in an experience of labour as a kind of rape. The exposure, and the loss of dignity and control experienced in giving birth may leave the woman feeling damaged, helpless and frightened by sex, or the man feeling unable to have sex because of his experience of his partner's labour as damaging and disturbing. Real experiences of rape and sexual abuse can surface and be deeply distressing as the lack of control in labour mirrors the previous violations.

After the birth it can be a long time before the sexual relationship is re-established to the satisfaction of both partners. Psychosexual difficulties can often be traced back to the first pregnancy and this is thought to be because pregnancy powerfully reactivates unconscious feelings that have been repressed since childhood (Raphael Leff 1993: 171).

Cultural ideas about motherhood and social constructions of femininity undoubtedly impact on the woman's experience of herself as a sexual being. The separation of motherhood and madonna images from sexual desire can make it difficult for either or both partners to feel that the 'mother' can still be sexually desiring or desirable. The idealisation and denigration of motherhood exert contradictory pressures on the woman and her concept of herself. Changes in reproductive technology, awareness of the fetus as a separate identity because of scans (Pollack Petchesky 1997, Piontelli 2000), the ability of postmenopausal women to have babies, lesbian parents and artificial insemination all radically alter our understanding of parenting, and the relationship of sex to conception seems more and more tenuous. The lack of a woman–centred perspective on female desire is evident in discussions of sexuality and pregnancy as it is elsewhere. Books, such as Dr Stoppard's (1998) *Healthy Pregnancy*, present sexual activity during pregnancy as more about heterosexual bonding than about the desire for pleasure.

> Sex becomes another legitimate activity to prime the pregnant body for childbirth, much like aerobics or yoga. Sexual pleasure and activity is legitimate if in the service of hormonal balance, muscular readiness and emotional well-being. (Huntley 2000: 357)

With all of these pressures, from social and cultural expectations to primitive anxieties resurfacing from childhood, pregnant women often feel a need to talk to someone. Often they feel ashamed and disturbed by what they regard as irrational fears and as a result they feel unable to speak to friends or partners. Midwives are in the ideal position to listen to these anxieties and provide confidential advice and reassurance.

CULTURAL DIFFERENCES

This chapter is written from a Western perspective. In other cultures sexuality is conceptualised very differently, and the rules governing sexual interactions are extraordinarily varied, as historians and anthropologists have shown. What is shared across cultures is that:

> All societies find it necessary to organise the erotic possibilities of the body – impose who restrictions and why restrictions, provide permissions, prohibitions, limits and possibilities. (Plummer 1984, cited in Weeks 2000: 130)

The body is a boundary marker in all cultures and women's bodies, in particular, are used to maintain the cultural identity of different groups through rules about marriage, kinship patterns and sexual relationships (Caplan 1987: 15). There are very diverse ideas about gender roles in different cultures, sexual relationships between men are accepted in some, and the moral judgements made about various sexual practices such as anal sex and masturbation also differ. The advent of HIV has forced health promotion practitioners to try to find ways of making services, written materials and campaigns more culturally appropriate. Homosexuality, as an identity, is a Western category rejected in other cultures by men who have sex with men; consequently, materials need to be designed which address sexual practices in culturally sensitive ways. Anthropologists have enabled us to understand the vast diversity of human sexuality, and as a result have opened our eyes to our own cultural assumptions. The other side of this, however, is that our inability to be knowledgeable about what is acceptable and what is taboo in all cultures can seem overwhelming. In fact, all of us accept some aspects of our cultures and resist and reject other aspects, and each of us has a unique relationship to our culture. Also, there are as many differences within cultures as between them and knowing the norms of different groups will not necessarily help us to understand individuals within the group (Pollen 1993).

Cultural differences are often problematic for us because they make us aware of the values and judgements we make without conscious thought. One practice that is especially disturbing to the Western world is female genital mutilation. Officially, it is condemned because of the damage to health, but we know that many women continue to support the practice. In order to work with such women it may be helpful to be aware of what women relinquish by stopping the practice as well as what they might gain. A study by Janice Boddy that explored its significance for women in Northern Sudan is useful in this respect. She came to understand that the practice was an assertive symbolic act for the women, enhancing their femininity and their social status. In this context, it is easier to relate it to Western practices and note similarities in the way:

> Feminine selfhood is . . . attained at the expense of female well-being. (Boddy 1997: 322)

Comparisons can be made with cosmetic surgery and the increased number of requests by women for caesarean births, where the main reason given is the desire to retain an attractive body and maintain self-esteem (Kitzinger 2000).

CONCLUSION

This chapter has attempted to introduce some of the main theories of sexuality and demonstrate that the assumption that there is a universal, natural, human sexuality based around gender differences fails to do justice to the complexity of sexual desire. Through greater understanding of the varieties of sexualities it is hoped that midwives will feel better prepared to raise discussions about sexuality, or at least will feel interested in learning more about a subject that is of such importance to most of us, and can contribute so much to our health and happiness.

KEY POINTS

- ↬ In order to deliver appropriate sexual healthcare, it is important to understand theories of sexuality and gender.
- ↬ Scientific research has focused on attempts to measure the influences of biology and the environment on human sexuality.
- ↬ This research reflects the political and ideological needs of the historical period in which it is undertaken.
- ↬ Medicine plays a major role in defining healthy and unhealthy sexuality, and these definitions reflect moral value judgements.
- ↬ Freud's theories provide insights into the role of childhood experiences and fantasy in sexuality.
- ↬ Contemporary images of female sexuality continue to present contradictory scripts. The 'coital imperative' and good/bad girl scripts influence the way in which women feel about their own sexuality.
- ↬ Pregnancy has a major impact on sexuality, often stirring up powerful feelings and fantasies.
- ↬ Different societies have radically different ways of conceptualising both gender and sex.

GLOSSARY

Determinism: The theory that human sexuality is determined by a necessary chain of causation.

Scripts: 'Scripts specify, like blueprints, the whos, whats, whens wheres and whys for given types of activity . . . It is like a blueprint or roadmap or recipe, giving directions.' (Gagnon,1977: 6) This theory of sexual behaviour is developed by Gagnon in the book referred to.

REFERENCES

Baker C. (1992) Female sexuality. In: Nicolson P, Ussher J, editors. *The Psychology of Women's Health and Health Care.* Basingstoke: Macmillan Press Ltd.

BBC News. (2007) *Anger at 'lenient' rape sentence.* London: BBC; 26 June 2007. Available at: http://news.bbc.co.uk/2/hi/uk_news/6237480.stm (accessed 6 Jan 2009).

Benjamin J. (1998) *The Bonds of Love: psychoanalysis, feminism and the problem of domination.* New York: Random House.

Blanchard R. (1990) Gender identity disorders in adult men. In: Blanchard R, Steiner BW, editors. *Clinical Management of Gender Identity Disorders in Children and Adults.* Washington, DC: American Psychiatric Press. pp. 47–76.

Boddy J. (1997) Womb as oasis: the symbolic context of pharaonic circumcision in rural northern sudan. In: Lancaster RN, di Leonardo M, editors. *The Gender/Sexuality Reader.* London: Routledge.

Boyle M. (1992) The abortion debate: an analysis of psychological assumptions underlying legislation and professional decision-making. In: Nicolson P, Ussher J, editors. *The Psychology of Women's Health and Health Care.* London: Macmillan Press Ltd.

Butler J. (1990) *Gender Trouble.* London: Routledge.

Caplan P, editor. (1987) *The Cultural Construction of Sexuality.* London: Routledge.

Chodorow NJ. (1994) *Femininities, Masculinities, Sexualities.* London: Free Association Books.

Connell RW, Dowsett GW, editors. (1992) *Rethinking Sex: social theory and sexuality research.* Melbourne: Melbourne University Press.

Dawkins R. (1978) *The Selfish Gene.* St Albans: Granada.

Dobson R. (2008) *UK Parliament rejects the 'need for a father' in IVF treatment* [online]. Available at: www.bionews.org.uk/new.lasso?storyid=3845 (accessed 6 Jan 2009).

Fausto-Sterling A. (1997) How to build a man. In: Lancaster RN, di Leonardo M, editors. *The Gender/Sexuality Reader.* London: Routledge.

Freud S. (1905) Three essays on the theory of sexuality. In: Strachey J, editor. *The Standard Edition of the Complete Psychological Works of Sigmund Freud, Vol. 7.* London: Hogarth Press and The Institute of Psychoanalysis; pp. 1953–74.

Gagnon JH. (1977) *Human Sexualities.* Glenview, Il: Scott, Foresman & Co.

Hamer D. (1994) *The Search for the Gay Gene and the Biology of Behaviour.* New York: Simon and Schuster.

Harding C, editor. (2001) *Sexuality, Psychoanalytic Perspectives.* Hove, East Sussex: Brunner-Routledge.

Hawkes G. (1996) *A Sociology of Sex and Sexuality.* Buckingham: Open University Press.

Heise LL, editor (1995) Violence, sexuality and women's lives. In: Parker RG, Gagnon JH, editors. *Conceiving Sexuality.* London: Routledge.

Holland J, Ramazanoglu C, Scott S, et al. (1990) *Women Risk and AIDS Project Papers 1–8.* London: Tufnell Press.

Holland J, Ramazanoglu C, Sharpe S, et al. (1998) *The Male in the Head.* London: Tufnell Press.

Horney K. (1967) *Feminine Psychology.* New York: Norton; pp. 133–46.

Hunter MS, O'Dea I. (1997) Menopause bodily changes and multiple meanings. In: Ussher JM, editor. *Body Talk.* London: Routledge.

Huntley R. (2000) Sexing the belly: an exploration of sex and the pregnant body. *Sexualities.* 3(3): 347–62.

Jackson M. (1987) 'Facts of life' or the eroticisation of women's oppression? Sexology and the social construction of heterosexuality. In: Caplan P, editor. *The Cultural Construction of Sexuality.* London: Routledge.

Joffe H. (1997) Intimacy and love in late modern conditions. In: Ussher JM, editor. *Body Talk.* London: Routledge.

Kinsey AC, Pomeroy WB, Martin CE, *et al.* (1948) *Sexual Behaviour in the Human Male.* Philadelphia: WB Saunders.

Kinsey AC, Pomeroy WB, Martin CE, *et al.* (1953) *Sexual Behaviour in the Human Female.* Philadelphia: WB Saunders.

Kitzinger S. (2000) Who would choose to have a Caesarean? *Br J Midwifery.* 9: 284–5.

Laqueur T. (1997) Orgasm, generation and the politics of reproductive biology. In: Lancaster RN, di Leonardo M, editors. *The Gender/Sexuality Reader.* London: Routledge.

Le Vay S. (1993) *The Sexual Brain.* Cambridge, MA: MIT Press.

Lewis J. (1997) 'So how did your condom use go last night, Daddy?' Sex talk and daily life. In: Segal L, editor. *New Sexual Agendas.* London: Macmillan Press Ltd.

Luria Z, Friedman S, Rose MD. (1987) *Human Sexuality.* New York: John Wiley & Sons.

Maguire M. (2001) Women's sexuality in the new millennium. In: Harding C, editor. *Sexuality, Psychoanalytic Perspectives.* Hove, East Sussex: Brunner-Routledge.

Malinowski B. (1963) *Sex, Culture and Myth.* London: Rupert Hart-Davis.

Masters WH, Johnson VE. (1966) *Human Sexual Response.* Boston, MA: Little, Brown and Co.

Meston CM, Buss DM. (2007) Why humans have sex. *Arch Sex Behav.* 36: 477–507. Available at: http://homepage.psy.utexas.edu/homepage/Group/BussLAB/pdffiles/why%20humans%20 have%20sex%202007.pdf (accessed 6 Jan 2009).

Money J. (1975) Ablatio penis: normal male infant sex reassigned as a girl. *Arch Sex Behav.* 4: 65–72.

Money J. (1994) *Sex Errors of the Body and Related Syndromes: a guide to counselling children, adolescents and their families.* 2nd ed. Baltimore, MD: Paul Brookes.

Nicolson P, Ussher J, editors. (1992) *The Psychology of Women's Health and Health Care.* London: Macmillan Press Ltd.

Piontelli A. (2000) 'Is there something wrong?': the impact of technology in pregnancy. In: Raphael-Leff J. *Spilt Milk: perinatal loss and breakdown.* London: Institute of Psychoanalysis.

Pollack Petchesky R. (1997) Fetal images. In: Lancaster RN, di Leonardo M, editors. *The Gender/ Sexuality Reader.* London: Routledge.

Pollen R. (1993) Cultural perceptions and misconceptions. In: Montford H, Skrine R, editors. *Contraception Care.* London: Chapman & Hall.

Raphael-Leff J. (1993) *Pregnancy: the inside story.* London: Sheldon Press.

Rich A. (1980) Compulsory heterosexuality and lesbian existence. *Signs.* 5(4): 631.

Richardson D. (2000) *Rethinking Sexuality.* London: Sage.

Sample I. (2008) *Gay men and heterosexual women have similarly shaped brains, research shows.* Manchester: Guardian; 17 June 2008. Available at: www.guardian.co.uk/science/2008/jun/16/ neuroscience.psychology (accessed 6 Jan 2009).

Segal L. (1994) *Straight Sex.* London: Virago.

Seidler VJ. (1987) Reason, desire and male sexuality. In: Caplan P, editor. *The Cultural Construction of Sexuality.* London: Routledge; p. 89.

Sobo EJ. (1995) *Choosing Unsafe Sex: AIDS-risk denial among disadvantaged women.* Philadelphia: University of Pennsylvania Press.

Stoppard M. (1998) *Healthy Pregnancy.* London: Dorling Kindersley.

Symons D. (1979) *The Evolution of Human Sexuality.* Oxford: Oxford University Press.

Thornhill R, Palmer C. (2000) *A Natural History of Rape.* Cambridge, MA: MIT Press.

Tiefer L. (1997) Medicine, morality and the public management of sexual matters. In: Segal L, editor. *New Sexual Agendas.* London: Macmillan Press Ltd.

Ussher JM. (1997a) *Body Talk*. London: Routledge.

Ussher JM. (1997b) *Fantasies of Femininity*. Harmondsworth: Penguin.

Vance CS, editor. (1984) *Pleasure and Danger: exploring female sexuality*. London: Routledge and Kegan Paul.

Vance CS. (1991) Anthropology rediscovers sexuality: a theoretical comment. *Soc Sci Med*. 33(8): 875–84.

Weeks J. (1985) *Sexuality and its Discontents: meanings, myths and modern sexualities*. London: Routledge and Kegan Paul.

Weeks J. (2000) *Making Sexual History*. Cambridge: Polity Press.

Whittier DK, Simon W. (2001) The fuzzy matrix of 'My Type' in intrapsychic sexual scripting. *Sexualities*. 4(2): 139–65.

Willig C. (1997) Trust as risky practice. In: Segal L, editor. *New Sexual Agendas*. London: Macmillan Press Ltd.

CHAPTER 3

Women, poverty and childbirth

Caroline Squire and Kate H Beverley

Far from being consigned to history, poverty remains a fact of life for millions of people living in the UK in the twenty-first century. Although the relationship between poverty and poorer health and life expectancy has been known for *around* 160 years, progress towards its eradication has arguably been faltering and fragmented because of differing political interpretations of the causes of poverty. This chapter focuses on material explanations of poverty and analyses the issues and limitations inherent in policy approaches, both in the recent past and contemporaneously. The impact of poverty on the health of poor mothers and their babies is explored, with a focus on lone mothers and teenage mothers, together with the challenges presented for midwifery practice. The chapter concludes with a review of some innovative approaches to practice.

INTRODUCTION

Two hundred and fifty years ago in Britain poverty was a crime punishable by death in some circumstances. The poor fared little better in the nineteenth and twentieth centuries, as industrialisation and capitalism brought their emphasis on competition and success in an increasingly complex world of work. The expectation was that an individual should 'work to live'. If a person did not work, or their work did not pay enough, they could not expect to have the means to live, or live well. In a less direct way than was the case during the eighteenth century, poverty was 'punishable' by suffering and even death, as poverty-related diseases and illnesses took their toll. This legacy has persisted into the twenty-first century. Poor people die younger than rich people and babies of poor mothers are twice as likely to die as babies of rich mothers.

How can differences in life outcomes among people living in a society be understood and explained? Is it a matter of genetics and biology, consistent with Darwin's 'Theory of Natural Selection', where all species, including humankind, evolve and refine themselves through a process that guarantees the survival of the fittest; where the weak and flawed who cannot 'keep up' simply die off, incrementally creating a gene pool that grows stronger and healthier in the course of successive generations? Such an approach arguably presents a rather gloomy view of human life, suggesting, as it does, that there is little to be done to improve the life circumstances and health chances of the members of human societies. Poverty would, in this view, be considered as a 'fault' located within the poor person, attributable to some moral or genetic flaw. Either way, the cause of poverty would be seen as resting with the individual.

There are signs that this viewpoint has some influence in our times. There is constant debate in the media and in parliament about the extent to which 'The State' should help people who are poor or unemployed, including 'Lone Mothers'. One of the accusations levelled by some politicians, is that Britain has become too much of a 'Nanny State'. In other words, too much is being done to help too many people, and instead they should 'stand on their own two feet'. Another way of putting this is to say that only the fittest deserve to survive, and by their own efforts.

This chapter will challenge naturalistic and individualistic explanations such as these, in its exploration of socio-political and economic factors that combine to increase the odds of unfavourable pregnancy and childbirth experiences and outcomes for significant numbers of women in contemporary Britain. The analysis will include a focus on two groups of women who are at particular risk during pregnancy because of poverty: lone mothers and teenage mothers. Poverty as a concept will be explored, focusing on some difficulties regarding its measurement and definition. The efficacy of political–economic and health policy responses to the presence of poverty, and its health-damaging effects in the lives of women and their children, will be evaluated. The chapter will conclude with a discussion of the challenges presented by poverty for midwifery practice.

DEFINING AND MEASURING POVERTY

Poverty is not an historical relic. It has not been eradicated. Certainly, the advent of welfare policies, ushered in by the Liberal Reforms of 1904 and culminating in the Welfare State, 1948, improved the lot of many people in British society – though, as will be seen later in the chapter, policy has tended to favour men over women. Most theorists distinguish between *absolute poverty*, where a person lacks the means necessary to sustain life, and *relative poverty*, where people struggle with a standard of living below that of the majority within a given society. Absolute poverty is a grim reality for those living in the so-called 'developing world', where daily suffering and death, as a result of malnutrition, diseases contracted through exposure to contaminated water, and conflict, are commonplace.

In contrast, the 'relatively poor' find themselves excluded from participation in ways of life which are taken for granted by others in society – having a home of one's own, an inside toilet, a refrigerator, a car, a garden, or sufficient income to afford a 'healthy lifestyle', whether in terms of food or leisure activities. Whether their poverty is classed as 'absolute' or 'relative' possibly matters little to those experiencing it. Poverty may be experienced as a condition of economic disadvantage and insecurity as well as a social condition of shame and corrosion reflected in powerlessness and lack of voice (Lister 2004). Poverty carries a degree of stigma, which may mean that some poor people are reluctant to take on this identity, also closing off the possibility of benefits that might help:

> What is more, people at the bottom of the income distribution in Britain may not see themselves as poor, particularly if they make comparisons with those elsewhere in the world who face starvation and destitution, or even with those elsewhere in Britain who are worse off than themselves – relative judgements of poverty are shared by the poor too. (Alcock 1997: 8–9)

According to a recent report more than 5 million people are currently living in *absolute poverty* in Britain (Gordon and Townsend 2001). The study used a definition of *absolute poverty* based on a statement by the United Nations in 1995, which identified the key characteristics as lack of basic human needs such as health, sanitation, shelter, safe drinking water and food, along with access to education and benefits. Gordon and Townsend found that 17% of households in Britain considered that their income was below the level needed to prevent conditions of *absolute poverty*. Within this overall statistic are the 54% of single parents who stated that their income was insufficient to ensure that basic needs could be met.

A significant feature of this study was its use of participants' own perceptions of their lived experiences as the basis for measuring poverty. Such an approach differs radically from that usually adopted, where the emphasis is on external indicators of poverty or wealth (e.g. income level), and enables altogether new data to emerge, when contrasted with the more orthodox findings discussed a little further on in this section. Both objective and subjective perspectives have a significant contribution to make to studies of poverty (Alcock 1997). Both women and men experience poverty, but significantly more women than men have consistently featured in poverty statistics (Lister 2004, Doyal 1998). This is borne out in the data generated by successive governments,

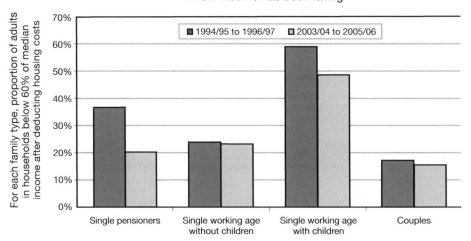

The two groups where women predominate – single pensioners and lone parents – are precisely the groups where the proportion who are in low income has been falling

Source: Households Below Average Income, DWP; UK; the data is the average for 2003/04 to 2005/06; updated June 2007

FIGURE 3.1 Distribution of poverty: change over time by family type

examples of which are provided in the statistical Figures 3.1 and 3.2. Figure 3.1 pro-vides a breakdown of the distribution of poverty within particular groups in society where women predominate by family type, while Figure 3.2 shows the rates from 1994 to 2006 of the rates of adults living in poorer households.

From Figure 3.2 it can be seen that the areas where women predominate in terms of low income have fallen during the years 1994–2006. This seems positive but, neverthe-less, lone women still predominate in terms of existing on low incomes and experiencing poverty.

Again, it is positive that the gap between men and women living in low income households is diminishing, but there is still a long way to go.

Children also experience poverty and child poverty is often related to women in poverty. In 2005, UNICEF published a report on child poverty in rich countries. The UK was found to have one of the highest child poverty rates in the rich world – 15.4% of the child population where relative poverty is defined as households with income below 50% of the national average.

Income has traditionally been used as a primary indicator of poverty and its effects (Lister 2004; Alcock 1997). Until recently this was problematic because of the assump-tion that, in households with a married couple (and children, if any), the female partner would be dependent financially on the male breadwinner's income. A married woman's paid contribution to the family income was thus rendered invisible, and the husband's socio-economic status ('social class') was automatically conferred on his wife. However, in 2001 a new system, the National Statistics Socio-economic Classification, was intro-duced by the UK Government (National Statistics Office 2002), and this tool, unlike its predecessor, promises to render women more visible in their own right, within the

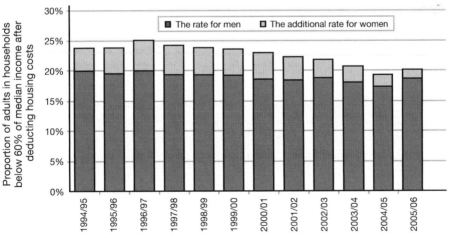

FIGURE 3.2 Distribution of poverty: change over time – all adults

data (Macfarlane 2002). The introduction of a new methodology will, however, make it difficult to measure or estimate trends over time, since data collected using the 'old' classification will not compare directly with that generated in studies using the new approach.

There has been a lack of consensus about the minimum income level below which poverty obtains, which has acted somewhat like a 'smokescreen', arguably extending debate, but contributing little to definitive action. Oppenheim (1997) is critical of the use made by some politicians, of data which indicate that significant numbers of poor have moved up the income ladder, and points out that such movement is often very temporary, given the insecurity of much low-paid work. Generally, studies of poverty by British researchers have made use of 'proxy' measures of poverty, in the form of 'deprivation indexes'. These are designed to account for the complex nature of poverty-deprivation, by assessing the degree to which a poor individual's ordinary life experiences vary from agreed 'social norms'. The present Government has brought such *social exclusion* effects of poverty and deprivation to the heart of its analysis and policy. Alcock (1997) offers the comment that:

> . . . a full picture of the problem of poverty within a society needs to address these fine grains of the experiences of deprivation, which the simplified definitions and statistical measures necessarily overlook . . . This broader focus on deprivation thus requires the development of an appreciation of what we do or do not do . . . Townsend has probably been the most articulate proponent of the notion of relative deprivation . . . He distinguished three different forms of relative deprivation:
>
> - lacking the diet, clothing and other facilities that are customary and approved in society
> - falling below the majority or accepted standard of living
> - falling below what could be the majority standard given a better redistribution or restructuring of society. (Alcock 1997: 85–6)

The lack of an agreed tool for measuring and defining poverty may also be understood as contributing to its perpetuation, though there is something of a 'chicken and egg' dilemma: have the politics of poverty failed because of 'academic' problems of measurement and definition, or has the acceptance of an agreed definition and tool for its measurement been constrained by the politics of poverty?

> Poverty is a term which is rarely heard on the lips of policy makers . . . The debate has been characterised by bland euphemisms – 'low income', 'below-average income', 'the bottom ten per cent' – terms which obscure the reality of deprivation, poverty and hardship. (Scottish Poverty Information Unit 1997: 2)

Human beings do not exist in a vacuum. The individual is situated within a complex system of interrelationships with other people, only some of which are directly experienced as part and parcel of everyday life, but which nevertheless exert an influence. Thus, for example, can the decision made by a financial business in the City to push up the price of some commodity or another result in less food on the table for a lone mother and her children.

CONSTRUCTING SOCIETIES AND ENGENDERING POVERTY

Arguably, therefore, poverty is not simply a case of 'the roll of the dice', nor is it an inevitable part of the human condition. Sociological analysis demonstrates that the dice may be loaded to start with, because of the existence of inbuilt social inequalities. Health, well-being and illness are profoundly influenced by the ways in which particular societies are structured, and the structure of a society is manufactured from political and economic ideas and decisions. As industrialisation and capitalism have evolved, the 'world of work' (the Labour Market) has become increasingly diverse and specialised, with concomitant income variability and disparity. Differences between individuals and groups within a society are thus manufactured by the unequal distribution of wealth and material resources, which in turn has an impact on potential status and power. The data in Table 3.1 illustrates the persistent inequalities in the distribution of wealth within the UK.

Gender divisions also form part of social stratification and, along with ethnicity, class, race and age, are supported by ideologies which include political systems of thought. The roles traditionally ascribed to women within evolving British society have ensured their unequal representation within the social system, whether in terms of restricted access to the labour market and lower rates of pay, or disparities in pensions

TABLE 3.1 Distribution of personal wealth in the UK 1991–2001

United Kingdom	Percentages				
	1991	*1996*	*1999*	*2000*	*2001*
Marketable wealth					
Percentage of wealth owned by[1]					
Most wealthy 1%	17	20	23	22	23
Most wealthy 5%	35	40	43	42	43
Most wealthy 10%	47	52	55	55	56
Most wealthy 25%	71	74	74	74	75
Most wealthy 50%	92	93	94	94	95
Total marketable wealth (£ billion)	1711	2092	2842	3093	3363
Marketable wealth less value of dwellings					
Percentage of wealth owned by[2]					
Most wealthy 1%	29	26	34	32	33
Most wealthy 5%	51	49	59	58	58
Most wealthy 10%	64	63	72	72	72
Most wealthy 25%	80	81	86	88	86
Most wealthy 50%	93	94	98	98	97

1 Distribution of personal wealth. Estimates for individual years should be treated with caution as they are affected by sampling error and the particular pattern of deaths in that year.

2 Adults aged 18 and over.

Source: Inland Revenue (accessed June 2008)

and welfare benefits (Equal Pay Task Force 2001, Watson and Doyal 1999, Abbott and Wallace 2005). Figures 3.3 and 3.4 illustrate the differentials in income between women and men, using current data, and thus providing insight into the contemporary situation within the UK.

Low income (<£7 per hour) is the same in this Office of National Statistics (ONS) survey between men and women in full-time work, but the disparities lay in the part-time sector with an almost 4:1 ratio of women to men in the very low paid arena. Part-time work contains other issues of lacking security and is made up, in part, of lone women with children who find themselves experiencing difficult lives of stress and vulnerability.

This table demonstrates the trend in distribution of low pay between men and women. It has been static since 2005 with twice the number of women being paid less than £7 compared to men. These figures comprise both part- and full-time employment.

Women do most of the caring and nurturing roles within the home, providing childcare and housework, or caring for a family member who is sick or disabled (Doyal 1995, Land 1999). These responsibilities can impact negatively on women's availability and capacities within the world of paid work. Thus, women are disproportionately represented within the lowest paid jobs, and are also much more likely than men to be in part-time work (Twomey 2002, Byrne 2005).

While issues of gender inequality were addressed in the latter part of the twentieth century, women remain disadvantaged relative to men in terms of their labour market position. This is confirmed by data from the Spring 2008 Labour Force Survey,

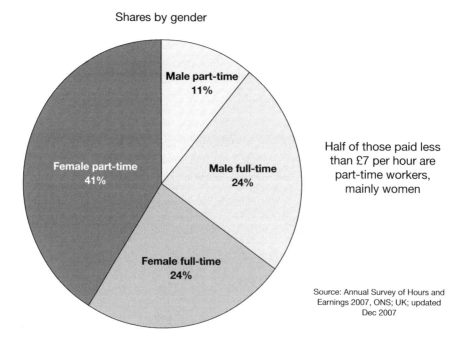

Shares by gender

Male part-time 11%

Female part-time 41%

Male full-time 24%

Female full-time 24%

Half of those paid less than £7 per hour are part-time workers, mainly women

Source: Annual Survey of Hours and Earnings 2007, ONS; UK; updated Dec 2007

FIGURE 3.3 Percentage distribution of shares by gender

Numbers in low pay: over time (proportions) The Poverty Site (2008)

The proportion of employees aged 22 and over who are low paid fell between 2002 and 2005 but has not fallen since. In 2007, 28% of the women – and 14% of the men – were paid less than £7 per hour.

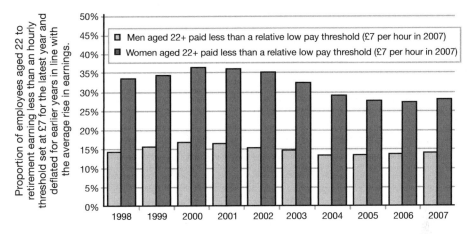

Source: NPI calulations based on ONS estimates; UK; updated Dec 2007

FIGURE 3.4 Pay inequalities between men and women: 1998–2007

published by the Government. The data also attest to the fact that there is wide variation among women from different social classes. Those in the lower classes (*social class* being defined as *occupational grouping*) experience a proportionately greater burden of material disadvantage both relative to men belonging to the same social class, and to women and men in higher social classes.

Women belonging to particular minority ethnic groups may be exposed to yet further disadvantage. The African-Caribbean, Pakistani, and Bangladeshi communities are disproportionately represented within the lower social classes, which may reflect exposure to the effects of institutionalised discrimination within the labour market, and within the social system more generally (Nazroo 1998, National Statistics Office 2008). While not all poor women develop poverty-related illness, or health problems during pregnancy and childbirth, they are at greater risk than are non-poor women, given the now well-established relationship between poverty and health inequalities (Acheson 1998, O'Dowd and Coombes 2008).

Where women are in paid employment outside the home they tend to have jobs which are part-time and have low pay (Twomey 2002, Abbott and Wallace 2005). This reflects women's involvement in childcare and other domestic labour roles. They may choose part-time work to facilitate these additional roles, or they may find themselves denied access to full-time employment perhaps because of discrimination by employers, on the grounds that caring responsibilities are likely to interfere with work performance. Most women who have paid employment have jobs in the service sector: hairdressing, retail, nursing, midwifery, education. These roles mirror the domestic and childcare work that women perform in an unpaid capacity at home, and are considered 'women's work' because of the presumption that such work requires skills that 'come naturally' to women (Crompton 1997, Doyal 1995). It is perhaps because of this 'feminisation' that such jobs attract low rates of pay.

Women in jobs that are mainly held by men tend to occupy the lower strata. Senior positions (especially management roles) are overwhelmingly reserved as 'jobs for men'. There is evidence, too, that women are denied promotion or career development by employers who take the view that, at some point, most women will take a break to have children, and that this justifies denying women the same opportunities as their male counterparts (Equal Pay Task Force 2001, Abbott and Wallace 2005).

Until very recently there was limited help available to women who wished to do paid work in addition to their childcare roles (Watson 1999). On the whole, employers have provided neither flexible working patterns, nor childcare facilities. The costs of purchasing private care may have the effect of trapping some women, particularly lone mothers, in a cycle of deprivation and unemployment, with all the associated risks for the health of these women and their children (Byrne 2005).

THE POLITICS OF POVERTY

Some political theorists (for example, Margaret Thatcher) have argued that the State should have a minimal role in ensuring the well-being of its citizens. Others (for example, Aneurin Bevan, the architect of the Welfare State, which was established in Britain in 1948) have argued an equally passionate case for a radical redistribution of wealth, to ensure that all members of a society have at least the minimum requisites. Welfare approaches, at least in part, go some way towards wealth redistribution. The main political parties in Britain traditionally have espoused fundamentally differing welfare strategies, broadly characterised as either *Individualist* or *Collectivist*, though more recently the high costs of welfare have resulted in some 'blurring' of the traditional boundaries.

Jordan (1996) puts forward a strong case for an approach which acknowledges that any human society will inevitably include individuals who are disadvantaged when it comes to competing for work. He gives as examples the very young (children), those who are disabled or sick, those who are old and those who lack skills or qualifications. Doyal and Gough (1991) in suggesting the existence of a number of *universal human needs*, propose that a new approach to social policy is needed, if the old inequalities are to be extinguished. Their 'Theory of Human Need' rejects both what might be called *Social Darwinism* (briefly discussed earlier) with its emphasis on *Individualism*, and *State Collectivism*, which emphasises *the social (collective)*.

Doyal and Gough contend that *autonomy* and *health* are fundamental human needs. From their perspective, traditional approaches to welfare policy have compromised autonomy. On the one hand they have ignored some individuals who, for whatever reason, cannot themselves meet their basic living needs. On the other, there is the problem that personal choice and freedom may be limited where policy dictates too much how people should live their lives. The problems relating to health inequalities, already referred to, will be further explored later on in the chapter.

The creation of the British Welfare State in 1948 seemed to break new ground. There was an explicit recognition that British Society as a whole owed a responsibility to each citizen for ensuring that she or he should have at least the basic requirements with which to sustain life. This included provision for those who were without employment, or whose income was limited. Successive governments after 1948 have restructured the welfare system according to their particular political philosophies. The result has been that a balance between individualism and collectivism, such as to ensure *autonomy*, has arguably never been achieved – certainly never sustained.

There is also evidence to suggest that the very essence of the traditional concept of 'welfare' was founded upon approaches which compounded, and even exploited, women's disadvantaged structural position within society.

> Because of their part-time and discontinuous employment patterns, women have less access than men to private and occupational pension and sickness schemes . . . The privatisation of 'care' through policies of community care has meant a greater burden of care falling upon 'carers', many of whom fail to qualify for the invalid care allowance . . . generally women have had rather 'less to lose' from welfare state restructuring and reductions than men. As has been well documented, the social security system was created with the needs of men rather than those of women in mind . . . (Millar 1997: 106)

Thus women have found themselves denied equitable pension rights because they did not work full-time (housework and mothering being excluded from definitions of work, because 'real' work happens outside the home). There is a paradox here, given that it is women who largely perform 'welfare work' whether in the home or in the labour market. Where welfare work is happening outside the home, women are doing this in addition to their other roles (Abbott and Wallace 2005). Formal acknowledgement and valuing of these contributions made by women, in the form of flexible working hours or workplace child-care facilities, have been largely absent from traditional welfare policy (Lister 2000, Lewis 2000). There have very recently been some inroads made, with the extension of pension rights and paid sick leave and holiday leave to part-time workers with commitment from the Government in tackling poverty to help lone parents and children (Department for Work and Pensions 2006a, Department for Work and Pensions 2006b).

Women are vulnerable both to poverty and poverty-related illnesses in unique and complex ways, not least among which is the mediation and reproduction of inequalities by welfare approaches that are gendered (Alcock 1997, Graham 1998, Kent 2000, Byrne 2005).

SOCIETY, POVERTY, HEALTH AND ILLNESS: LESSONS FROM RECENT HISTORY

Society can make people sick, or it can enable them to flourish and be well. Sociologists have been able to demonstrate that patterns of illness or wellness existing in a society such as Britain cannot be explained in purely biological terms. They argue that social factors, such as income levels and type and location of housing, have a direct effect in producing biological events that result in illness. This is not a new revelation; it has been known for at least 160 years. Chadwick, in 1842, published his 'Report on the Sanitary Conditions of the Labouring Population of Great Britain' and provided the earliest clear evidence that health varies with social class. Scambler (2003) observes that the work of Chadwick and others demonstrated the 'vicious circle' of poverty and disease, whereby poor people develop diseases, which in turn reinforce or compound their poverty.

The evidence that there is a strong relationship between material living conditions and poorer health and earlier death leads again to questions about the structure of human societies. The same health inequalities have persisted over the 160 years since Chadwick's study. Contemporary British society is constructed, then, in ways that ensure inequalities among and between people. To ignore this fundamental fact, and state that each person as an individual must assume responsibility for her/his own survival and well-being, seems something of a double standard. Social stratification ensures that some people start out with better material resources and access to opportunities than others.

Doyal and Gough (1991) assert that society should be accountable where the social conditions which foster poverty and deprivation, and their consequences for health, are a product of political-economic decisions. Their position then seems to echo that of Jordan, whose work was discussed earlier. There have been a succession of studies by social scientists in Britain over the last 22 years, which have sought to present evidence to guide political policy towards a radical response to health inequalities (Townsend and Davidson 1982, Whitehead 1987, Townsend, Phillimore and Beattie 1988, Drever and Whitehead 1995, Acheson 1998). The problem remains that politicians of differing political persuasions interpret the research in different ways.

POVERTY, PREGNANCY AND CHILDBIRTH

There is evidence that poverty and deprivation play a significant part in the poorer health of women:

> One in twenty mothers in Britain – particularly lone mothers on income support – go without food to meet the needs of their child. (Scottish Poverty Information Unit 1997: 3)

The findings of a research study carried out 18 years ago resonate closely with those generated by more recent research. Rutter and Quine (1990) demonstrated a relationship between poor housing and higher rates of miscarriage and infant mortality, housing type and quality being used as indicators of poverty and deprivation. Poverty, with its combination of disadvantages, impacts negatively on the health of women and their children – whether during pregnancy or in the years following birth. Women not in full-time paid employment outside the home, or who are working only part-time, spend more time in the home. Thus, while both women and men may be living in shared poor housing, women's exposure to these conditions may be greater, and thus render them more vulnerable to the cumulative effects of, for example, inadequate heating, damp, overcrowding, distance from shops and inoperative lifts in high-rise blocks. Contemporary research in this field is yielding a depressingly familiar picture (Lewis 2007, Sugrue, Kenner and Finkelman 2007) and many others. This attests to the absence of effective anti-poverty strategies up to the present time.

Lone mothers constitute the majority of lone parents and, as demonstrated in Figure 3.1, figure significantly in the statistics for households below average income. Women who are lone mothers are very likely to be poor, and they and their children are therefore at greater risk of ill health. Far from attracting compassionate welfare policy responses, in recent years lone motherhood has become stigmatised. One of the most pervasive stereotypes is that which represents the lone mother as a manipulator who deliberately becomes pregnant in order to secure housing. The evidence presented here rather gives the lie to that view. Currently the percentage of lone mothers within the population as a whole remains high as can be seen from the data presented in Figure 3.5.

There has been a trend towards housing lone mothers in hostel accommodation, which confers additional risks during pregnancy. More than a decade ago, Payne (1991) cited a survey by the London Food Commission, Maternity Alliance and Shelter, which demonstrated that hostel living was associated with a number of negative health effects on women and children. This included a greater than average incidence of premature births and babies born with low birthweights. Research carried out some years later reinforced the association between poverty, deprivation (including housing type and location) and increased rate of low birthweight babies (Wilcox, *et al.* 1995). Sawtell (2002) reports on the findings of a small-scale study carried out by Maternity Alliance in 2001, in which the experiences and perceptions of women living in temporary accommodation were explored. Almost half of those interviewed were lone mothers, and women from black and minority ethnic groups were disproportionately represented. The conditions in which women (some of whom were pregnant) and their children were living are graphically described by Sawtell:

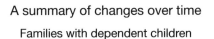

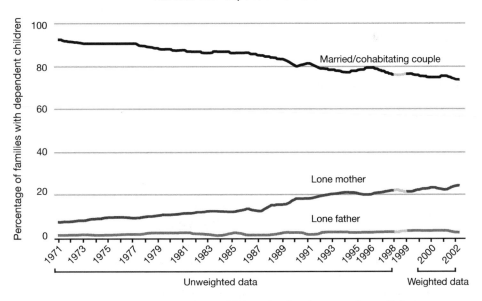

FIGURE 3.5 Families with dependent children by family type: Great Britain, 1971–2002: a summary of changes over time. (Source: The 2002 General Household Survey)

> Eighteen of the women were living in bed and breakfast (B and B) accommodation, six were in hostels and four were in temporary flats. With the exception of those in flats, most were living in one room and sharing amenities such as the kitchen, bathroom and toilet. All three types of accommodation were generally of very poor quality. Overcrowding, sharing of amenities, and infestation with mice or cockroaches were common concerns for the women. One woman estimated she was sharing a toilet with 19 others. The accommodation was often in areas of London that the women did not know, where they felt unsafe and where they did not have pre-existing local networks. (Sawtell 2002: 518)

These conditions caused the women concern about *their* health, including psychological effects, and also the health of their children. They had a sense of their deprivation, and were aware also that, at some level, this felt punitive. There has been a great deal of stigmatising political rhetoric about lone mothers over the last two decades, with lone mothers seen as 'the generative mechanism of welfare dependency and underclass status', which exists not only during their lifetime but also the lives of their children who will lack the male breadwinner role model (Byrne 2005: 99). In Hunt's (2004) study of mothers in the West Midlands, an emergent theme was that if a man was not economically supportive to the family unit, then a mother was best off without him – 'no wage, no use' (Hunt 2004: 143).

Nutrition is of enormous importance during pregnancy and where a mother is breastfeeding. There is evidence that poor nutrition may be causally linked to congenital abnormalities, and there is an increased incidence among pregnant women who are enduring poverty and deprivation (Acheson 1998). Payne (1991) observed that the state maternity allowance was insufficient to meet the cost of the recommended nutritional intake during pregnancy. As such, it was unlikely to enable women who had to rely on that allowance and other state benefits to afford to eat healthily. In 2005, the Department of Health launched a scheme called 'Healthy Start' to help families from low income and disadvantaged households, in England, Scotland, Wales and Northern Ireland, by giving vouchers for free milk and fresh fruit and vegetables to children and pregnant women. The scheme (Department of Health 2005) is to encourage earlier and closer contact with health professionals who can give advice on pregnancy, breastfeeding and healthy eating. This scheme was evaluated in 2006 in Devon and Cornwall. It was found that the scheme was more successful where Sure Start programmes existed and it has been hampered by senior professionals, such as Heads of Midwifery, who did not prioritise the scheme. Part of the scheme involves midwives discussing at booking the availability of vouchers to women of low income, including pregnant adolescents. But it was found that many midwives did not have a clear idea of the scheme.

Teenage pregnancies leading to maternities account for a very small percentage of all pregnancies. Teenage mothers are at particular risk of poverty, given that they are more likely to be unemployed, since they are at the very beginning of life as an independent adult, and pregnancy may have interrupted a nascent career or job development pathway (MacKeith and Phillipson 1997).

Despite the efforts of the Government and healthcare professionals, teenagers have had only marginally reduced numbers of conceptions over the past 10 years though more now choose to terminate their pregnancies – *see* Figure 3.6. Clearly, similar numbers of teenagers are currently having unprotected sexual intercourse compared

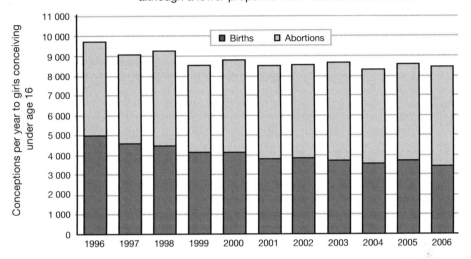

Source: Health Statistics Quarterly, ONS and ISD Scotland; Great Britain; updated Feb 2008

FIGURE 3.6 Teenage pregnancy rates 1996–2006

with 10 years ago, at the same time as the rates of heterosexual transmission of HIV are increasing as well as rates of sexually transmitted diseases.

It would seem that teenage mothers are disadvantaged not only by age but also by poverty and social exclusion – *see* Figure 3.7. As a group of people, they are over-represented in the Confidential Enquiry into Maternal Deaths (Lewis 2007) and may experience the childbirth outcomes associated with poverty, such as a higher rate of perinatal death and preterm birth (National Statistics Office 2008). There are also concerns about the risks to the children of young mothers including low school attainment, antisocial behaviour, substance abuse and early sexual activity. Many young teenage mothers drop out of school early, and more than half never resume their education, even though they are below the statutory school leaving age.

The Government's Teenage Pregnancy Strategy (Department for Children, Schools and Families 2008) was launched in 1999 as an attempt to tackle both the causes and the consequences of teenage pregnancy. The strategy's targets were to:

•◆ halve the under-18 conception rate by 2010, and establish a firm downward trend in the under-16 rate

•◆ increase the proportion of teenage parents in education, training or employment to 60% by 2010, to reduce their risk of long-term social exclusion.

The reduction of teenage pregnancy is a priority for the Government and in its latest response to the 4th Annual Report of the Teenage Pregnancy Independent Advisory Group, the Department for Children, Schools and Families is optimistic that the strategy to reduce teenage conception and pregnancy rates is being successful. However,

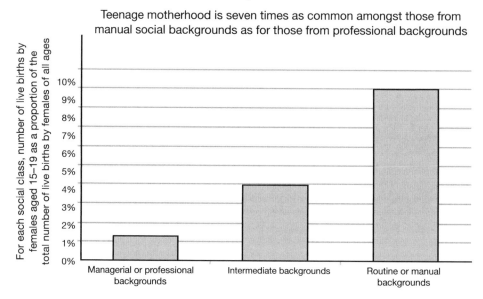

FIGURE 3.7 Percentage of teenage mothers according to social class background

close scrutiny of the number of conceptions to teenagers reveals little change and there is clearly much work to be done.

Hanna (2001) in describing the experiences of five teenage mothers in Australia, could be expressing the reality of life as a teenage mother in Britain today:

> It was concluded that becoming a sole-supporting mother during the teenage years was a difficult struggle for the young women, because of their youth, their lack of preparation for motherhood and their reliance on welfare supports. In addition, they experienced negative public attitudes directed towards them wherever they went, and this included their visits to community child health centres . . . (Hannah 2001: 456)

In their paper, Salmon and Powell (1998) draw on a wide range of research and policy literature to provide a review of the problems and challenges raised by poverty for mainstream midwifery practice. They echo Payne's analysis of a decade earlier in warning that women struggling to meet basic living needs may not be able to make the healthy lifestyle choices during pregnancy that midwives exhort them towards. Midwives need to take the facts of poverty on board fully, or they will run the risk of actually increasing the burden of anxiety for poor pregnant women. Lockey and Hart (2004) suggest that midwives develop an 'inequalities imagination' in order to provide good quality care that is empathetic and not judgemental. This would involve being able to work effectively and flexibly with women from a wide variety of backgrounds and with different personalities and needs in order to address health inequalities and involve the women themselves in the planning of their care – key aspects of current Government policy.

What a dreadful paradox, if the very substance of antenatal advice produces stress, which in turn may go on to bring about adverse physiological effects damaging to the health of both mother and her unborn child. What of women, working to a limited budget and perhaps having to juggle the demands of a job and childcare, who do not live near a big supermarket offering a range of healthy foods at affordable prices? The reality for many is that they have to rely on what is available locally, and such traders cannot usually afford the price mark-downs of the retail giants.

Thus, simply reciting the 'mantras' of health education advice to women, without being empathetically aware of how difficult it might be from some women's standpoints to achieve is, arguably, at best patronising and at worst dangerous. If experienced as moral censure (i.e., it makes a woman feel conflicted or guilty) it may possibly so alienate a woman as to ensure her non-attendance at future antenatal appointments. Reisch and Tinsley (1994) found that poverty itself may have a significant effect on the health beliefs of poor women who are pregnant, influencing their uptake of antenatal services. Armed with such knowledge and insight, midwives are better able to establish a relationship with poor women, which is based on respect and empathy. Getting to know and understand the beliefs that a poor woman may have about how she should behave healthwise during her pregnancy is a prerequisite for introducing any change. The alternative is simply to deal in pre-judgements which assume that non-compliance is the result of 'deviance' or ignorance, and as such constitutes a recipe for failure from the outset.

Crafter (2002) urges midwives to be realistic about the complex processes involved in attitude change. Expectations about timescales within which change can take place need to be informed by insights from psychological frameworks, and not simply aligned with political target dates. Being able to unravel the 'paradoxical messages', which are part of what might be referred to as 'the current professional rhetoric' that a midwife is expected to operate out of, is a key skill if she is to avoid reproducing this in her/his practice:

> It is important to address this issue of mixed messages because they can create confu-
> sion and inconsistency, and undermine the confidence of both women and midwives
> . . . Furthermore, if midwives do not acknowledge that they may be the agents of
> giving mixed messages to women, and women do not understand the paradoxes of
> what they see and hear, our good relationships may flounder. (Crafter 2002: 59)

The image of a woman depriving herself and her unborn baby of adequate nourish-
ment, because she puts her family's needs first in a situation where there is not enough to go round, is a dreadful one. It is the stuff of which a tear-jerking scene in a Dickens' novel is made. However, it is real life for some in contemporary Britain (Salmon and Powell 1998, McLeish 2002) and the situation is not getting better with reported price increases for wheat, bread and dairy products, the staples of those with low income (Borger 2008). The Acheson Report includes a section on the health and nutrition of women and children, and a focus on health during pregnancy, and makes recommendations for improving these. Emphasis is not only on short-term improvements to the health of pregnant women and their unborn babies. The importance of a 'healthy start in life' for the prevention of illnesses much later in life (such as coronary heart disease, mental illness and diabetes) is strongly argued.

Goodman (1999) contends that midwives need to use the report's findings as leverage for achieving increased involvement in planning and decision-making about health and social policy, both at local and national levels. It is possible that the 'Sure Start' initiatives introduced in 2001, referred to earlier in this chapter, came about, at least in part, as a result of lobbying of the kind Goodman urges.

Being poor is not just about physical effects. Self-esteem, which is a core component of well-being, may be reduced by the experience of poverty, particularly in a social climate where being poor is regarded as a 'moral failing'. The relationship between low self-esteem and depression among poor women has been well documented (Brown and Harris 1978, Graham 1993, Byrne 2005). Recent research suggests that postnatal depression may actually start during pregnancy. It is reasonable to assume that poor women are likely to be at greater risk of developing depression during pregnancy, given the limitations and uncertainties with which they may have to deal. They may not be able to rely on support or material help from family or friends, either because their social support network is limited, or because these people also are poor (Walker 1994, Oakley 1992).

CONCLUSION

Midwives can make a difference to the quality of a woman's experience of pregnancy and childbirth, and to the future health and well-being of her baby. In order to practise effectively, they require sound understanding and knowledge of poverty and its effects. Insights from sociology can inform good midwifery practice by replacing naturalistic and individualistic assumptions about poverty, learned in the course of socialisation, with knowledge of its social basis. At the very least such knowledge should enable midwives to avoid simply reinforcing the stigma attached to poverty by engaging in non-judgemental ways with women who are poor. At very best it may inspire some midwives to challenge those in positions of leadership and influence within midwifery to lobby for social and political change. Meanwhile, the impact of poverty on pregnancy remains an issue of social justice (Hunt 2004).

REFERENCES

Abbott P, Wallace C. (2005) *An Introduction to Sociology: feminist perspectives*. 3rd ed. London: Routledge.

Acheson D. (1998) *Independent Inquiry into Inequalities in Health Report*. London: HMSO.

Alcock P. (1997) *Understanding Poverty*. 2nd ed. Basingstoke: Macmillan.

Borger J. (2008) *Crisis talks on global food prices*. Manchester: Guardian. 27 May 2008. Available at: www. guardian.co.uk/environment/2008/may/27/food.internationalaidanddevelopment (accessed 11 Mar 2009).

Brown G, Harris T. (1978) *The Social Origins of Depression*. London: Tavistock.

Byrne D. (2005) *Social Exclusion*. 2nd ed. Maidenhead: Oxford University Press.

Crafter H. (2002) The practical aspects of health promotion in pregnancy. *MIDIRS Midwif Digest*. 12(Suppl. 1).

Crompton R. (1997) *Women and Work in Modern Britain*. Oxford: Oxford University Press.

Department for Children, Schools and Families. (2008) *Government Response to the 4th Annual Report of the Teenage Pregnancy Independent Advisory Group*. Available at: www.dcsf.gov.uk (accessed 8 Jan 2009).

Department for Work and Pensions. (2006a) *UK National Action Plan on Social Inclusion 2006–2008.* London: The Stationery Office.

Department for Work and Pensions. (2006b) *Tackling Poverty: a progress report.* London: The Stationery Office.

Department of Health. (2005) *Healthy Start.* Available at: www.dh.gov.uk (accessed 8 Jan 2009).

Doyal L, editor. (1998) *Women and Health Services.* Buckingham: Open University Press.

Doyal L, Gough I. (1991) *A Theory of Human Need.* Basingstoke: Macmillan.

Doyal L. (1995) *What Makes Women Sick: gender and the political economy of health.* Basingstoke: Macmillan.

Drever F, Whitehead M. (1995) Mortality in regions and local authority districts in the 1990s. *Popul Trends.* **82**: 19–26.

Equal Pay Task Force. (2001) *Just Pay: a report to the Equal Opportunities Commission.* Manchester: Equal Opportunities Commission.

Goodman M. (1999) The poor health of poor women. *Pract Midwife.* **2**(1): 4–5.

Gordon D, Townsend P. (2001) Breadline Europe: the measurement of poverty. In: Catchside K, editor. *Millions Live in Poverty in the UK.* Available at: www.news.bbc.co.uk/1/hi/health/1207241.stm (accessed 23 Dec 2008).

Graham H. (1998) Health at risk: poverty and national health strategies. Chapter 1. In: Doyal L, editor. *Women and Health Services.* Buckingham: Open University Press.

Graham H. (1993) *Hardship and Health in Women's Lives.* Hemel Hempstead: Harvester Wheatsheaf.

Hanna B. (2001) Negotiating motherhood: the struggles of teenage mothers. *J Adv Nurs.* **34**(4): 456–64.

Hunt SC. (2004) *Poverty, Pregnancy and the Healthcare Professional.* London: Books for Midwives.

Jordan B. (1996) *A Theory of Poverty and Social Exclusion.* Cambridge: Polity Press.

Kent J. (2000) *Social Perspectives on Pregnancy and Childbirth for Midwives, Nurses and the Caring Professions.* Buckingham: Open University Press.

Land H. (1999) The changing world of work and families. In: Watson S, Doyal L, editors. *Engendering Social Policy.* Buckingham: Open University Press.

Lewis G, editor. (2007) *Saving Mothers' Lives: reviewing maternal deaths to make motherhood safer – 2004–2005.* The Seventh Report of the Confidential Enquiries into Maternal Deaths in the United Kingdom. Confidential Enquiry into Maternal and Child Health (CEMACH). London: CEMACH.

Lewis J. (2000) Gender and welfare regimes. In: Lewis G, Gewirtz S, Clarke J, editors. *Rethinking Social Policy.* London: Sage.

Lister R. (2000) Gender and the analysis of social policy. In: Lewis G, Gewirtz S, Clarke J, editors. *Rethinking Social Policy.* London: Sage.

Lister R. (2004) *Poverty: key concepts.* Cambridge: Polity Press.

Lockey R, Hart A. (2004) Improving consultation with disadvantaged service users. *Br J Midwif.* **12**(12): 784–9.

Macfarlane A. (2002) Measuring health inequalities in pregnancy and its outcome. *MIDIRS Midwifery Digest.* **12**(Suppl. 1).

MacKeith P, Phillipson R. (1997) Young mothers. In: Karger I, Hunt SC, editors. *Challenges in Midwifery Care.* Basingstoke: Macmillan.

McLeish J. (2002) All I ate was toast: poverty and diet in pregnancy. *MIDIRS Midwifery Digest.* **12**(Suppl. 1).

Millar J. (1997) Dimensions of poverty and social exclusion: gender. In: Walker A, Walker C, editors. *Britain Divided: the growth of social exclusion in the 1980s and 1990s.* London: Child Poverty Action Group.

National Statistics Office. (2002) *Social Trends 32.* Available at: www.statistics.gov.uk/downloads/theme_social/Social_Trends32/Social_Trends32.pdf (accessed 23 Dec 2008).

National Statistics Office. (2008) *Social Trends 38.* Available at: www.statistics.gov.uk/downloads/theme_social/Social_Trends38/Social_Trends_38.pdf (accessed 6 Jan 2009).

Nazroo JY. (1998) Genetic, cultural or socio-economic vulnerability? explaining ethnic inequalities in health. *Sociol Health Illn.* **20**(5): 710–30.

O'Dowd A, Coombes R. (2008) News: Government will not meet its health inequalities targets in England. *BMJ.* **336**(7645): 633.

Oakley A. (1992) *Social Support and Motherhood.* Oxford: Blackwell.

Oppenheim C. (1997) The growth of poverty and inequality. In: Walker A, Walker C, editors. *Britain Divided.* London: Child Poverty Action Group.

Payne S. (1991) *Women, Health and Poverty.* Hemel Hempstead: Harvester Wheatsheaf.

Reisch LM, Tinsley B. (1994) Impoverished women's health locus of control and utilisation of prenatal services. *J Reprod Infant Psychol.* **12**: 223–32.

Rutter DR, Quine L. (1990) Inequalities in pregnancy outcome: a review of psychosocial and behavioural mediators. *Soc Sci Med.* **30**: 553–68.

Salmon D, Powell J. (1998) Caring for women in poverty: a critical review. *Br J Midwif.* **6**(2): 108–11.

Sawtell M. (2002) Lives on hold: homeless families in temporary accommodation. *MIDIRS Midwifery Digest.* **12**(Suppl. 1).

Scambler G, editor. (2003) *Sociology as Applied to Medicine.* 5th ed. London: WB Saunders.

Sugrue NM, Kenner C, Finkelman A. (2007) Women and poverty: the link with neonatal mortality. *J Perinat Neonatal Nurs.* **21**(4): 276–7.

The Poverty Site. (2008) *UK: Low income by gender.* Available at: www.poverty.org.uk (accessed 25 June 2008).

Townsend P, Davidson N. (1982) *Inequalities in Health: The Black Report.* Harmondsworth: Penguin.

Townsend P, Phillimore P, Beattie A. (1988) *Health and Deprivation: inequality and the north.* London: Croom Helm.

Twomey B. (2002) *Women in the Labour Market: results from the Spring 2001 Labour Force Survey.* London: National Statistics Office. Available at: www.statistics.gov.uk/articles/labour_market_trends/Women_in_the_labour_market_mar2002.pdf (accessed 23 Dec 2008).

UNICEF. (2005) Child poverty in rich countries 2005. *Innocenti Report Card No. 6.* Florence: UNICEF Innocenti Research Centre.

Walker C. (1994) Managing poverty. *Sociol Review.* April: 5–9.

Watson S, Doyal L, editors. (1999) *Engendering Social Policy.* Buckingham: Open University Press.

Watson S. (1999) Introduction. In: Watson S, Doyal L, editors. *Engendering Social Policy.* Buckingham: Open University Press.

Whitehead M. (1987) *The Health Divide.* London: Health Education Council.

Wilcox M, Smith SJ, Johnson IR, *et al.* (1995) The effect of social deprivation on birthweight, excluding physiological and pathological effects. *Br J Obstet Gynaecol.* **102**(11): 918–24.

CHAPTER 4

The family

Val Dunn-Toroosian

In industrialised societies, forms or models of families are changing rapidly, but one form, the nuclear family, is generally portrayed by the media as normative, because it is regarded as well adapted to the demands of modern societies. Family life has become a topic for political debate, and various policies have been devised to try to support families. In this chapter, the diversity of family structures and some of the social and demographic changes that impact on family structure and type are explored. Marriage remains popular in the UK, and is considered together with an examination of the roles of women in this context. A brief exploration of children's perceptions of families will be included. Some sociological theories emphasise tensions and conflicts within the family, whereas others view family structure and roles as the product of social consensus. The various sociological approaches with regard to the family are compared, and there is a particular focus on feminist perspectives, with their emphasis on women's experiences of oppression within the family.

INTRODUCTION

The idea of 'family' is an elusive one, as the word is used in a variety of different senses, and it tends to hold different meanings for different people. Families are supposed to signify security and love, and for the majority of individuals they do so. Family and marriage are also viewed as two of the most familiar, fundamental and enduring social institutions in virtually all societies (Giddens 1997). However, the debate continues as to whether the nuclear two–parent family is a central ideal type, or whether it is essentially a socially constructed concept and as such is influenced by the cultural and historical social practices in which it is situated.

Furthermore, families are unlikely to conform to any stereotypical image. In industrialised and Western societies, families are changing rapidly. Modern Britain, for example, is characterised by a range of different family and household structures, but the media always seems to portray a particular type of family. It is therefore hardly surprising that politicians have a traditional view of the family and fail to acknowledge the increasing disparity between family realities and family ideology. This chapter will explore the diversity of family structures and some of the social and demographic changes that impact on family structure and type. The various roles and responsibilities and the gendered division of household tasks will also be discussed with reference to the various theoretical perspectives.

First, the terms 'family' and 'social institution' require clarification.

The family

Families may be regarded as dynamic sets of social relationships, where each individual makes a unique contribution that combines with others to form the whole family unit. Giddens defines the family as 'a group of persons directly linked by kin connections, the adult members of which assume responsibility for caring for children' (Giddens 1997: 140).

Family members can be interrelated by biological, legal or functional relationships, which means that they are essentially a crucial support system, both structurally and emotionally, and they can be nuclear, intergenerational or extended in configuration (Kristjanson 1992). The United Nations definition of the family unit is based on 'the conjugal family concept', which is a traditional and unrealistic perspective of modern family life, as it assumes that most families are based on marriage and it therefore excludes huge numbers of families that do not necessarily fit within this narrow definition. According to 1987 recommendations:

> The family should be defined in the narrow sense of a family nucleus – that is, the persons within a private or institutional household who are related as husband and wife or as parent and never-married child by blood or adoption. Thus a family nucleus comprises a married couple without children or a married couple with one or more never-married children of any age or one parent with one or more never-married children of any age. (Hantrais and Leteblier 1996: 8)

It must also be acknowledged that every family functions within and is uniquely influenced by its cultural and social context. Different demographic structures, cultural traditions and economic characteristics of various ethnic groups will necessarily influence family composition. Thus lifestyle differences may be due to ethnicity, social class or religious beliefs, and families will differ not only across cultures but also within a given culture. For example, indigenous white British families do not all function in the same way. There will be variations in household type, family structure and the division of domestic labour.

More recently, sociologists have begun to argue that family is best understood as a set of practices as opposed to an institution. Which means that family is more appropriately viewed as something that we 'do' rather than something we are 'in' (Morgan 2006). This reflects the view that our social experiences are not only shaped by social structures but by our actions as well.

Social institution

Social institutions are a way of referring to particular social groupings that are common to the majority of people in society. They are often viewed in terms of the social need or function that they serve. According to Giddens: 'Social institutions are the "cement" of social life. They provide the basic living arrangements that human beings work out in their interactions with one another and by means of which continuity is achieved across the generations' (Giddens 1995: 387).

This definition of a social institution seems to aptly describe a view of the family, which is not only recognised as the most complex but also the most familiar of the social institutions. It is the primary socialising agency, responsible for transmitting the values of a society and fostering the growth of children into competent adulthood. It is also the main context within which children receive care and protection. Furthermore, *the family*, where common residence, marriage and parenthood are frequently seen as central features, represents the first experience of social life, and for many individuals it will be the most enduring social group to which they will belong (Murdoch 1949, cited in Hantrais and Letablier 1996). Most people have some experience of family life, and irrespective of whether it was good or bad the experience will undoubtedly influence what they think a real family should be. These personal experiences can result in judgemental attitudes, which are detrimental to effective client care.

FAMILY MODELS

People's experience of family shifts over time. Experience and life events will alter the composition of many children's families before they reach adulthood. These experiences make individuals re-examine their perception of family and the role of family. As long ago as 1982 Rapoport, *et al.* (cited in Giddens 2006) acknowledged the diversity of family forms and identified types of diversity as: organisational, cultural, class and life course cohort, and Giddens (2006) added sexual diversity.

FAMILY STRUCTURES

- Extended family
- Nuclear family
- Symmetrical family
- Mono-gender family
- Lone-parent family
- Matrifocal family
- Reconstituted family
- Cohabitation family

Because of the great diversity of family types and structures that exist within a given society, Gittins (1993) suggests that the use of the term 'families' rather than 'the family' is more appropriate, as it demonstrates cognisance of this reality. However, despite the many variations, there are underlying similarities in cultural perceptions of family life. The evidence suggests that, for more people, family is regarded as a kin relationship (biological, legal or functional), and links are maintained by frequent telephone calls, correspondence and visits. The family provides mutual structural and emotional support (Hantrais and Letablier 1996) and sociologists and anthropologists agree that the family serves to locate children socially and it is a major socialising agent. 'Kinship' is a term often employed by sociologists and anthropologists when exploring what constitutes 'families', and it is defined as the ties that exist between individuals. 'Ties' can be described as a special social relationship that creates the social and/or biological attachment between individuals. In some cases, friendship ties can provide much more social support than biological ties with brothers, sisters and other family members.

A broad distinction can be made between what sociologists and anthropologists refer to as the *nuclear family* and the *extended family*. These are the two main types of family. Most other family structures, namely lone-parent families, reconstituted families, mono-gender families, symmetrical families, cohabitation and matrifocal or matriarchal families, can fit within these two distinctions.

Nuclear families

According to Giddens (2006), nuclear families consist of one or two parents and their children (biological or adopted) living in the same household. Despite the decline in nuclear families, and it not being the reality for a large number of households, the nuclear family remains the most common and popular image of a family in Great Britain, and in the Western world (Office for National Statistics 2005, Bernardes 1997). It is still held up to be the ideal against which other family forms are measured.

TABLE 4.1 Percentage of dependent children living in different family types in the UK

Great Britain	Percentages				
	1972	1981	1997[1]	2001[1]	2007[1]
Couple Families					
1 child	16	18	17	17	18
2 children	35	41	37	37	36
3 or more children	41	29	25	24	22
Lone mother families					
1 child	2	3	6	6	7
2 children	2	4	7	8	8
3 or more children	2	3	6	6	6
Lone father families					
1 child	–	1	1	1	1
2 or more children	1	1	1	1	1
All children[2]	100	100	100	100	100

1 Data are at Q2 each year.
2 Excludes cases where the dependent child is a family unit; for example, a foster child.
Source: Census, General Household Survey, Labour Force Survey, Office for National Statistics

According to Jones (1994), this model is considered to be the typical and ideal family unit in UK culture, and this view is reinforced by current political ideology. Despite acknowledging the significant changes that the family has undergone in recent decades, the Government still asserts that the traditional patriarchal family (within a marriage) provides the most reliable framework for raising children (Home Office 1998). However, it is clear that the 'cereal-box' family, as it is sometimes referred to, is not the norm for a large number of children, and reinforcing the traditional family as the ideal can have detrimental consequences for children who are being raised in non-traditional families. The reality is that household composition has undergone significant transformation in recent decades. The percentage of two-parent family households with dependent children has fallen, while the proportion of lone-parent households with dependent children has increased. Although divorced lone mothers have traditionally been the most numerous category, the last decade has seen a sharp increase in the incidence of births outside marriage. However, despite recent social and demographic changes, in April to June (Q2) 2007, 76% of children lived in a family unit headed by a couple, compared with 92% in 1972. However, notably there has been an increase of 2% of couple families since 2001 (Table 4.1) (Office for National Statistics 2008).

Extended families

The extended family, which is a multigenerational unit, includes three generations or more living in the same household or in close proximity, or having continuous contact. It may include grandparents, brothers and sisters and their partners, aunts, uncles, nieces or nephews. Extended families predominate in most non-industrialised parts of the world. They are also more likely to conform to the traditional model of family life, with a male breadwinner who is the head of the household. They are often patriarchal units characterised by a dominant male and (usually) subordinate female and children, with unequal distribution of power and status. Female heads of households are less common except where the women are single, divorced or widowed and there are no other adult members present (Haralambos and Holborn 2008).

Symmetrical families

Young and Willmott (1973) believe that there has been a growth in the symmetrical family, which is characterised by more egalitarian role sharing. The symmetrical nuclear family is said to be home-centred, self-reliant and self-contained. Women take up paid employment and their partner participates in the household chores and child-rearing. Free time is spent around the house sharing chores. However, contemporary sociological evidence suggests otherwise. There certainly is a trend for more women to be in employment, but often it is either part-time or flexible working hours in order to enable them to fulfil their childcare and household responsibilities. Therefore they carry the double burden of labour in the home and in the waged economy (Jones 1994, Haralambos and Holborn 2008). Women undertake the bulk of household chores, and only a very small minority of men participate in domestic work on an equal basis. This finding holds regardless of whether wives or partners work outside the home or are full-time homeworkers. Women's share of total waged employment increased throughout the European Union (EU) during the 1980s, and in the UK women are now almost outnumbering men in the labour market, albeit in part-time and low-paid jobs. Despite these changes, men's level of participation in the home and family life has not changed significantly (Mintel Report 1994, Office for National Statistics 2001). This evidence dispels the myth of the 'new man'.

Lone-parent families

Another significant demographic change is the increasing number of single-parent families; they may be headed by either the male or female parent, but the vast majority of single-parent families are headed by a lone mother. Approximately 21% of dependent children are raised by their mother, while lone fathers account for just 2% of all families with dependent children (*see* Table 4.1). The majority of lone-parent families result from separation or divorce, but they may also be the result of bereavement or individual choice. Statistics show a rise in the number of births outside marriage and an increase in the number of divorces following the implementation of the Divorce Reform Act in 1971 (Office for National Statistics 2001). The UK has a greater proportion of children in single-parent and stepfamily households than most of Europe (Jones and Millar 1996, UNICEF 2007). However, there appears to be an ethnic difference here. Nearly 50% of black families are lone-parent families, compared with only 8% of Indian families (Office for National Statistics 2002).

In 2001, lone-parent households were more common among African-Caribbeans than among any other ethnic group in Great Britain. About half of Other Black and Black Caribbean households with dependent children were headed by a lone parent (52% and 48% respectively), and 36% of Black African households were headed by a lone parent, notably a lone mother (Office for National Statistics 2001). Lone-parent families are less common among Indian, Bangladeshi, Pakistani and Chinese households (*see* Table 4.2) (Office for National Statistics 2007). Even though there has been a notable increase in white lone-parent families, a decline is noticed among black families between 1991 and 2001.

TABLE 4.2 Lone parent households with dependent children:[1] by ethnic group[2]

Great Britain	Percentages	
	1991	2001
Black Caribbean	20.2	17.7
Black African	20.6	17.2
Bangladeshi	8.3	8.7
Pakistani	7.2	8.6
White	5.0	6.2
Chinese	5.3	5.6
Indian	4.5	4.8

1 Living in 'one family and no others' households.

2 Of the household reference person (*see* reference persons' box above).

Source: Census 2001, Office for National Statistics; Census 2001, General Register Office for Scotland

The Innocenti Report Card 7 uses data on the proportion of children living in single-parent families and stepfamilies as a measure of well-being, but it is acknowledged that this may seem unfair and insensitive as many children in single-parent and stepfamilies grow up happy and secure (UNICEF 2007). However at a statistical level there is evidence to associate growing up in single-parent families and stepfamilies with greater risk to well-being, including dropping out of school early and resultant low paid jobs. On the whole though, one should be wary of taking single risk factors in isolation as they are likely to have only a slight effect (Kolvin, *et al.* 1990, cited in Rutter, *et al.* 1998). Not only single-parenthood, but associated economic disadvantage is an important factor in determining well-being. In general, economically disadvantaged women are more likely to become single mothers and rates of separation or divorce are highest among the poorest families (Somerville 2000). Poverty rates are significantly higher among ethnic minority groups.

Matrifocal families

Matrifocal families (female-headed families or matriarchal families) often consist of a woman with her dependent children, and sometimes their grandmother. Such families are common in low-income black communities in New World societies; in the USA, 29% of all black families are headed by women (Haralambos and Holborn 2008). In the UK, 49% of black families are lone-parent (generally mother-headed) families (Office for National Statistics 2002). According to Haralambos and Holborn (2008), female-headed families are more common in black communities for the following reasons:

- Historically in West Africa 'polygyny' (a form of extended family consisting of one husband and two or more wives) was practised. Perhaps this continues to influence black family structures.
- Economic deprivation may lead to desertion by the husband or partner because he cannot fulfil the responsibilities of paying the bills, being head of the household and being the main breadwinner.
- Poverty is the primary cause of matrifocal families, and they have become the subculture of poverty.

Patrick Augustus' autobiographical novel *Baby Father*, which was serialised by the BBC, explores the lives of young black men who have children with more than one woman and boast about it. Darcus Howe once said 'We are black men; that means we make babies all the time' (Alibhai-Brown 2000). This is one of the worst stereotypes of black men. It portrays them as extremely irresponsible, but there are a number of complex reasons why young men behave in this way. Some men never agreed to be fathers (which is not a valid excuse), and are therefore resentful and feel no responsibility towards either their child or the mother of the child. The women involved are referred to as 'Baby Mothers' in the above-mentioned novel.

However, despite the statistics, matrifocal families are neither the norm nor the ideal within black communities. They are usually the result of the breakup of a nuclear family. This would suggest that many matrifocal families are the products of both culture and poverty. It is well documented that financial stressors are a significant factor in family breakup.

Stepfamilies

Households composed of one biological parent and a step-parent living with dependent children from more than one marriage or a non-marital relationship are referred to as stepfamilies, reconstituted, multiparental families or reordered families. Children whose biological families have not broken up, but who live with both parents and their step-brothers or stepsisters, also belong to a reordered family (Hantrais and Letablier 1996).

The evidence indicates that the number of stepfamilies or reconstituted families in the UK is increasing for a variety of reasons, and the rising divorce rate is but one of these. There is also an increase in the number of children being born premaritally (Office for National Statistics 2008). However, lone-parent status is often a temporary state, as most individuals still marry or remarry. Studies indicate that 50% of divorced or separated men will remarry within two years, and that 50% of divorced or separated women will do so within five years (De'Ath 1992). This evidence suggests that stepfamilies or reconstituted families are also on the increase. According to the National Children's Bureau, 2.5 million out of 12.5 million dependent children are in stepfamilies, and 300 000 children are born into stepfamilies (Foley, *et al.* 2001). These figures are still an underestimate, as they do not take into account cohabiting couples with stepchildren, who do not have to register their union or their separation in the UK.

In 2006 more than 10% of all families with dependent children in Great Britain were stepfamilies (*see* Table 4.3). It is socially expected that children will remain with their mother if a partnership breaks up, and Government statistics indicate that 84% of stepfamilies consist of a natural mother and a stepfather (Office for National Statistics 2008).

Stepfamilies are far more complex than biological families, and all family members have to make huge adjustments in order to make them work. Most stepchildren will spend time in at least two homes and have four adults trying to parent them. In families where grandparents are involved the numbers increase and the dynamics become even more complex. Thus there are sometimes three sets of parents and three sets of rules to observe and accommodate. Carers/parents often have very different rules, standards and goals for effective childrearing, which can sometimes cause confusion or conflict for the children, especially with regard to the issues of behaviour and discipline. Sibling rivalry may be exaggerated, and children may be concerned that the parents love their

TABLE 4.3 Stepfamilies[1] with dependent children[2]

Great Britain	Percentages				
	1991/92	1996/97	2000/01	2001/02	2006[3]
Child(ren) from the woman's previous marriage/cohabitation	86	84	88	83	84
Child(ren) from the man's previous marriage/cohabitation	6	12	9	9	10
Child(ren) from both partners' previous marriage/cohabitation	6	4	3	8	6
Lone parent with child(ren) from a previous partner's marriage/ cohabitation	1	–	–	–	–
All stepfamilies	100	100	100	100	100

1 Family head aged 16–59.

2 Dependent children are persons under 16, or aged 16–18 and in full-time education, in the family unit, and living in the household.

3 In 2005 GHS data collection changed from financial to calendar year.

Source: General Household Survey (Longitudinal), Office for National Statistics

brothers or sisters more than them. For some families there may be a need to appear like an 'ordinary' family, thus underplaying or denying the complexities of their family arrangement (De'Ath 1992).

Gay families

Gay families may consist of two adult females or two adult males who are caring either for their own children from a previous heterosexual relationship, or for adopted children. New reproductive technologies or surrogate motherhood may have been utilised (Haralambos and Holborn 2008). There is still much controversy about gay families arising from the belief that homosexuality is undesirable and therefore not the ideal environment in which to raise children. There is concern that children may be stigmatised, taunted or bullied by intolerant peers, and therefore it is suggested that gay families must be discouraged (King and Pattison 1991). However, there is no real evidence to show that children in such households are worse off. The quality of the relationship between the children and their carers is the major outcome determinant, not the carer's sexuality.

It is also known that because the current laws discriminate against gay couples as adoptive parents, most children of gay couples are from a previous heterosexual relationship. Therefore relationships between children and their parents, good or otherwise, are already established. Children more often remain with their mother following a marital breakup, and consequently lesbian mothers living with dependent children are more common than gay fathers living with dependent children (Haralambos and Holborn 2008). The evidence also suggests that homosexual fathers very rarely gain sole custody of their children, partly because few of them apply to do so, but also because those who do are usually denied. Lawyers are hesitant to advise clients to apply for custody, because if a heterosexual family is available that option is likely to be favoured (King and Pattison 1991). Social disapproval of and prejudice against gay fathers raising children is much more acute than for gay mothers, and this attitude seems to be reinforced by the courts.

In most Western societies, gay couples are not allowed to marry, and they are not considered to be 'proper' families by some. In the UK, Section 28 of the Local Government Act 1988 explicitly states that a local authority shall not 'promote the teaching in any maintained school of the acceptability of homosexuality as a "pretended" family relationship' (Secretary of State for Environment and Transport 1988).

Parents and Friends of Lesbians and Gays (PFLAG),[*] which is a national organisation in the USA that offers support and understanding to these families, points out that same-sex families should be given the same recognition and support as is afforded to traditional families. These families are often under huge emotional strain, and they need support from society for the family unit. They see the family as:

> . . . two or more persons who share resources, share responsibility for decisions, share values and goals, and share commitments to one another over a period of time. The family is that climate that one comes home to; and it is that network of sharing and commitments that most accurately describes the family unit, regardless of blood, legalities, adoption or marriage. (PFLAG; www.pflag.org/about/family.html)

---

* Parents and Friends of Lesbians and Gays (PFLAG) Family Values; www.pflag.org/about/family.html

In British Columbia, Canada, the Government has recognised homosexual relationships as being 'on a par' with heterosexual relationships with regard to child support, custody and access. These changes to the Family Relations Act gave same-sex couples the same rights as heterosexual couples. These changes and the general trend for more inclusive legislation are further affirmed by Callahan, who argues that:

> Gay or lesbian households that consist of intimate communities of mutual support and that display permanent shared commitments to intergenerational nurturing share the kinship bonding we observe and name as family. (Callahan 1997, cited in Haralambos and Holborn 2008: 507)

In the UK, Section 28, a law that prevents local councils from promoting or encouraging homosexuality through publications or campaigns or in schools, was brought in by Margaret Thatcher in 1988. The present New Labour Government promised to repeal the law in England and Wales as a measure against intolerance, and so teachers would not be prevented from tackling homophobic bullying in schools (Stonewall Survey 1996), to which Section 28 has contributed significantly. This met with strong opposition from the Conservatives, and was voted down in February 2000. However, in Scotland, Section 28 has been repealed and education authorities are free to discuss alternative lifestyles. In May 1996, South Africa became the first country in the world to enshrine equality, regardless of sexual orientation, in the constitution (Achmat 1998).

The Civil Partnership Act came into effect across the UK in December 2005. The Act grants same-sex couples rights and responsibilities identical to civil marriage. When a couple enters into a civil partnership it demonstrates that they have the same commitment to each other as a heterosexual married couple. In 2006, 1600 civil partnerships were formed (*see* Table 4.4). London and the South East were the most popular regions in which to register a partnership (Office for National Statistics 2008).

Even though gay couples have been adopting children for many years, prior to the 2005 Act they could not do so jointly. Only married couples and single people, including gay people, could adopt. In the case of cohabiting and gay couples, one partner could be the legal parent and the other had to apply for a joint residence order with the legal parent to gain parental responsibility. The new Act provides for an adoption order to be made in favour of single people, married couples and, for the first time, civil partners, same-sex couples and unmarried couples. It replaced the Adoption Act 1976. Supporters argued that children need a legal parental relationship with both parents regardless of their parent's relationship. Conservative Iain Duncan Smith refused to support the law because statistically gay and unmarried couples are more likely to separate. Research shows that cohabiting couples are twice as likely as married couples to split up before their child's third birthday. This holds true even when accounting for income and other socio-economic factors (Family Breakdown Working Group 2006). The Church is opposed to homosexual adoption on the basis that they are more fragile and unstable. However, Tony Blair has stated that Catholic adoption agencies are not exempt from the new law (Wilson 2007). Most adoption agencies now welcome gay parents, and statistically, gay couples are more likely to have 'difficult-to-place' children. There is an abundance of evidence to support the view that children raised in a stable two–parent family fare best, but there is very limited evidence to support arguments for or against homosexual parenting. The numbers of families with homosexual parents are too small to produce valid evidence on outcomes. There is some anecdotal evidence on positive and negative outcomes for children; some studies, claiming that children with homosexual parents are more likely to subsequently adopt a homosexual lifestyle, are flawed because of the small sample size.

According to Giddens (1999) in the Reith Lectures, up to the beginning of the twentieth century, due to the absence of effective contraception, sexuality in the traditional family was dominated by reproduction. With the advent of the pill, sexuality was separated from reproduction, and was no longer defined in relation to marriage and legitimacy. This being the case, the increasing acceptance of homosexuality may become evident. As Giddens (1999) says, 'sexuality which has no content is by definition no longer dominated by heterosexuality'.

TABLE 4.4 Civil partnerships:[1] by sex, 2005–06

United Kingdom	Numbers	
	Male	Female
Dec	1287	666
Jan	1308	529
Feb	1004	578
Mar	886	564
Apr	957	592
May	813	564
Jun	820	617
Jul	919	674
Aug	792	679
Sep	794	634
Oct	552	419
Nov	410	308
Dec	393	300

1 Data do not include civil partnerships of UK residents taking place abroad but will include non-UK residents who form a partnership in the UK.

Source: Office for National Statistics; General Register Office for Scotland; Northern Ireland Statistics and Research Agency

THE CONSEQUENCES OF SINGLE PARENTHOOD

The New Policy Institute, as part of its monitoring of poverty and social exclusion, found the following differences among ethnic groups in Great Britain. These include:

- The highest rate of poverty is among Bangladeshis (65%), followed by Pakistanis (55%), black Africans (45%), black Caribbeans (30%), Indians (25%) and white British (20%) who have the lowest rate.
- People from minority ethnic groups are much more likely to be in income poverty than white British people.

- 70% of those in income poverty in inner London are from minority ethnic groups, as are 50% in outer London.
- Three factors – differences in age, family type and work status – account for only half of the 'excess' income poverty rates among minority ethnic groups.
- There is a prevalence of lone parents within the black Caribbean and the black African population. For both ethnic groups family type is an important factor in rates of poverty. Work status also has an effect (Palmer and Kenway 2007).

According to O'Neill (2002) and Morgan (2006), for many mothers, fathers and children, the 'fatherless family' has meant poverty, emotional heartache, ill health, increasing dependence on state benefits and a lack of stability. An overwhelming weight of evidence indicates that the traditional family based upon a married father and mother is still the best environment for raising children, and it forms the soundest basis for the wider society. Children from these households have less antisocial behaviour, have better mental and physical health and generally are more likely to fare better in life than children raised in non-traditional families. This is not to say that all children from non-traditional families will have poor outcomes (Rutter, *et al.* 1998, O'Neill 2002, Bjornberg 1997, cited in Morgan 2006).

Many early theories made links between socially disadvantaged backgrounds, and delinquency and crime. However it has become clear that the association between crime and social disadvantage is not as strong or as consistent as assumed. This being said, social disadvantage and poverty do create increased risk for delinquency (Bolger, *et al.* 1995, cited in Rutter, *et al.* 1998). In fatherless families, reduced parental attention and supervision have a significant impact.

To date, British social policy has concentrated on eliminating poverty and reducing inequalities because of the belief that deficiencies in children's backgrounds can be countered by anti-poverty strategies. To address this issue the Government set a specific target to reduce child poverty by half by 2010 (HM Treasury 2006). However it is increasingly apparent that family structure is far more disadvantageous for many young people than parental unemployment or poverty. According to Utting (1995), there is evidence to suggest that much of the stress and adversity that impacts on the lives of parents and their children is preventable. Cohabiting couples are six times more likely to break up after the birth of a child than married couples. Therefore it is imperative that there are services to support the stability of cohabiting parents with dependent children. Unless coordinated family support services, such as parent education, and other policies that aim to strengthen all types of families are put in place, the increasing number of lone parents and the encouragement the present tax and benefit system gives to lone parenthood will continue to have a negative impact on the wider society and on economic dependence (Morgan 2006).

Politicians and the media have recently spoken out about family structure in the USA and the UK. According to USA presidential hopeful, Senator Barack Obama (now President Obama), 'What makes you a man is not the ability to have a child. Any fool can have a child. That doesn't make you a father. It's the courage to raise a child that makes you a father.' He referred to a 'national epidemic of absentee fathers' stating that 'more than half of all black children live in single-parent households . . . the foundations of our families are weaker because of it.' His message was that fathers should be made to take responsibility for their children (Bosman 2008).

David Cameron, the Conservative leader, echoed Barack Obama's thoughts over family breakdown and race. He warned that too many black fathers have abandoned their responsibilities to their children, and it is now time for a 'responsibility revolution' to change patterns of behaviour. His sentiments are supported by black church leaders and leading British African-Caribbean figures who are concerned about family breakdown and social breakdown. However, the Conservative leader goes on to say the discrimination and economic disadvantage experienced by black people must be recognised and changed, but at 'the same time we will never solve the long-term problems unless people also take responsibility for their own lives' (Wintour, *et al.* 2008).

Cameron has spoken out where Labour ministers have been anxious to play down the idea that the absence of fathers is a major influence on crime rates. By avoiding the issue of families and responsibility '. . . you leave out a whole important area of reform'. His view is that poverty will not be solved by increasing tax credits. The causes of poverty, which he identifies as drugs, alcohol and family breakdown, need to be addressed.

Educationalist Tony Sewell notes that the black Caribbean community has a higher level of absent fathers than any other group and questions why, when we're told that women can do everything, the absence of fathers is having a devastating effect on teenage black boys, turning large numbers to drugs and violence. He sees it as a matter of 'unchannelled masculinity'. In all societies, the driving forces of young men are sexual and aggressive, and marriage and fatherhood serve to channel these energies (Sewell 2008, Giddens 2006).

Personal responsibility is crucial, but more needs to be done to improve childcare support, unemployment, training and skilling of all lone parents, especially absent fathers, in order to give them the opportunity to meet their responsibility of raising their children. Singling out black fathers may be construed as racist. Absent fathers is a much bigger social issue and the negative outcomes and impact on society is equally relevant to all ethnic groups. The civil rights group *Fathers 4 Justice* claim that British law favours the mother when couples break up and make it difficult for fathers to stay involved in raising their children.

FUNCTIONS OF THE FAMILY

Sociologists are in general agreement that the family has several core functions that may be seen as essential to the reproduction and maintenance of society. These functions also play a significant part in ordering society and in determining individual life chances. Within the family, children learn discipline, acceptable ideas about right and wrong and the limits of tolerated behaviour. Fletcher (1988) divided these into essential and non-essential functions, the essential functions being reproduction, sexual activity and the provision of a home. Each family also takes responsibility for childcare, primary socialisation, informal healthcare, economic provision and maintaining the household. Traditionally, the family fulfilled many of the functions that today are provided by State-sponsored institutions, and the family is expected to utilise these services. Some examples include healthcare, education and the health surveillance role of health visitors.

The functions of the family have changed over time. The modern family is now seen more as a unit of consumption, whereas the pre-industrial family was regarded as a unit of production. Some writers assert that the role of the family is being eroded, and they bewail the breakdown of the traditional family. However, Fletcher (1988) suggests that the family has retained its central roles and that these have actually increased and intensified. Significantly, political leaders in the UK also urge the return to earlier family values (focusing specifically on the assumed evils of single parenthood), since an adequately functioning family is believed to contribute to the orderly maintenance of an industrial society (O'Neill 2002, Morgan 2006). The Government has pledged to support families and children because they believe that a secure family life gives a child a good start in life and the best chance of succeeding (Home Office 1998).

The 'deviant' or 'problem' family is defined by the powerful as one that is a burden on society, either because it relies on welfare support or because such families are perceived as being unable to 'control' their children, thus failing in their responsibility for socialisation. Again, mothers in particular bear the brunt of the criticisms. The case of a mother who was jailed for failing to prevent her children from playing truant made the media headlines (Staff and Agencies 2002).

An increase in industrialisation demanded a more mobile workforce, and this contributed to a change in family structures and role relationships, such as an increase in the number of symmetrical nuclear families (Young and Willmott 1973) and a reduction in the number of extended families. These changes are of interest to the State because there is a reduced role for grandparents in supporting young working families with dependent children, and this in turn creates a need for the State to provide adequate childcare facilities, as well as care for the elderly and dependent.

The notion of the family is reinforced by social policy, which is based on the assumption that everyone is in a traditional family. The family ideology in State policy asserts that:
- men are primarily breadwinners
- women are their dependants
- a woman's primary role is that of housewife and mother.

There is a dichotomy here. Conservative politicians in particular would prefer mothers not to work, as they need to be at home to care for and protect their children. On the other hand, they do not want single mothers to be claiming income support.

MARRIAGE

Marriage, according to Giddens (2006: 207), is 'a socially acknowledged and approved sexual union between two adult individuals'. This is a predominantly Western definition, as there are some cultures in which individuals marry before adulthood. Of course this calls into question the way in which the terms 'adult' and 'child' are defined. Although falling in love is the most obvious reason for marrying in Western societies, marriage is also of great social significance, in that it is an effective way of ensuring societal continuity through reproduction and socialisation.

Most EU member states recognise the family as an important social institution and are committed to its protection, focusing in particular on the 'legitimate' family sanctioned by marriage. Where there is a strong Roman Catholic influence or where marriage is a defining feature of family life, divorce reform has been difficult to institute. For instance, Ireland had not legalised divorce by the early 1990s (Hantrais and

Letablier 1996). The Family Law (Divorce) Act of 1996 legalised divorce.

Women are socialised at an early age that their main role is to be a mother, and that men must first have a career and secondly be a father. Women are therefore likely to leave work in order to bear and raise children. Once she is married, a woman's career is less important than that of her husband. Perrone (2001) has examined the sacrifices that both men and women are forced to make when attempting to juggle career and family life. She notes that in the USA men are becoming more active in parenting and homemaking as more women pursue full-time careers. However, women are more likely than men to describe sacrifices made with regard to promotion or pay in order to enable them to lead a more balanced life. It seems irrelevant that today most mothers are in paid employment out of necessity. They have to juggle both of their roles, and therefore they are disproportionately represented in low-paid jobs (Abbott and Wallace 1992, Crittenden 2001). Their choice of hours and employment is governed by domestic and childcare responsibilities (Abbot, Wallace and Tyler 2005). Furthermore, 'duty' is a sentiment that is often expressed within marriage, and women are made to feel guilty or deviant if they put their career before their family. It is also a reality that women can be poor even within an affluent household, because men generally control the finances and women receive a relatively small share of the household resources. They may also make sacrifices for their children, and are then left with even less to spend on themselves. This economic dependence reinforces the inequality between men and women (Abbot, Wallace and Tyler 2005).

Once they are married, women are expected to undertake the housework and childcare. Ann Oakley, in her classic study, *The Sociology of Housework*, concluded that housewives worked up to 72 hours a week, and were not rewarded by a wage or even status (Oakley 1974). Household labour, which is classified as non-market work, is deemed to be insignificant by male economists, even though studies show that non-market work contributes around 40–60% of production in many countries (Crittenden 2001).

Until the 1960s, the rights of mothers were legally subordinated to those of the partner and/or father. However, legislation is adapting in recognition of the fact that the male partner is often not the sole or even main breadwinner, and therefore he is not the undisputed head of the family in economic terms. Men and women are jointly responsible for managing family affairs, and legal subordination of women and children has been removed in most EU states. For example, the concept of parental authority was introduced to replace paternal authority. In the UK, the 1989 Children Act introduced the concept of parental responsibility, which could be shared with another person – for example, the father. After separation or divorce and in consensual unions, when unions are dissolved, the mother is presumed to be more capable of caring for the child than the father (Hantrais and Letablier 1996). This fact goes some way towards explaining why there are more lone mothers than lone fathers.

Social practices, such as the wife and children using the father's surname after the couple are married, confirm male dominance within the family. However, the sharing of parental authority and responsibility, division of property and the right of women to retain their maiden name after marriage and to choose their children's surname are some factors that symbolise a trend towards greater gender equality in some countries. In the UK, the father's surname generally takes precedence, but parents can give their child either the father's or the mother's surname.

Marriages are legally registered and confer certain rights and responsibilities on spouses. However, English law does not automatically give cohabitees the same rec-ognition, and when these consensual unions break up, if property was jointly owned, property disputes have to be settled through property law. Most EU member states have now formally recognised the rights of cohabiting couples, and heterosexual con-sensual unions can be registered. Case law has made provision for issues with regard to inheritance, division of jointly acquired property and parental authority on separation. However, some countries (e.g. Greece, Luxembourg and Ireland) have still not formally accepted consensual unions, and this places cohabitees, especially women, in a very vulnerable position (Hantrais and Letablier 1996).

A number of countries have extended their legislation on heterosexual cohabitees to homosexual couples. In the UK The Civil Partnership Act grants same-sex couples rights and responsibilities identical to civil marriage. Sweden has done so, and in the Netherlands same-sex partners can draw up cohabitation contracts to cover property rights and taxation, just like unmarried heterosexual partners (Collins 1992).

The terms 'legitimate' and 'illegitimate' are used to indicate whether a child was born in or out of wedlock. These are old-fashioned, value-laden terms that reflect soci-ety's attitude to marriage and childbearing. Furthermore, they reinforce the New Right view and the Conservative pro-family movement, derived from Christian morality, that the traditional family (with wives economically dependent on their husbands) is the ideal, and that marriage binds the family together. However, it is encouraging to note that discrimination between children born in wedlock or extramaritally is now being abolished by most governments, so that where paternity is recognised, regulations gov-erning care, maintenance and inheritance are the same for both. This arrangement may, though, inadvertently disadvantage the resident married partner. The UK, Germany and Sweden have acknowledged the rights of children born extramaritally since 1969 (Hantrais and Letablier 1996).

Because of the nature of role division in families, with women taking the greater role in childcare and housework, they are disadvantaged in the labour market. Due to the fact that they interrupt their careers to raise children, and because of family com-mitments, women may also have relatively less education, training and work experience and so be forced to take low-paid, low-status jobs. Feminists have repeatedly called for mothers to be paid, thus giving them some economic independence and raising their status. In the UK, women's average gross income was £119 a week, compared with £247 for men (Office for National Statistics 2001), and in the USA women earn 75% of what men earn (Crittenden 2001). Motherhood is considered by Crittenden (2001) to be the greatest obstacle to economic equality for women. On the whole, women draw the short straw in marriage in all respects. They are disadvantaged even with regard to their morbidity and mortality. It is well documented that women have a higher morbid-ity rate than men (Acheson 1998, McDonough and Walters 2001), although this may be accounted for by sex-role socialisation and structural disadvantage, but married women have a still higher morbidity rate than their unmarried counterparts, especially with regard to mental health (Abbot, Wallace and Tyler 2005).

CHILDREN'S PERCEPTIONS OF FAMILIES

Children's beliefs and ideas about what constitutes a 'family' have rarely been sought, and social policies that impact on their care and welfare are implemented by adults, without listening to what they want. Children's image of family composition does not mirror the traditional nuclear family form, which is often held up as the standard against which to measure all other family forms. Children's understanding of family is influenced by both social and cultural factors. Rigg and Pryor (2007) found in their New Zealand study that children were unanimous about the importance of family and being loved. The children referred to family as anyone you consider to be family, or as immediate family and relatives. Children and adolescents mentioned affective factors such as love, care, nurturing and support as the predominant criterion when defining family. This was followed by biological factors and cohabitation (Rigg and Pryor 2007). The prominence of affective factors was also reported by other researchers (Brannen, *et al.* 1999, Diez-Martinez Day and Remigy 1999, Morrow 1998) Very few differences were found in children's endorsement of family groupings across various ethnic groups. However, cultural context has a significant impact on adolescent's perceptions and older children emphasised the quality of the relationships. One teenager in Morrow's 1998 study intimated that a family is a group of people that all care for each other and help each other through life. They will cry together, laugh together, argue together and some may live together as well.

It is clear that a range of people including friends are important in providing emotional support to children. According to Dunn and Deater-Deckard (2001), where children experience the separation of their parents, grandparents and friends are key sources of support, and children who feel emotionally close to their maternal grandparents are less likely to have adjustment problems. Friendships become more important for older boys and girls. Overall, children and adolescents' views of the family embrace the diversity of today's society. The roles and quality of relationships and the provision of emotional and material security are more important than family structure (Morrow 1998). They generally have an inclusive and realistic view of what constitutes a family (Morrow 1998, Rigg and Pryor 2007).

Where parents had separated, many children said they missed their non-resident parent very much and longed to see more of them, and they frequently mentioned the unreliability of non-resident fathers, which caused much distress. However, children who had been given a role in the decision-making process about arrangements were more likely to feel positive about their 'divided' lives. Dunn and Deater-Deckard (2001) and Morrow (1998) also noted that children wanted to be heard but not to have ultimate control of decisions.

SOCIOLOGICAL PERSPECTIVES

Families are said to be the building blocks of society, and they remain the basic unit for the protection and rearing of young children. They provide emotional and financial support for both adults and children and have several core functions, which are important in terms of the reproduction and ordering of society. Thus it is important to explore their roles and functions from different sociological perspectives.

Interpretive sociology studies the meaning that is given to everyday life by those involved in its construction. The cultures in which people live have a profound effect on what is perceived as 'common sense' or 'reality', and this is just as true for family life. The definitions that are used for family life are the product of shared meaning. Goffman (1969, cited in Steel and Kidd 2001) states that people are actors and that they act out their social roles as public performances. Each role has a script, which includes cues about what to expect from others with whom one interacts. Some roles are *ascribed* (that is, given at birth, e.g. female), whereas others are *achieved* (that is, gained through life experiences, e.g. parent). According to interpretive sociology, these roles and corresponding scripts give meaning to social life (Steel and Kidd 2001).

The functionalists and the New Right adopt a *consensus* perspective, which means that they uphold consensus-based family values. Feminism and Marxism are *conflict* perspectives, which view 'family values' as part of the problem in relation to power, control, status and inequality.

From a *functionalist* perspective, social roles are culturally determined and adopting these roles contributes to the smooth running of society. The importance of integration and harmony between the various parts of society that are *functionally* related is emphasised. In general, functionalists define the family by the 'needs' it fulfils in society. Functionalists believe that roles give people their place in society and thus ensure 'normal' functioning of family and society. Families have an important role in the primary socialisation of children, who will conform to the norms and values of society. A distinction is made between male and female roles with regard to the division of domestic labour. Roles are segregated along traditional gender lines. Functionalists talk of a female expressive role, which implies that females are more suited to caring, nurturing and providing emotional support.

The male instrumental role provides financial support and is the breadwinner. A gendered division of labour is perceived as best serving the needs of industrial society (Abbot, Wallace and Tyler 2005).

The anthropologist George Murdoch (1949) regards biological differences as the basis of sexual division of labour in all societies, since this is the most efficient way of organising society. Woman's biological function of childbearing confines them to the home, and their physique limits them to less strenuous tasks. Men can wander further from home and perform heavier tasks. These were studies of 'primitive' family units, but one can still draw parallels in today's families (Haralambos and Holborn 2008).

Parson (1951, cited in Haralambos and Holborn 2008) viewed the family as serving universal (biological) human and social needs, and emphasised the necessity for a gendered division of labour so that care and nurturing (expressive role) and material resources (instrumental role) can be provided.

The *New Right* takes a similar perspective to the functionalists. Its adherents are clear that men's role is as head of the family and economic provider. The woman is the homemaker and responsible for childcare (Abbott and Wallace 1992). However, today many couples rebel at the notion of traditional marital roles.

The New Right and Conservative administrations since the 1970s have emphasised support for the stable patriarchal nuclear family with a dependent female and a dominant male. The Conservative Family Campaign was established in 1986 to restore the traditional patriarchal family and revive fundamental Christian values. Moral decline and family breakdown are considered to be the cause of economic and military decline in the UK. Conservative members of parliament have, in public speeches, blamed a variety of social ills, namely delinquency, vandalism, juvenile crime and a decline in educational standards, on the weakened position of parents. In a 1988 speech, Margaret Thatcher famously said that 'family breakdown . . . strikes at the very heart of our society'. A major problem, as they see it, is poor single-parent (single-mother) families (Abbott and Wallace 1992, Jones and Millar 1996). This was an era of 'lone-parent' bashing, and even though New Labour has played this down, their rhetoric continues to idealise nuclear families and marriage.

Feminists believe that functionalists support patriarchy by claiming that men and women are biologically suited to different roles in the family, and that therefore their ideology is problematic. Feminist sociologists argue that the family is the main means by which women are oppressed in modern Britain, and they have looked primarily at the gender roles within families. For them the unequal division of domestic labour is a matter of real concern. The heavy burden of housework and childcare leads to the 'captivity' of women in traditional gender roles. The stereotypical view of the family has assisted the subordination and exploitation of women and other dependants, and perpetuates the domination of men (Abbot, Wallace and Tyler 2005). Feminism has also emphasised the heavy emotional and financial price that is paid by women in families with traditional gender roles where they have little autonomy or emotional support and are responsible for most domestic labour (Finch and Groves 1983). The majority of men take on a minor share of childcare and household chores, but on the other hand may work long hours with much overtime. These expectations make it difficult for women to compete on equal terms with men in the labour market. Their occupational choices are constrained by family roles and responsibilities. As mentioned earlier, most working married women take employment and hours that are governed by the need to juggle domestic and childcare responsibilities and work. Oakley (1974) also emphasised the extent to which housework is built into the feminine role. Women are disproportionately represented in part-time, low-paid jobs and in social class five, living in poverty with dependent children (Oakley 1974, Abbott and Wallace 1992, Office for National Statistics 2001, O'Neill 2002, Palmer and Kenway 2007).

Feminists view domestic labour as real and physically demanding work, and as such they consider that it should be paid. Oakley (1974) also points out that housework is unrecognised and underrated, and radical feminists consider that men benefit from women's unpaid work, so they have an interest in maintaining the status quo – *see* Figure 4.1 for a lighthearted look at women's work. Marxist feminists, on the other hand, emphasise that women's exploitation in the family serves the interests of capitalism. Marxist analysis tends to concentrate on the way in which families encourage and reproduce hierarchical and non-egalitarian relationships. They maintain the status quo by providing tomorrow's labour force, and by offering a secure place for relaxation and rest. Through socialisation and day-to-day relationships, rebellious spirits are quelled. Therefore the family is seen as detrimental to the development both of the individual (woman) and of society. Feminists and Marxists are in agreement that the family oppresses women (Abbot, Wallace and Tyler 2005). Capitalism also oppresses women by excluding them or making it difficult for them to participate in the public sphere of waged labour, and by exploiting their labour in the domestic sphere. However, women's oppression pre-dates capitalism. It is argued that it is the patriarchal social system, with all of its structural constraints, that oppresses women.

The ideology of 'familism' supports this position, and Dalley (1988, cited in Jones 1994) states the following:

> The ideology of familism is based on the assumption that the family, and particularly the nuclear family, with breadwinner male and dependent female and children, is the

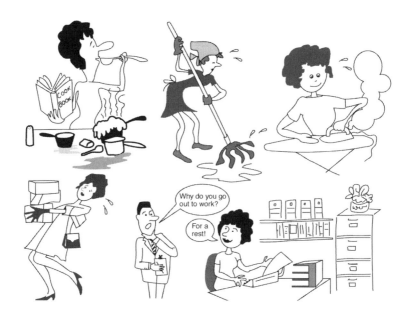

FIGURE 4.1 Women at Work (reproduced with the permission of Nelson Thornes Ltd from *Sociology Alive!* by Stephen Moore, first published 1987).

normal and natural unit for nurturing and caring. It is the standard against which all forms are measured and, importantly, judged. Accordingly, non-family forms are deemed to be deviant and/or subversive. (Dalley 1988, cited in Jones 1994: 93)

Postmodernism suggests that the world is shaped by pluralism, religious freedom, consumerism, mobility and increasing access to news and entertainment. The postmodern is inclusive, and dismisses the existence of an absolute reality acknowledging instead that there are multiple realities. By definition, therefore, the postmodern family is less uniform and includes a variety of family forms, as described earlier. Furthermore, the purposes and functions of families have changed and are more diverse. Shorter (1975) may have been the first to describe the emerging postmodern family. He noted the following three important characteristics:

Adolescent indifference to the family's identity; instability in the lives of couples, accompanied by rapidly increasing divorce rates; and destruction of the 'nest' notion of nuclear family life with the liberation of women. (Shorter 1975)

According to Elkind (1995), the postmodern family values autonomy, and is parent–centred, basing decisions on the needs and aspirations of both parents. 'Maternal love' is believed to be a social construction that can be expanded to include 'paternal love', and shared parenting replaces the 'universal' construction of mother as sole carer. These trends are often seen as the breakdown of the family.

All industrialised countries have seen a change in families from the predominantly

TABLE 4.5 Summary of sociological perspectives on the family

Sociological perspectives	Description (view)	Division of labour	Functions	Paid employment (earnings, dependence)
Consensus perspectives				
Functionalists	Traditional, patriarchal nuclear family with dominant man and dependent woman and children seen as the ideal. Other family forms are undesirable	Gendered division of domestic labour is taken for granted. Male breadwinner, female housewife who cares for children and breadwinner. Female has expressive role and male has instrumental role	Seen as a necessary institution in society. Emphasis is on the benefits of families, namely procreation, socialisation, economic and emotional support. Traditional nuclear family is most suited to the needs of industrialised society	Men need a family wage, as their prime responsibility is earning to support the family. Women do not need a family wage. They work for non-essentials, their prime responsibility is as a homemaker, and therefore they usually have low-paid or part-time jobs
New Right	Similar to functionalist. They take a moralist view and they emphasise heterosexual marriage as central to a family unit	Social/gender roles are prescribed and have biblical origins	Women should be at home caring for the children and pampering the male breadwinner. All social ills are blamed on the woman rebelling against her traditional role	New Right feel that women should not take up paid employment
Conflict perspectives				
Feminists	Feminists argue against the view that any specific family form is 'natural' or 'normal'. They focus attention on the diversity of families, and they draw on anthropological evidence to demonstrate a wide variety of kinship systems across the world	Women have the major responsibility for domestic labour (the essential repetitive tasks), while men 'help out'. Even when in full-time employment, women bear the double burden because domestic labour is not viewed as 'real' work	The family is the main means of oppression and subordination of women and children. It reinforces and perpetuates women's subordinate roles, while men exploit women's unpaid domestic labour	Motherhood, domestic responsibilities and childcare restrict the choice of jobs. Therefore women are predominantly in low-paid, part-time work. Restricted work opportunities mean that economic and political power lies with men

(cont.)

Conflict perspectives (cont.)

Sociological perspectives	Description (view)	Division of labour	Functions	Paid employment (earnings, dependence)
Marxists	Similar to feminists. They question the assumption that the traditional nuclear family is best for the individual	The unequal division of domestic labour oppresses women, and women's traditional role within the family helps to maintain the status quo – and provides a healthy, happy workforce	Families meet the needs of a capitalist society at the expense of the individual (female). Capitalists exploit women's unpaid labour as carers and homemakers. Marxists view the family, where socially acceptable behaviour and social responsibility are learned, as an agent of social control	Capitalism makes it difficult for women to compete with men in the workplace

extended institutional family to the small self-contained modern or postmodern family. For many postmodern children there is dual socialisation by family and childminder or nursery. This can create new problems, because while some children thrive, others are unable to adjust to the demands of a daily transition from one environment to the other.

Functionalists tend to ignore the harmful effects of family life and the inequalities of domestic life, while feminists question commonsense and conventional sociological assumptions of the family. Thorne (1982) states that feminists argue against the view that any specific family form is natural. Family forms are socially constructed around assumptions about people's roles, and there is no biological reason for the gendered division of labour. Families have 'power relationships that can and do result in conflict, violence and the inequitable distribution of work and resources' (Abbot, Wallace and Tyler 2005). Family crime, a term that is used to define violence and abuse in domestic life, is seen as less serious than 'real crime', even though domestic violence accounts for 25% of all violent crime (Saraga and Muncie 2001). (*See* Table 4.5 for a summary of sociological perspectives on the family.)

Roles and relationships within the family are not becoming more democratic and symmetrical, and equality remains an illusory goal. The Omnibus Survey (Office for National Statistics 1999) clearly illustrated that the family is still essentially patriarchal. In the UK, the average male spends more time eating out, watching television and gardening than his female partner, and does less than a quarter of the cooking and routine housework, even though he is less likely to be the sole or even main breadwinner. The proportion of women in employment increased during the latter half of the twentieth century, while for men the proportion has declined. However, men do spend more time on gardening, caring for pets and home improvements, and on average they work longer hours than women in waged labour (Office for National Statistics 2001).

CONCLUSION

This chapter has explored the diversity of family forms, noting the various demographic changes and cultural influences on families, and considering some sociological perspectives. Roles within the family have also been explored, especially the division of domestic labour.

Family structures have become more diverse and complex during the last decade, but despite these changes families will continue to play a very important role in people's lives. The family does not have a static, fixed definition and will survive in a plurality of family forms. A postmodern family perspective will become more common. Cohabitation is a popular prelude to marriage, and this trend will continue as social attitudes become increasingly tolerant, but evidence suggests that it will not replace marriage. Dual-earner families, stepfamilies and single-parent families are also on the increase. Homosexual families and families using new advances in reproductive technology create another set of issues, and introduce debates about biological versus social definitions of kinship.

There are some advantages to traditional families. Two-parent families are less vulnerable to socio-economic deprivation and health problems than lone-parent families. This does not mean that they are necessarily better than alternative family structures, which even in today's climate tend to be devalued. There is greater social acceptance that children can and indeed do flourish in non-traditional family environments, even though Government policy and ideology continues to promote the idea of a traditional nuclear heterosexual two-parent family as the ideal. However, it should not be forgotten that the traditional family is essentially patriarchal, with subordinate women and children, and domestic violence towards women and children is a consequence of unequal power relationships and male authority.

KEY POINTS

- ∞ There is a great diversity of family structures and family types in UK society.
- ∞ Ideologies of the family, such as familism, patriarchy and the gendered division of domestic labour, impact on women's lives.
- ∞ Families play an important role in ordering society. Marriage remains a popular social institution.

REFERENCES

Abbot P, Wallace C, Tyler M. (2005) *An Introduction to Sociology: feminist perspectives*. 3rd ed. London: Routledge.

Abbott P, Wallace C. (1992) *The Family and the New Right*. London: Pluto Press.

Acheson D. (1998) *Independent Inquiry into Inequalities in Health*. London: The Stationery Office.

Achmat Z. (1998) *Africa gay rights win in South Africa*. London: BBC News; 9 October 1998. Available at: http://news.bbc.co.uk/1/hi/world/africa/190268.stm (accessed 24 Dec 2008).

Alibhai-Brown Y. (2000) *We are black men: that means we make babies*. Manchester: Guardian; 13 April 2000; p. 8.

Benson H. (2006) *The Conflation of Marriage and Cohabitation in Government Statistics – a Denial of Difference Rendered Untenable by Analysis of Outcomes*. Bristol: Bristol Community Family Trust.

Bernardes J. (1997) *Family Studies*. London: Routledge.

Bosman J. (2008) *Obama takes on absent black fathers in speech*. USA: International Herald Tribune; 16 June 2008. Available at: www.iht.com/articles/2008/06/16/america/fathers.php (accessed 24 Dec 2008).

Brannen J, Heptinstall E, Bhopal K. (1999) *Connecting Children: care and family life in later childhood*. Andover: Routledge Falmer.

Collins H. (1992) *The Equal Opportunities Handbook: a guide to law and best practice in Europe*. Oxford: Blackwell.

Crittenden A. (2001) *The Price of Motherhood: why the most important job in the world is still the least valued*. New York: Henry Holt and Company.

De'Ath E. (1992) Stepping into family life. *Health Visit*. **65**(1): 15–17.

Diez-Martinez Day E, Remigy MJ. (1999) Mexican and French children's conceptions about family: a developmental approach. *J Compar Fam Studies*. **30**: 95–112.

Dunn J, Deater-Deckard K. (2001) *Children's Views of Their Changing Families*. York: Joseph Rowntree Foundation.

Elkind D. (1995) School and family in the postmodern world. *Phi Delta Kappan*. **77**: 8–14.

Family Breakdown Working Group. (2006) *The State of the National Report: fractured families*. Chair: Samantha Callan. London: Social Policy Justice Group.

Finch J, Groves D. (1983) *A Labour of Love: women, work and caring*. London: Routledge and Kegan Paul.

Fletcher R. (1988) *The Shaking of the Foundations: family and society*. London: Routledge.

Foley P, Roche J, Tucker S, editors. (2001) *Children in Society: contemporary theory, policy and practice*. Basingstoke: Palgrave, in association with Open University Press, Buckingham.

Giddens A. (1995) *Sociology*. 2nd ed. Cambridge: Polity Press.

Giddens A. (1997) *Sociology*. 3rd ed. Cambridge: Polity Press.

Giddens A. (1999) *Family*. London: BBC Reith Lectures. Available at: http://news.bbc.co.uk/hi/english/static/events/reith_99/default.htm (accessed 18 Feb 2009).

Giddens A. (2006) *Sociology*. 5th ed. Cambridge: Polity Press

Gittins D. (1993) *The Family in Question*. 2nd ed. Basingstoke: Macmillan.

Hantrais L, Letablier M-T. (1996) *Families and Family Policies in Europe*. London: Longman.

Haralambos M, Holborn M. (2008) *Sociology Themes and Perspectives*. 7th ed. London: Collins Educational.

HM Treasury (July 2006) *Child Poverty Review*. London: The Stationery Office.

Home Office. (1998) *Supporting Families: a consultative document*. London: The Stationery Office.

Jones H, Millar J, editors. (1996) *The Politics of the Family*. Aldershot: Avebury.

Jones L. (1994) *The Social Context of Health and Health Work*. Basingstoke: Macmillan.

King MB, Pattison P. (1991) Homosexuality and parenthood. *BMJ*. **303**: 295–7.

Kristjanson LJ. (1992) Conceptual issues related to measurement in family research. *Can J Nurs Res*. **24**: 37–52.

Mason A, Palmer A. (1996) *Queer Bashing: a national survey of hate crimes against lesbians and gay men*. London: Stonewall.

McDonough P, Walters V. (2001) Gender and health: reassessing patterns and explanations. *Soc Sci Med*. **52**: 547–59.

Mintel Report. (1994) *Men 2000*. London: Mintel.

Morgan P. (2006) *Family Policy, Family Changes: Sweden, Italy and Britain compared*. London: The Institute for the Study of Civil Society, CIVITAS.

Morrow V. (1998) *Understanding Families: children's perspectives*. London: National Children's Bureau.

Murdoch GP. (1949) *Social Structure*. New York: Macmillan.

Oakley A. (1974) *The Sociology of Housework*. Oxford: Martin Robertson.

Office for National Statistics. (1999) *National Statistics Omnibus Survey*. London: The Stationery Office.

Office for National Statistics. (2001) *Social Trends No. 31*. London: The Stationery Office.

Office for National Statistics. (2002) *Social Trends No. 32*. London: The Stationery Office.

Office for National Statistics. (2005) *Social Trends No. 35*. London: The Stationery Office.

Office for National Statistics. (2007) *Social Trends No. 38*. London: The Stationery Office.

Office for National Statistics. (2008) *Social Trends No. 40*. London: The Stationery Office.

O'Neill R. (2002) *Experiments in Living: the fatherless family*. London: The Institute for the Study of Civil Society, CIVITAS.

Palmer G, Kenway P. (2007) *Poverty Among Ethnic Groups: how and why does it differ?* York: Joseph Rowntree Foundation. Available at: www.jrf.org.uk/bookshop/eBooks/2042-ethnicity-relative-poverty.pdf (accessed 6 Jan 2009).

Rigg A, Pryor J. (2007) Children's perceptions of families: what do they really think? *Children & Society*. **21**: 17–30.

Rutter M, Giller H, Hagel A. (1998) *Antisocial Behaviour in Young People*. Cambridge: Cambridge University Press.

Saraga E, Muncie J. (2001) Family crime. In: McLaughlin E, Muncie J, editors. *The Sage Dictionary of Criminology*. London: Sage.

Secretary of State for Environment and Transport. (1988) *Local Government Act 1988*. London:

HMSO. Availabe at: www.hmso.gov.uk/acts/acts 19/Ukpga_19880009_en_5.htm (accessed 6 Mar 2009)

Sewell T. (2008) *Scandal of the absent fathers*. London: Daily Mail; 16 Feb 2007. Available at: www.dailymail.co.uk/news/article-436527/Scandal-absent-fathers.html (accessed 24 Dec 2008).

Shorter E. (1975) *The Making of the Modern Family*. New York: Basic Books.

Somerville J. (2000) *Feminism and the Family: politics and society in the UK and USA*. Basingstoke: Palgrave Macmillan.

Staff and Agencies. (2002) *No place for a mother. Truancy is bad: prison won't solve it*. Manchester: Guardian; 15 May 2002: p. 17.

Steel L, Kidd W. (2001) *The Family*. Basingstoke: Palgrave.

Thorne B. (1982) *Feminist Rethinking of the Family: an overview*. New York: Longman.

UNICEF. (2007) Child poverty in perspective: an overview of child well-being in rich countries. *Innocenti Report Card 7*. Florence: UNICEF Innocenti Research Centre.

Utting D. (1995) *Family and Parenthood: supporting families, preventing breakdown*. York: Joseph Rowntree Foundation.

Wilson G. (2007) *Blair retreats over opt-out for gay adoption*. The Telegraph; 26 January 2007. Available at: www.telegraph.co.uk/news/uknews/1540480/Blair-retreats-over-opt-out-for-gay-adoption.html (accessed 18 Feb 2009).

Wintour P, Watt N, Topping A. (2008) *Cameron: absent black fathers must meet responsibilities*. Manchester: Guardian; 16 July 2008. Available at: www.guardian.co.uk/politics/2008/jul/16/davidcameron.conservatives1 (accessed 24 Dec 2008).

Young M, Willmott P. (1973) *The Symmetrical Family*. Harmondsworth: Penguin.

CHAPTER 5

'Race', ethnicity, culture and childbirth

Dave Sookhoo

Pregnancy and childbirth are unique life events. They cannot be reduced to primarily biological events since the social and cultural contexts are central to the subjective and collective experiences of women. Personal factors, such as the woman's age, ethnicity, social class, religion and culture, may influence the experiences of pregnancy and childbirth. This chapter explores the concepts of 'race', ethnicity and culture in respect to pregnancy and childbirth. The issues of access to maternity services, stereotyping and racism are explored within the context of midwifery service provision and practice. The challenge of caring for someone whose cultural beliefs and practices are not similar to one's own raises questions about the cultural competence of healthcare professionals, particularly the midwife.

INTRODUCTION

In health sciences, as elsewhere, the definition and meanings of terms such as 'race', 'ethnicity', and 'culture' have been extensively debated. The mosaic or maze approach does not clarify the situation. The use of these terms, sometimes without any clarification of the context or the perspective being adopted, does little to eliminate the confusion that can arise, particularly when the terms are used synonymously or assumed to be implicit in their sense. The common sense approach does not help either because sometimes these terms have been used to advance particular political and economic viewpoints with ideological values attached, in the process of illuminating issues that are deemed to be of significance. The values that are implied may be real and may enhance or impede understanding. In the health sciences and health service provision, the gulf between what may be presented as an intellectual argument and what may be experienced during real life encounters can be overwhelming. The need to address more fundamental and sensitive issues of practical value becomes a professional imperative in order to influence difference in the care of women and the newborn.

This chapter examines the definition and terms, sets them in the context of the evolutionary framework and attempts to illustrate their usefulness and limitations with evidence from the literature. Much of the discourse will be conceptually based and applied to midwifery to inform practice. As our communities become increasingly multicultural, or as the *Parekh Report* (Runnymede Trust 2000) puts it with reference to the United Kingdom, a 'community of communities', the pluralism that we embrace becomes self-evident even in our everyday lives. The terms are difficult to define and not without pitfalls or risks of putting across oversimplifications of complex issues.

'RACE'

Any discourse about ethnicity today requires that we also engage, from a historical perspective, with 'race' in order to bring clarity to the context within which these terms are used. The complex use of the term 'race' can be traced back to the nineteenth century, when it was used to express the 'interweaving of biology, culture and language' (Tonkin, *et al.* 1996). Today, it is generally accepted that 'race' as a concept is a social construct. The use of the word 'race' between quotes has come to emphasise this acceptance of its use in debates about races and racial groups, with the understanding that race does not exist (Sarup 1996, van Dijk, *et al.* 1997). To say that race does not exist may imply a simplistic approach. However, the evidence suggests that genetically there is no such thing as race (Royal and Dunston 2004, Bhopal 1998b, McKenzie and Crowcroft 1994). However, among certain populations, the biological component tends to assume significant importance with respect to diseases that have a basis in genetic transmission, such as sickle cell disease and thalassaemia. In the context of the appropriateness of healthcare services provision, such racialisation of diseases impacts on the political ideologies and sensibilities of resources allocation, and cultural competence in care and genetic counselling.

Ahmad (1993) has argued that an ideological stance has permeated the use of the term 'race', thus projecting a racialisation of health and illness within health research. The use of 'racial' or 'ethnic' groups as primary categories and reliance upon these categories in an attempt to put forward robust explanatory models plays down the role of inequalities based on stratification by class, income, education, occupation and employment. When this happens 'issues of institutional and individual racism as determinants of health status or healthcare become peripheral . . .' (Ahmad 1993: 19).

Although there is a much more critical appreciation of the anomalies associated with the use of the term 'race', the sometimes negative attitudinal and behavioural values that it may convey cannot be ignored nor can it be said that there is any lack of evidence for such precedence. Events within the UK in the last decades have suggested, and serve as reminders, that racism and institutionalised racism are real challenges to all of us as citizens and healthcare professionals.

Racism

Everyday experiences of racism reported by individuals from minority ethnic groups vary by gender, age and social class (Virdee 1995). Racism is the attitudes of racists and 'not an inevitable feature of the ethnic minority' (Bradby 1995: 413). The acknowledgement of the existence of racism itself suggests that the healthcare professionals themselves are contextualised within a frame that racism affects everyday lives (Beishon, *et al.* 1995). As far as patients are concerned, the services are bound to reflect some of the wider societal issues about racism. Misunderstanding of others, their cultural values and beliefs often arise simply because the overt behavioural acts are judged at face value, without any analysis of the underlying motives and intent. However, institutional racism has been a fact of everyday life for many non-white people from minority ethnic groups (Macpherson 1999). It is recognised that planned, concerted and outcome-oriented action is urgently required to address racism in the NHS (NHS Executive 1998).

Thus, although not often recognised as such by professionals and service providers, to service-users the concerns and experiences of 'racism', behavioural and attitudinal dispositions and actions are real and demeaning (Bassett 1994). Hence, in health and social care services, racism is a real concern for people accessing these services, and the eradication of racism is high on the agenda for action. Midwifery care is one such area of practice for action on tackling racism (Hunt and Richens 1999).

ETHNICITY

Ethnicity is a multidimensional concept (Christian, *et al.* 1976, Nazroo 1997, Culley 2000). Ethnic identity is not a fixed entity. It is socially constructed and is given particular emphasis in diverse contexts. Ethnicity is a term often used in place of race. However, this has not escaped the attention of those who see it as problematic as the latter. It is a difficult term to define and pin down, as the ethnicity of individuals is not fixed. It is fluid and situational as described by Senior and Bhopal (1994). Ethnicity is generally taken to mean shared origins in terms of geographical regions, shared and distinct culture and traditions that are maintained over generations, common language or religion, that all give the person a distinct sense of identity and group affiliation (Brass 1996, Nash 1996).

Similar to the use of 'race' as a category, which is meaningless but may be dangerous, the use of ethnicity as a category has been criticised for its vagueness, but more importantly, the misinformation or distortion that it presents. Ethnicity is often attributed to 'others'; it is about 'them' and 'their ethnicity', not appreciating that we all belong to ethnic groups and that we all have an 'ethnicity'. In the white European context, white ethnic groups are often 'invisible' (McAuley, *et al.* 1996). There are further problems when terms are used synonymously with nationality. The picture is further complicated when religion and geographical regions are introduced in defining the ethnic groups.

The use of ethnicity as a variable in health data is problematic (Ahmad 1993, Bradby 1995, Senior and Bhopal 1994, Sheldon and Parker 1992). De Bono (1996) has argued that there is an equally pressing need to accurately describe the ethnicity of 'white' populations. The use of ethnicity as a variable has major flaws and disadvantages because of its imprecise and fluid nature. As Ahmad (1993), Smaje (1995), and Nazroo (1997) have argued, ethnicity-related data tend to camouflage the real materialist inequalities and outcomes of discrimination.

Ethnic monitoring and health needs assessment

The needs of the population we serve at local level and the demographics are essentially what generate the planning for care. The issues involved in needs assessment of minority ethnic groups are well established in the literature (Rawaf and Bahl 1998).

In general, there is concern about the accuracy and completeness of data collection at local levels in maternity units (Kenney and Macfarlane 1999). The maternity services data may not be adequately or accurately collected. Incomplete information is of concern with regard to effective management of the systems of care. It represents a gap in knowledge about the health needs of the community and minority ethnic women. The audits for accuracy of data and their availability need to be improved (Kenney and Macfarlane 1999). The limitations of ethnic statistics relate to the accuracy with which the categories are filled, how the information is obtained and from whom, and the completeness of the data. The implementation of the Race Relations (Amendment) Act 2000 in April 2001, heralds a new era in tackling indirect discrimination. The Act removes exceptions to indirect discrimination by institutions and agencies including the NHS and higher education (The Home Office 2001). Thus, health and social care will be required to demonstrate legally acceptable standards for information and workforce planning. However, the relevance of any data lies in its interpretation and its influence upon the context of local services provision.

The concept of ethnicity as fixed or static, referring to a stable set of cultural traits or attributes, is misleading and may be instrumental in leading to stereotyping. Therefore, it is useful and less narrow to think of ethnic and cultural identities of individuals as transitions through social and cultural adaptation and acculturation. Conceptualisation of ethnicity may benefit from a broader perspective through analysis of, first, the multidimensional and dynamic nature of ethnic identity, and second, the transitions that ethnic identities undergo over time. This may be exemplified by what Bhachu (1991) has tried to show with respect to Punjabi Sikh women. She has emphasised the self-determinative role of Punjabi women. This is a contrast to the view, often erroneously held, and generalised, that women of South Asian background are oppressed and have little or no opportunity for self-determination.

Intergenerational differences, between the beliefs and practices of women about care during pregnancy, childbirth and following delivery, have been reported by Katbamna (2000). She illustrates these with the interview data from her study with Bangladeshi (Muslim) and Gujarati (Hindu) women. The differences are greater among women who have lived in the UK for longer and have been acculturated to the norms of life in the UK. Although there are similarities, Katbamna (2000) suggests that the differences between Bangladeshi and Gujarati women were also due to socio–economic reasons, family structure, and religious beliefs.

STEREOTYPES AND CULTURAL RELATIVISM

Ethnocentric attitudes held by healthcare professionals may prevent them from establishing relationships with their patients/clients unless those relationships are founded on equality and mutual respect. Generalised beliefs held about others may or may not be true. Stereotypical thinking and behaviours may serve many functions such as bolstering the person's self-esteem in what may be considered situations of threat as in being in the presence of others not of the same group (Hilton and von Hippel 1996). However, stereotypes reflect misguided or ill-informed beliefs about people of different ethnic origins, about their traits, attitudes and behaviours. They tend to be negative or arouse negative images about out-group members, and are perpetuated through various means. The media in particular, with their access to large sections of the population, the institutions, and social networks may all be influential in promoting stereotypes. It has been observed that racist views are common in the media (van Dijk, *et al.* 1997).

Stereotypes held by midwives such as those reported by Bowler (1993), demonstrate the need for education and more understanding of the values and beliefs of others in our care. Bowler (1993) reported four themes that emerged from a qualitative study of midwifery care of women of South Asian descent:
1 difficulty in communication
2 women's lack of compliance with care, and abuse of services
3 a tendency to 'make a fuss about nothing'
4 lack of maternal instinct.

Earlier research by Larbie (1985) had shown that women from African-Caribbean backgrounds had also experienced similar stereotyping and discrimination. It becomes apparent from these studies that racism may take the form of *cultural racism*, which is associated with the belief that the cultural values, beliefs and practices of others are inferior to one's own. Such racism, based on cultural and religious discrimination, is prevalent throughout the health services (Weller, *et al.* 2001).

Cultural relativism
Cultural relativism holds that cultures are unique; that cultures must be evaluated according to their own values and standards; that specific cultural practices are exempt from criticism by outsiders; and that such judgement by outsiders is primarily based on ethnocentric standards (Baker 1997, Haviland 1993). Cultural relativism emerged as a way to confront racism and ethnocentric views, and promote respect and tolerance for the other. However, as Brannigan (2000) has argued, there are ethical issues that arise from adopting positions of cultural relativism, not least as a consequence of an uncritical acceptance of the cultural practice of others. Therefore it is important to generate (through dialogue and reflection) a critical understanding of the explanations of cultural practices, and their impact on the perceptions and experiences of women in pregnancy and childbirth. However, there are ethical problems with this stance.

Suspending any judgement about others is not easy and represents deeper cognitive processes and attitudinal integration. In the context of a system of care, it is easy to forget some of the perspectives that govern professional practice. From the consumer's perspective, not knowing the acceptability or otherwise of certain practices is unacceptable not just in a cultural, moral context, but also more seriously in the legal context of professional practice. Values and beliefs can be challenged. Otherwise, the relativistic position leads to a cul-de-sac (Baker 1997).

WOMEN'S EXPERIENCES
The cultural perspectives of birth cannot be ignored (Thomson 1997). Kitzinger (2000) has illustrated how birth is perceived in different cultures. The experiences of women concerning pregnancy, childbirth and motherhood vary according to their perceptions of their pregnancy, and how they feel and negotiate their relationships with others during these transitions. The experiences of women suggest a great divide between the professional and the lay perceptions. MacVicar (1990) recognised that the information and expectations of women during pregnancy and the antenatal visits were at odds, simply because the women's understandings were not the same as the midwives'.

When confronted with people from other ethnic and socio-cultural backgrounds than our own, 'difference' seems to be the most common aspect in the discourse about ethnic groups (van Dijk, *et al.* 1997). The experiences of women from minority ethnic backgrounds suggest that assumptions are made about them on the basis of skin colour, how they present, their traditional dress, language spoken, and their apparent willingness to respond to requests or perceived lack of cooperation.

Maternity services have been criticised for not being flexible enough in the past (Larbie 1985, James 1997). The problem seems to lie in the resistance to change and the lack of empowerment and choice extended to women in general and not just women from minority ethnic backgrounds. The medical model and the ethnocentric views of pregnancy and childbirth promote conformity. When conformity is not perceived, then the pattern of behaviours or attitudes are interpreted as deviations from the accepted norms. There is no doubt that various stereotypes may characterise women with disability or female circumcision, and lead to stigmatisation of some women (Thomas 1997). Bowes and Domokos (1996) have suggested that the participation of women in decision making is limited, and expressions of emotions and pain are frowned upon, giving the distinct impression that the voices of Pakistani women are muted during labour. Thus, in the spirit of emancipation and empowerment of women, the raising of muted voices represent an even greater social challenge for women themselves, advocates and care providers.

The Audit Commission report highlighted postnatal maternity services as an area of expressed dissatisfaction by service users (Audit Commission 1997). It is contended that what often underpins the dissatisfaction with postnatal services is the imbalance between an unfair overemphasis on the women's characteristics and a less-than-critical evaluation of the inappropriateness of many aspects of the maternity services (Phoenix 1990, Parsons, *et al.* 1993). For example, access to maternal services remains problematic for some women from minority ethnic groups (Hayes 1995, Healthcare Commission 2008). It is not as simple as it is made out to be. In many instances, access involves structural barriers that disadvantaged women have to overcome. Explanatory models may include not only ethnicity but also the interactions between many other factors such as educational and socio-economic status.

Generally, the services fail women from several points of view. Language appears to have been a major problem for a long time and a recurrent theme (Robinson 2004, Cross-Sudworth 2007). Bangladeshi women in Katbamna's study frequently referred to language as a barrier to communication with healthcare professionals. Inadequate interpreter services often means that patients rely on relatives to act as interpreters. Brooks, *et al.* (2000) report that in a sample of 277 women, 31% did not speak or understand English and about one-third of the sample were not aware of the interpreter services provided. This may reflect local variations where the minority ethnic population is highly represented. One would expect that the use of interpreters and advocates would be widespread in maternity services. Where interpreter services are provided, women should be informed of their availability and usefulness. Service providers need to address those issues that are well known and documented and ensure that ineffective communication does not remain a major contributor to a less-than-acceptable level of quality care provision.

Antenatal classes and screening

Narang and Murphy (1994) showed that only about half of the women in their study had any understanding and knowledge of the tests and screening procedures and only a few knew the reasons for the tests. The lack of knowledge was indicative of the information and decision making during the management of their pregnancy. The Healthcare Commission report pointed out that women of Asian and black origin saw a health professional later during the antenatal phase and were more likely to be booked within the recommended 12 weeks (Healthcare Commission 2008). Black African and Bangladeshi women in particular reported being booked later than 12 weeks.

Atkin, *et al.* (1998) concluded that ethnic and racial stereotypes adversely influence policy decision making in the provision of antenatal screening for the haemoglobinopathies, with the consequence that choice is often limited, and there appears to be an inability to provide culturally sensitive care. They also found that referral to screening services tended to be *ad hoc* with poor understanding among healthcare professionals about the value and purpose of genetic screening. Recent findings reported that women of Asian and black origin felt they had less choice in deciding where they would have their baby and were less likely to have a scan at 20 weeks in their pregnancy (Healthcare Commission 2008).

Knowledge of the socio-cultural aspects of minority ethnic women's sexuality and associated taboos may, in part, provide explanations for any perceived lack of responses to the uptake of antenatal examinations and procedures. Assumptions about what is expected from a professional viewpoint may underestimate elements of embarrassment, anxiety, and fear that are perceived by women. The person whose integral self feels threatened in the environment of risk discourse, may not be attuned to the 'medicalised body', that is so much a part of professional attitudes. However, as Crawford (1984: 95) has argued, 'Cultural meanings are not only shared or given, they are fragmented and contested'. This requires that assumptions are always critically appraised in each case. Women's feeling of loss of control over their pregnancy and childbirth is a serious issue for the self-esteem of women. Lack of self-esteem, traumatic experiences and a sense of disempowerment may lead to depression (Kitzinger 2000).

Men's involvement

The part played by men in the transitions of women through pregnancy, childbirth, and parenthood is welcome and there is evidence to suggest that more men from various ethnic groups are taking part in antenatal classes and are present during the birth of their children. However, the beliefs and cultural issues surrounding the presence of men during what, in traditional cultures, is very much a woman's event (Kitzinger 2000), may influence whether or not the husband or partner chooses to attend during labour.

Husbands and partners are encouraged to attend the birth. When the man does not wish to attend the birth, this is often attributed to lack of interest or concern. However, such negative stereotypes of men are not warranted. In some instances such attitudes and behaviour may be explained from a perspective of the legitimate wishes of women in the social context of gender relationships. Somali women's experiences in hospital in Sweden suggest that there are women who, due to the cultural and socially differentiated roles during pregnancy and childbirth, are not comfortable with the expectation that their husbands/partners will be present at childbirth (Wiklund, *et al.* 2000). The cultural influences on body modesty may represent a critical issue for what is perceived as modesty, and the deeper issues of the self, disclosure and the ethics of the social and medicalised body.

Technology and interventions

The medical model's emphasis on risk management and surveillance sometimes fails to give enough credence and attention to the psychological and social needs of women (Oakley 1984). The NHS environment of childbirth may be alien to many women who were not born in the UK. It can be overwhelming even to those who *are* familiar with the services. The system of care and the specialised approach to maternity care with technological interventions and screening procedures may reinforce the feeling of loss of control, particularly when language is also a barrier to accessibility of services. As Sandelowski (1999) suggests, technological systems maintain the knowledge and power differentials between patients and professionals, and serve the process by 'muting' the voices of women.

The lack of support is another aspect that is not taken into account. For those women who have extended families and friends, the experience may differ from those who do not have such support. Assumptions about support and its availability prevail, with respect to an immigrant community (Choudhry 2001) and in relation to support during pregnancy and postnatal care (Katbamna 2000). Based on these assumptions, there is often a lack of understanding of women's care needs.

Management of labour

Bowler (1993) described how midwives perceived pain in women of South Asian descent in labour in a stereotypical manner and did not respond by providing more analgesia when required. This was due in part to blaming the women or being punitive. The stance was very much one where the midwives believed that it was the woman's fault for not attending antenatal classes where they would have been taught 'how to breathe' and since they did not attend, they suffered pain. Such an approach, needless to add, is unacceptable in the management of pain. The lack of analgesia is a recurrent theme in the literature (Bowler 1993, Cheung 1994). However, in some circumstances the woman herself may see the notion of pain during childbirth as natural and acceptable. Zaidi (1994) suggests that Muslim women may accept pain during childbirth as part of the will of Allah (God).

Postpartum care

It is common practice to place the newborn on the mother's abdomen immediately after birth. However, placing the newborn on the mother's abdomen without first washing it, is seen in some cultures and according to religious beliefs as not acceptable because blood is seen as 'contamination'. This may explain in part the observation that some women from Indian, Pakistani and Bangladeshi backgrounds do not or are reluctant to hold their babies immediately after birth (Midwives Information and Resources Services 1998). Breastfeeding is another area of care that may reveal differences in beliefs and practices. Littler (1997) has reported how the perceptions and beliefs held by women about colostrum influence their breastfeeding behaviour. This may be observed particularly in Bengali women. What is pertinent about Littler's findings is that a lack of knowledge on the part of midwives about the cultural and religious beliefs of Bangladeshi women perpetuates the stereotypes held by midwives. Zaidi (1994) provides a brief but useful guide to the care of Muslim women. Much can be learned from the experiences of migrant women who have moved from one culture to another with a more sophisticated and complex healthcare system and diversity of healthcare professionals (Abuidhail and Fleming 2007).

Rest and recovery

There is a common belief that after labour and childbirth, women need much rest and care. A long period of rest is traditionally expected. This has been reported among Asian and Chinese women (Cheung 1997, Gervais and Jovchelovitch 1998, Katbamna 2000, Davis 2001). This may well be misinterpreted as the women being 'lazy' (Bowler 1993). However, in a culture-specific approach, this is seen as giving time for recovery and balancing the body (Davis 2001, Chu 2005).

SOME SOCIO-CULTURAL ISSUES

Stillbirth and infant mortality

Stillbirth and infant mortality rates among mothers from certain ethnic groups tend to be higher than the average for mothers born in the UK (Balarajan and Raleigh 1993). The rates are higher among Pakistanis, followed by Bangladeshis, African-Caribbean, and Indians. In *Social Inequalities* (Drever, *et al.* 2000), it is reported that 5 out of every 1000 babies born to mothers who were themselves born in the UK, will die in the first year of life. For mothers born outside the UK, this figure rises to 6 in 1000 and for those mothers born in Pakistan or the Caribbean to 10 out of 1000. Health inequalities are very much the by-products of poverty and social deprivation, and materialist explanations shed light on the rates of infant death among different ethnic groups (Andrews and Jewson 1993). Among ethnic groups, the socio-economic status of Pakistani and Bangladeshi communities tends to be the lowest (Berthoud 1997, Chandola 2001). Distinctions should be made between the diverse groups subsumed under the label 'Asian'. In relation to health, the Indian group is better off than the Pakistani or the Bangladeshi groups and the Bangladeshi group does worst (Nazroo 1997). This may well be a direct reflection of settlement patterns and time of arrival combined with education and occupational opportunities. Other ethnic groups such as Somalis, Vietnamese, Ethiopians and Albanians may show similar trends. Poverty has long been one of the major critical factors in health inequalities among the population in general and among various ethnic groups (Haines 1997, Nazroo 1998).

Family size and family structures

Family size varies and it would appear that the Pakistani and Bangladeshi ethnic groups on average have family sizes larger than others (Nazroo 1994, Katbamna 2000). This is in part explained by the attitudes held about family planning, having and not having children, and religious beliefs.

The family structures in various ethnic groups vary and the localities that people inhabit tend to emphasise proximity with kin. The joint family system emphasises the collectivist approach, which poses problems for the individualistically oriented system, especially in the context of one-to-one interactions (Laungani 1999). The role of women within certain family structures influences the perceptions of motherhood itself. Traditional views about pregnancy and childbirth may become superimposed on the role expectations of the pregnant woman with respect to other family members. As illustrated in Katbamna (2000) there is a need to be alert to the familial influences on the woman and her attitudes and responses in relation to the role and expectations in the extended family. There is always a risk of stereotyping, and one has to be aware that cultural norms are not fixed with respect to social mobility, personal biography, values and beliefs.

Religion

Religion plays an important part in the everyday lives of many people. People from the Indian subcontinent are diverse in their origins with regional variations in language, diet, religious beliefs and practices, and social structure (Bhopal 1998a). Indeed, one of the major criticism of the 1991 Census was that 'the strong differentiation of the South Asian groups by religion was not captured' (Aspinall 2000: 586). To Hilton (1996) it is inconceivable to think of ethnicity without giving equal consideration to religion. The Indian category conceals those of religious faiths such as Muslims, Sikh, Hindu, Christians and Jains. In relation to regional variations, people may see themselves as Gujeratis or Punjabis. The pattern of migration from East Africa also adds to the subtle differences that may be brought into the categories (Bhachu 1991).

Bhopal (1998a) reported variations between single and married women in their affiliation to religious beliefs and practices among women in South Asian communities. Married women are more likely to follow religious practices than single women, and Muslim women identified themselves by reference to Islam. These findings have implications for continuity of identity formation and identities in the context of place of birth. The *Parekh Report* (Runnymede Trust 2000) further showed that religion is helping redefine cultural identities among communities.

However, whilst they may not be immediately perceived as such, the religious beliefs and practices of people from non-European backgrounds appear to govern their lives much more by comparison. When professionals are not familiar with the diversity of religious beliefs and practices, it may give rise to misunderstandings and lack of sensitivity to women.

RESEARCH AND ANTI-RACIST PERSPECTIVES

There are issues in researching minority ethnic groups that present difficulties with the process, beginning with access, participation and response rate. It is well documented that the response rate and participation in research is low among people from minority ethnic groups (Bowler 1997). Part of the problem lies in the perceptions of what research is and is not. Bowler (1997) gives examples of how initial willingness to take part in research later turned into refusal because of the potential respondent's lack of understanding why their views were being sought and the importance of their views in informing service delivery. When doing research one has to be cognisant of the cultural factors that may influence respondents' decisions to participate. Bowes and Domokos (1996) see their approach as meeting the principles of anti–racist, sensitive research. It is critical to the process of research to ask the women what they perceive as problems rather than having predetermined ideas about what the problems are. Gerrish (2000) has provided useful ways of understanding ethnic categories and practical issues when doing research with ethnically diverse populations.

CULTURAL COMPETENCE

Effective communication and an understanding of the expectations and practices of women from diverse socio-cultural and religious backgrounds influences the degree of advocacy and empowerment that may be achieved. It is therefore important that when caring for women the midwife shows a level of cultural competence that builds on her role in advocacy and empowering. In order to become culturally competent, the midwife has to embrace skills and knowledge that would enable one-to-one communication based on an understanding of the social, cultural and religious needs of women.

Although culturalist analysis has come under criticism, the value of understanding cultures is not to be underestimated. It is through understanding of the culture in its context that one can begin to make sense of the comparative (Jahoda 1984, Alasuutari 1995). In ways that are not immediately apparent, the stereotyping of women appears to go hand in hand with the perpetuation of certain myths, and in the context of women-to-women interactions, the management of pregnancy and childbirth becomes a series of negotiations within an arena of power positions, mutual respect and rights.

The individualistic and the collectivist perspectives

Appreciation of the perspective of the individual or ethnic group may assist in identifying the needs of the individual and the family. The notion that the individualistic perspective prevails, no matter what meanings are attached to the event, mitigates against care that is appropriate for women who come from cultural groups that have a collectivist orientation to life and life events. Policies that are drawn up may not necessarily sit comfortably with the goal of providing culturally competent care, be it at the individual level (with the practitioner) or the collective level (with the institution), unless cultural assessment of women's needs are carried out.

CONCLUSION

This chapter has attempted to explore the issues of terminologies used in the literature and everyday practice with respect to the experiences of childbirth by women and men from diverse ethnic backgrounds. The women's experiences are unique; unlike diseases and their outcomes, pregnancy and childbirth have different moments for women, with transitions being defined by the experiences themselves. 'Race', ethnicity and culture are concepts frequently used in the discourse of pregnancy and childbirth. Their use should not be without some critical analysis, as argued by those who suggest that advancing any explanatory model based on these concepts simply detracts from addressing the socio-economic inequalities that reflect inequalities in health (Andrews and Jewson 1993).

However, migrant women tend to have similar experiences of midwifery services and health professionals across modern health systems (Rolls and Chamberlain 2004, Chu 2005, Essén, *et al.* 2005, Grewal, Bhagat and Balneaves 2008, Tsianakas and Liamputtong 2008). Whilst various explanations have been put forward for the experiences of women from different ethnic groups, of pregnancy, childbirth, and the associated mortality, no single explanation is conclusive by itself. Each has its merits and limitations. The explanations of service providers and the experiences of women suggest that there is much to consider in relation to appropriateness and satisfaction with the care that women report in receiving in maternity services. In part, the disadvantage associated with ethnicity and social positions may be based on social inequalities that cut across ethnic and cultural divides.

The experiences of women and their responses to the perceived needs of women, however, should be a matter of serious concern for the professionals who come into contact with women. Only through an understanding of the factors that contribute to the women's experiences, not only their biological condition but also the psychosocial and cultural needs, can the professional person begin to offer care in an equal partnership. Developing cultural competence (i.e. anti-racist anti-discriminatory practice) in caring for women through pregnancy, childbirth and the postpartum period, is an essential imperative for professional education and training in the pursuit of excellence in maternity care. The culture of midwifery itself requires further exploration and actions for the empowerment of midwives (Kirkham 1999).

REFERENCES

Abuidhail J, Fleming V. (2007) Beliefs and practices of postpartum infant care: a review of different cultures. *Br J Midwif.* **15**: 418–21.

Ahmad WIU. (1993) Making black people sick: 'race', ideology and health research. In: Ahmad WIU, editor. *'Race' and Health in Contemporary Britain.* Buckingham: Open University Press.

Alasuutari P. (1995) *Researching Culture: qualitative method and cultural studies.* London: Sage.

Andrews A, Jewson N. (1993) Ethnicity and infant deaths: the implications of recent statistical evidence for material explanations. *Sociol Health Illn.* **15**: 137–56.

Aspinall PJ. (2000) Should a question on 'religion' be asked in the 2001 British census? A public policy case in favour. *Soc Policy Admin.* **34**: 584–600.

Atkin K, Ahmad WUI, Anionwu EN. (1998) Screening and counselling for sickle cell disorders and thalassaemia: the experiences of parents and health professionals. *Soc Sci Med.* **47**: 1639–51.

Audit Commission. (1997) *First Class Delivery: improving maternity services in England and Wales.* Abingdon: Audit Commission Publications.

Baker C. (1997) Cultural diversity and cultural relativism: implications for nursing practice. *Adv Nurs Sci.* **20**: 3–11.

Balarajan R, Raleigh VS. (1993) *Ethnicity and Health: a guide for the NHS.* London: Department of Health.

Bassett C. (1994) Not just a black and white issue. *J Commun Nurs.* **6**: 12–14.

Beishon S, Virdee S, Hagell A. (1995) *Nursing in a Multiethnic NHS.* London: Policy Studies Institute.

Berthoud R. (1997) Income and standards of living. In: Modood T, Berthoud R, Lakey J, *et al.*, editors. *Ethnic Minorities in Britain: diversity and disadvantage.* London: Policy Studies Institute.

Bhachu P. (1991) Culture, ethnicity and class among Punjabi Sikh women in 1990s Britain. *New Community.* **17**: 401–12.

Bhopal K. (1998a) South Asian women in East London: religious experience and diversity. *J Gender Studies.* **7**: 143–56.

Bhopal R. (1998b) Spectre of racism in health and healthcare: lessons from history and the United States. *BMJ.* **316**: 1970–3.

Bowes AM, Domokos TM. (1996) Pakistani women and maternity care: raising muted voices. *Sociol Health Illn.* **18**: 45–65.

Bowler I. (1993) 'They're not the same as us': midwives' stereotypes of South Asian descent maternity patients. *Sociol Health Illn.* **15**: 157–78.

Bowler I. (1997) Problems with interviewing: experiences with service providers and clients. In: Miller G, Dingwall R, editors. *Context and Method in Qualitative Research.* London: Sage.

Bradby H. (1995) Ethnicity: not a black and white issue. A research note. *Sociol Health Illn.* **17**: 405–17.

Brannigan M. (2000) Cultural diversity and the case against ethical relativism. *Healthcare Anal.* **8**: 321–7.

Brass PR. (1996) Ethnic groups and ethnic identity formation. In: Hutchinson J, Smith AD, editors. *Ethnicity.* Oxford: Oxford University Press.

Brooks N, Magee P, Bhatti G, *et al.* (2000) Asian patients' perspective on communication facilities provided in a large inner city hospital. *J Clin Nurs.* **9**: 706–12.

Chandola T. (2001) Ethnic and class differences in health in relation to British South Asians: using the new national statistics socio–economic classification. *Soc Sci Med.* **52**: 1285–96.

Cheung N. (1994) Pain in normal labour: a comparison of experiences in southern China and Scotland. *Midwives Chronicle.* **107**: 212–16.

Cheung NF. (1997) Chinese *zuo yuezi* (sitting in for the first month of the postnatal period) in Scotland. *Midwifery.* **13**: 55–65.

Choudhry UK. (2001) Uprooting and resettlement experiences of South Asian immigrant women. *West J Nurs Res.* **23**: 376–93.

Christian J, Gadfield NJ, Giles H, *et al.* (1976) The multidimensional and dynamic nature of ethnic identity. *Int J Psychol.* **11**: 281–91.

Chu CMY. (2005) Postnatal experience and health needs of Chinese migrant women in Brisbane, Australia. *Ethnicity and Health.* **10**: 33–56.

Crawford R. (1984) A cultural account of health, control, release and the social body. In: McKinlay JB, editor. *Issues in the Political Economy of Healthcare.* London: Tavistock.

Cross-Sudworth F. (2007) Racism and discrimination in maternity services. *Br J Midwif.* **15**: 327–31.

Culley L. (2000) Working with diversity: beyond the factfile. In: Davies C, Finlay L, Bullman A, editors. *Changing Practice in Health and Social Care.* Buckingham: The Open University Press, and London: Sage.

Davis R. (2001) The postpartum experience for Southeast Asian women in the United States. *Am J Matern Child Nurs.* **26**: 208–13.

de Bono D. (1996) Describing race, ethnicity, and culture in medical research: 'white' populations also need to be accurately described. *BMJ.* **313**(7054): 425–6.

Drever F, Fisher K, Brown J, *et al.* (2000) *Social Inequalities. 2000 edition.* London: The Stationery Office.

Essén B, Johnsdotter S, Hovelius B, *et al.* (2005) Qualitative study of pregnancy and childbirth experiences in Somalian women resident in Sweden. *Br J Obstet Gynaecol.* **107**: 1507–12.

Gerrish K. (2000) Researching ethnic diversity in the British NHS: methodological and practical concerns. *J Adv Nurs.* **31**: 918–25.

Gervais M–C, Jovchelovitch S. (1998) *The Health Beliefs of the Chinese Community in England.* London: Health Education Authority.

Grewal SK, Bhagat R, Balneaves L. (2008) Perinatal beliefs and practices of immigrant Punjabi women living in Canada. *J Obstet Gynecol Neonatal Nurs.* **37**(3): 290–300.

Haines A. (1997) Working together to reduce poverty's damage. *BMJ.* **314**: 529–30.

Haviland WA. (1993) *Cultural Anthropology.* 7th ed. Orlando, FL: Harcourt Brace Jovanovich.

Hayes L. (1995) Unequal access to midwifery care: a continuing problem? *J Adv Nurs.* **21**: 702–7.

Healthcare Commission. (2008) *Towards Better Births: a review of maternity services in England.* London: Commission for Healthcare Audit and Inspection.

Hilton C. (1996) For debate: collecting ethnic group data for inpatients: is it useful? *BMJ.* **313**: 923–5.

Hilton J, von Hippel W. (1996) Stereotypes. *Ann Rev Psychol.* **47**: 237–71.

Hunt S, Richens Y. (1999) Unwitting racism and midwifery care. *Br J Midwif.* **7**: 358.

Jahoda G. (1984) Do we need a concept of culture? *J Cross-Cult Psychol.* **15**: 139–51.

James D. (1997) Maternity services: the Audit Commission reports: listen to women, especially after delivery. *BMJ.* **314**: 844.

Katbamna S. (2000) *'Race' and Childbirth.* Buckingham: Open University Press.

Kenney N, Macfarlane A. (1999) Identifying problems with data collection at local level: survey of NHS maternity units in England. *BMJ.* **319**: 619–22.

Kirkham M. (1999) The culture of midwifery in the National Health Service in England. *J Adv Nurs.* **30**: 732–9.

Kitzinger S. (2000) Some cultural perspectives of birth. *Br J Midwif.* **8**: 746–50.

Larbie J. (1985) *Black Women and Maternity Services: a survey of thirty young Afro-Caribbean women's experiences and perceptions of pregnancy and childbirth.* London: Health Education Council and National Extension College for Training in Health and Race.

Laungani P. (1999) Client centred or culture centred counselling? In: Palmer S, Laungani P, editors. *Counselling in a Multicultural Society.* London: Sage.

Littler C. (1997) Beliefs about colostrum among women from Bangladesh and their reasons for not giving it to the newborn. *Midwives.* **110**: 3–7.

Macpherson W. (1999) *The Stephen Lawrence Inquiry: report of an inquiry.* London: Home Office.

MacVicar J. (1990) Obstetrics. In: McAvoy BR, Donaldson LJ, editors. *Healthcare for Asians.* Oxford: Oxford University Press.

McAuley J, de Souza L, Sharma V, *et al.* (1996) Describing race, ethnicity, and culture in medical research: self-defined ethnicity is unhelpful. *BMJ.* **313**: 425–6.

McKenzie KJ, Crowcroft NS. (1994) Race, ethnicity, culture, and science. *BMJ.* **309**: 286–7.

Midwives Information and Resources Services. (1998) Infant feeding in Asian families. *MIDIRS Midwif Digest.* **8**: 358–61.

Narang I, Murphy S. (1994) Assessment of antenatal care for Asian women. *Br J Midwif.* **2**: 169–73.

Nash M. (1996) The core elements of ethnicity. In: Hutchinson J, Smith AD, editors. *Ethnicity.* Oxford: Oxford University Press.

Nazroo JY. (1997) *The Health of Britain's Ethnic Minorities.* London: Policy Studies Institute.

Nazroo JY. (1998) Genetic, cultural or socio-economic vulnerability? Explaining ethnic inequalities in health. *Sociol Health Illn.* **20**: 710–30.

NHS Executive. (1998) *Tackling Racial Harassment in the NHS: a plan for action.* London: Department of Health.

Oakley A. (1984) *The Captured Womb: a history of the medical care of pregnant women.* Oxford: Blackwell.

Parsons L, Macfarlane A, Golding J. (1993) Pregnancy, birth and maternity care. In: Ahmad WIU, editor. *'Race' and Health in Contemporary Britain.* Buckingham: Open University Press.

Phoenix A. (1990) Black women and the maternity services. In: Garcia J, Kilpatrick R, Richards M, editors. *The Politics of Maternity Care.* Oxford: Clarendon Press.

Rawaf S, Bahl V. (1998) *Assessing Health Needs of People from Minority Ethnic Groups.* London: Royal College of Physicians.

Robinson J. (2004) Are midwives less kind if you speak Urdu? *Br J Midwif.* **12**: 22.

Rolls C, Chamberlain M. (2004) From East to West: Nepalese women's experiences. *Int Nurs Review.* **51**: 176–84.

Royal CDM, Dunston GM. (2004) Changing the paradigm from 'race' to human genome variation. *Nat Genet.* **36**(11 Suppl.): S5–7.

Runnymede Trust. (2000) *The Future of Multi-ethnic Britain. The Parekh Report.* London: Profile Books.

Sandelowski M. (1999) Culture, conceptive technology, and nursing. *Int J Nurs Stud.* **36**: 13–20.

Sarup M. (1996) *Identity, Culture and the Postmodern World.* Edinburgh: Edinburgh University Press.

Senior P, Bhopal R. (1994) Ethnicity as a variable in epidemiological research. *BMJ.* **309**: 327–30.

Sheldon T, Parker H. (1992) Race and ethnicity in health research. *J Pub Health Med.* **14**: 104–10.

Smaje C. (1995) *Health, 'Race' and Ethnicity: making sense of the evidence.* London: King's Fund Institute.

The Home Office. (2001) *The Race Relations (Amendment) Act 2000. New Laws for a Successful Multi Racial Britain: proposals for implementation.* London: The Stationery Office.

Thomas C. (1997) The baby and the bath water: disabled women and motherhood in social context. *Sociol Health Illn.* **9**: 622–43.

Thomson A. (1997) The importance of culture in the provision of midwifery care. *Midwifery.* **13**: 53–4.

Tonkin E, McDonald M, Chapman M. (1996) History and ethnicity. In: Hutchison J, Smith AD, editors. *Ethnicity.* Oxford: Oxford University Press.

Tsianakas V, Liamputtong P. (2008) *Confinement Beliefs and Practices Among Afghan Immigrant Women Living in Australia.* Melbourne: Ausmed Publications. Available at: www.buildabook.com.au/index. php?main_page=product_info&products_id=390 (accessed 25 Dec 2008).

van Dijk TA, Ting-Toomey S, Smitherman G, *et al.* (1997) Discourse, ethnicity, culture and racism. In: van Dijk TA, editor. *Discourse as Social Interaction.* London: Sage.

Virdee S. (1995) *Racial Violence and Harassment.* London: Policy Studies Institute.

Weller P, Feldman A, Purdam K. (2001) Religious discrimination in England and Wales. *Home Office Research Study 220.* London: Home Office.

Wiklund H, Aden AS, Högberg U, *et al.* (2000) Somalis giving birth in Sweden: a challenge to culture and gender-specific values and behaviours. *Midwifery.* **16**: 105–15.

Zaidi F. (1994) The maternity care of Muslim women. *Prof Midwife.* **4**: 8–10.

CHAPTER 6

Refugee women

Caroline Squire and Jo James

In the UK, refugee women face overwhelming obstacles to their health and well-being. Many have been through traumatic events and experiences, and exile and loss (both cultural and material) will add to their suffering when they are here. The refugee experience in the UK is not a comfortable one. These women face bigotry, ignorance, disinterest, hostility and poverty. Pregnancy and childbirth represent a dangerous time for these individuals, who can be particularly vulnerable. In order to provide the support and care that a refugee woman needs, the healthcare professional must understand who she is, what she has been through and the challenges that she faces when bearing a child in her country of exile.

INTRODUCTION

Refugee women are among the most marginalised and misunderstood groups in the world today. They face not only the stigma of being refugees but also gender persecution, and they often suffer in a culture of silence because of their sex. Women and their dependent children represent 'the overwhelming majority of refugee caseloads in almost every country' (Marshall 2000). Many will find their way to the UK, either through cross-border flight or after languishing in a neighbouring country's refugee camp, sometimes for years. Although these women are survivors who will have shown remarkable fortitude and resourcefulness to get here at all, they are also vulnerable and often severely traumatised by their experiences. A high percentage of them will be pregnant – some when they arrive, and others soon afterwards. This in itself may seem odd. Why should women want to give birth at a time of such hardship and uncertainty? First, they may not be pregnant through choice. The great majority (approximately 80%) of refugee women are Moslem and come from a culture of short birth spacing (Wali 1995). Secondly, they may be pregnant due to lack of available contraception, or as a result of rape. Finally, women who are already in their host country may choose to become pregnant. Possibly (as one doctor who cares for refugees has suggested) this has to do with a reaffirmation of life and an attempt to move towards normality by entering into a life experience that encompasses both ritual and tradition, as well as a new beginning. Once they are in the UK, refugees experience deteriorating health, poor housing and poverty (Burnett and Fassil 2004, Yates, Crane and Burnett 2007, Palmer and Ward 2007). They are the subjects of resentment and sometimes violence. The policy of dispersal of refugees throughout the UK has led to problems with existing communities, an issue that was tragically illustrated by the murder of an asylum seeker in Glasgow in 2001.

Refugees are a diverse group, coming from extremely varied social and cultural backgrounds. It is important for healthcare workers to understand that the terms 'refugee' and 'asylum seeker' denote a situation rather than an identity and that refugees and asylum seekers should be treated as individuals with differing needs, hopes and fears. It is also imperative to appreciate that the needs of newly arrived asylum seekers are different from those who have been in the UK for some time (Burnett and Fassil 2004). However, there are certain common issues of which those caring for them need to be aware. It is vital to be able to understand and contextualise these experiences in terms of the pregnant woman if she is to receive the care that she needs. Van der Veer (1998) suggests that refugees are subject to trauma, which is similar to that experienced by immigrants, disaster victims and war veterans, but which is a unique amalgamation of all three.

One of the most important factors that contributes to an understanding of these women is a knowledge of the different statuses of refugees in the UK, as their living conditions and concerns will be significantly different – *see* Table 6.1. The asylum seeker does not have access to benefits, has no long-term security and faces the possibility of

TABLE 6.1 The differing asylum definitions (Bennett, Heath and Jeffries 2007)

Asylum seeker	A person who has submitted an application for protection under the Geneva Convention and is waiting for the claim to be decided by the Home Office
Refugee status (status altered in August 2005)	Accepted as a refugee under the Geneva Convention and granted five years leave to remain. Granted Indefinite Leave to Remain (ILR) – permanent residence in the UK – if they have not, through own actions, brought her/himself within the scope of the Refugee Convention's Exclusion and Cessation clauses and, therefore, triggered a review. Eligible for family reunion
Persons granted Humanitarian Protection (HP) or Discretionary Leave (DL): (replaced Exceptional Leave to Remain (ELR) in April 2003)	Refused asylum but the Home Office has granted HP or DL for five years because it has recognised that there are strong reasons why those persons should not return to their countries at the present time. Status reviewed if subject triggers a review under the Refugee Convention's Exclusion and Cessation clauses. Eligible for family reunion
Unaccompanied minor/separated child	A person who, at the time of making his/her application, is under 18 years of age or who, in the absence of documentary evidence, appears to be under that age, and who is: • applying for asylum in his/her own right • without adult family members or guardians to turn to in this country
Family reunion	One spouse and children under the age of 18

forced repatriation. She may still be preoccupied with survival, and could be heavily involved with asylum applications or appeals. The refugee, on the other hand, will have access to all of the benefits available to a UK citizen, and she will know that she can live and raise her child in the UK, and she will be adjusting to her new life and dealing with the loss of her homeland.

The aim of this chapter is to consider these women in terms of who they are, how they came to seek asylum, and how the experiences of persecution, war, loss, flight and exile may have affected them physically and psychologically. In addition, strategies will be discussed that will help professionals to care for these women and to ensure that the journey through pregnancy and childbirth does not traumatise them further.

WHO BECOMES A REFUGEE?

Member states of the United Nations are obliged to offer refuge to any person who steps on to their soil and requests asylum. It is then incumbent on that state to decide whether the person concerned will or will not be granted refugee status. The guide that is used to decide this is the 1951 United Nations Refugee Convention, which defines the refugee as follows:

> . . . (any person who) owing to a well-founded fear of being persecuted for reasons of race, religion, nationality, membership of a particular social group or political opinion, is outside the country of his nationality and is unable or, owing to such fear, is unwilling to avail himself of the protection of that country . . . is unable or, owing to such fear, is unwilling to return to it. (United Nations 1951, cited in United Nations High Commission for Refugees 1998)

The statistics kept by the Home Office are complex and detailed but Table 6.2 gives an idea of the outcomes following applications for asylum over the years 2003–06.

The 1951 United Nations Refugee Convention is noted for its lack of reference to gender as a reason for persecution. Women still have a low status in the world, and are often subjected to maltreatment, sexual abuse and domestic violence by their husbands or families. The practice of female genital mutilation also abounds in many countries. As governments came under greater pressure from refugee numbers in the late twentieth century, the convention was interpreted in an increasingly narrow fashion, culminating in the assumption that a refugee, by definition, could only be someone who had been persecuted by government forces. For the thousands of women fleeing persecution by their families and husbands this meant being sent back to appalling living conditions. However, in 1985 the problem of vulnerable women was finally recognised, and it was agreed that women who faced harsh or inhuman treatment and received no help from their government could become refugees under the convention. Despite this, the majority of host countries are still reluctant to grant asylum on these grounds (United Nations High Commission for Refugees 2000).

It is important for professionals caring for refugees to be aware that there is an assumption that every refugee is an escapee from war or civil unrest, and that they will be missing their home and desperate for the company of their own race. The woman who has sought refuge from gender-based persecution may be reluctant to engage with

TABLE 6.2 Summary of estimated outcomes of asylum applications (including appeal outcomes at Immigration Asylum Appeal (IAA) and Asylum and Immigration Tribunal (AIT) (Bennett, Heath and Jeffries 2007)

	2003	2004	2005	2006
Asylum applications	49 405	33 960	25 710	23 610
Recognised as a refugee and granted asylum	7 650	4 370	4 370	4 040
as a percentage of total applications	15%	13%	17%	17%
Not recognised as a refugee but granted HP or DL	5 245	3 720	2 850	2 185
as a percentage of total applications	11%	11%	11%	9%
Refused asylum, HP or DL, or withdrawn by appellant	33 635	23 860	16 000	13 375
as a percentage of total applications	68%	70%	62%	57%
Cases with decision not known	1 555	930	1630	3 090
as a percentage of total applications	3%	3%	6%	13%

anyone from her own country. She may also be living in fear of being returned, or of being found by a UK-based branch of her family.

However, most of these women will be fleeing from situations of war. This is because in modern warfare the civilian population is deliberately targeted. On average, civilians represented approximately 90% of casualties in late twentieth century wars (Chinkin 1993, Paulson 2003). In *The Times*, 14 July 2008, Halima Bashir tells movingly of her story of being gang-raped near Darfur by Sudanese Government-backed Janjawid Arab militia. In 2005, Halima arrived in the UK and was granted asylum but has no idea where her family are or even if they are alive. She cites her case of rape being used as a weapon of war. Women bear the brunt of this, as they continue to be particularly vulnerable in times of war or civil unrest. Nikolic-Ristanovic (2000) suggests that this vulnerability stems from a combination of the following factors.

- Women are usually unarmed and do not have access to weapons. Most of them do not know how to use a weapon.
- They are less mobile. For example, they may be pregnant, or caring for small children or elderly relatives.
- They are usually reluctant to leave their homes, as their role is to look after the home in the absence of men.
- They need to provide for their families, which may lead to dangerous expeditions for basic necessities, such as food, and also to prostitution.
- Women are often objectified as the property of their men. Attacking them is therefore often seen as a direct assault on the man concerned and on the honour of his family.
- Women will often stay in their homes until the last minute, when a final traumatic event, such as an attack, a rape or a threat to their children, causes them to flee. Many do this reluctantly, torn between their children and their husband, and

experiencing guilt about leaving their home and husband, who may return after the war. The account of Olivera, a Serb refugee, clearly illustrates this:

> I can't forgive myself for leaving with the children. You know, I was taught to be always by my husband's side. I thought 'What would happen if he has to go to fight and then gets killed? Would my children tell me that I had left and let him manage everything alone and get killed?' (Nikolic-Ristanovic 2000)

COMMON EXPERIENCES

Although, as a rule, generalisations are dangerous and should be avoided, they have a use in the refugee situation, if only to act as a paradigm in which to explore the many factors that will affect the pregnant refugee. As mentioned earlier, the refugee woman will have had a unique series of experiences that will have affected her prior to her encounter with the healthcare professional. Many of these women will be suffering from psychological trauma. Kielson 1979 (cited in Van der Veer 1998) suggests that the process of traumatisation of the refugee is a slow one and generally takes years. He divides it into three periods, namely the increasing political repression at home, the traumatic events that culminated in flight, and exile itself. This is a useful observation, as it shows how the woman has been moving towards becoming a refugee over a long period of time and will already be showing signs of long-term traumatisation. Seligman (1975) suggests that passivity is often observed as a result of trauma, and this view is supported by Gielis (1982), who introduced a concept of 'learned helplessness' caused by trauma. This has the following features:

- reduced motivation to react, including passive slow reactions, sluggish thinking, low expectations and no belief in the possibility of an improvement in the situation
- reduced capacity to learn that actions can lead to desired results
- negative feelings such as fear, depression, emptiness, and absence of desires
- self-reproach and low self-esteem.

This is particularly relevant with regard to the pregnant refugee, who could thus appear passive and uninterested in the outcome of her pregnancy as a result of this long-term trauma. So what factors lead to this level of trauma in the woman? Van der Veer (1998) has identified eight types of experience that the majority of refugees will undergo. Although no list could encompass the entirety of every individual refugee's experience, this is useful as a framework for exploring the effects of becoming a refugee on a pregnant woman.

- increasing political repression
- detention
- torture and rape
- other types of violence
- disappearance of relatives
- separation and loss
- hardship
- exile.

INCREASING POLITICAL REPRESSION

Wars do not start suddenly and refugees are not made instantaneously. Frequently, there is a slow political shift towards an opposing ethnic or political group. Many individuals initially experience the loss of privileges, with increasing restrictions being placed on their lives and work. They will see their own and their children's future slowly becoming less hopeful, and they may begin to be the subjects of abuse in the press and when they go out of the home. As the repression increases, there is a build-up of tension within the family, leading to an increase in domestic violence, and women will be under enormous stress as they work to keep their family safe in this environment. Living in a constant state of fear is both depressing and damaging to health, and there may also be a loss of faith and trust in others as neighbours and friends turn against them. Many refugees will find it difficult to trust anyone again. For the pregnant refugee in the UK, this loss of trust can be very difficult, as she will not automatically trust her care team, and she may require more time and understanding before she has confidence in them. Some women will also be very nervous in the presence of interpreters whom they do not know, as they often suspect them of being spies or members of opposing parties. It is vital for them to develop a rapport with an interpreter and remain with that person if possible. A high turnover of medical and midwifery staff will also worry the woman, as she has come from a world of disappearances and will wonder why different people are present at each appointment. It is vital that the voices of these women are listened to and heard, not only by midwives and other healthcare workers, but also at Government level to encourage the formation of more woman-centred strategies (Dumper 2005).

Detention

Many women will have been detained for a period of time prior to their flight. This may have been a sudden arrest or an expected event. However, the mother will have been separated from her family, and she may have missed important family events or ceremonies. She will be unable to fulfil her role of mother, and this will lead to feelings of guilt and self-reproach, particularly if the arrest is due to any actions on her part (e.g. handing out leaflets). Detention also signifies the loss of hope of any improvement in the political situation, and it is often the catalyst that makes a woman flee.

Torture and rape

Torture is common in repressive regimes. It frequently occurs during detention, and women are tortured as often as men. It would be impossible to determine how many refugee women have been tortured, as there is great stigma attached to it and many would never speak of their experiences, even to loved ones. However, United Nations High Commission for Refugees (UNHCR) figures have suggested that up to 80% of refugees have been tortured either in their own country or during flight.

One of the main aims of the torturer is to silence dissent by using techniques that take away the voice of the victim. These will involve physical violence in all of its forms: psychological violence (e.g. sensory deprivation), threats to the woman and her loved ones, particularly her children, the assault of loved ones in front of her, and sexual torture, including rape, mutilation of genitals and the administration of electric shocks to organs. Sadly, the list of ways that torturers have found to hurt their victims could go on for ever. However, this chapter will concentrate on some of the effects on the woman and her life afterwards. Rape will be discussed as a separate issue.

The physical sequelae of torture include scarring, chronic headaches, shoulder pain, back pain and haemorrhoids. Many women will suffer from chest complaints after having been imprisoned in damp cells. Some will complain of problems eating, possibly due to the forced ingestion of taboo substances such as faeces, oil and semen (Douglas 1966) during torture. These women will often have somatised complaints, which can be described as the physical manifestation of psychological pain. Hinshelwood (1996: 195) suggests that 'the body's language to communicate and live with the unspeakable is much more primitive and simple than the spoken word'. Survivors of torture often have difficulty sleeping and are plagued by nightmares and flashbacks.

Women who are pregnant at the time of torture frequently miscarry afterwards. The torturers will often convince them that they will never again bear healthy children because of the torture, and for women this is one of the most powerful long-term effects of torture. The following quote illustrates this clearly: 'Women who have been tortured feel the torture is inside them and that their insides are spoiled and, most particularly, their creative reproductive capacity' (Hinshelwood 1996: 195).

This sense of internal spoiling is not unusual, and it represents a major psychological stumbling block for the pregnant woman. Consider, for example, the moving story of Sylvia, who begged for a termination because of her belief that anything that came from inside her could only be evil and deformed (Agger and Jenson 1993). Hinshelwood (1996: 195) also writes of her client who believed 'her body to still be filled with blood and torturer's semen and dead fetus'. There are numerous descriptions of women asking for the removal of something evil that they felt was inside them and tangible. Hinshelwood (1996) suggests that a sensitive gynaecological examination can help to provide reassurance in these situations. Perhaps an ultrasound scan would also serve the same function if it was approached with this purpose in mind. Meeting medical staff and undergoing procedures can be particularly traumatic for the survivor of torture, because much torture is medicalised. Some of the instruments that are used for torture will look 'medical', and rooms will be given ironic, euphemistic names, such as 'intensive care' and 'operating theatres', by the torturers (Morris 2000).

This leads us on to the subject of rape and the devastating consequences of this for refugee women. In war situations, the incidence of rape increases dramatically (Seifert 1993), a fact that was most clearly demonstrated by the recent Balkan conflict. Before the war, rape was very rare, but during the war an estimated 20 000–50 000 women were known to have been raped (it is believed that the true figure is higher). Brownmiller (1993) suggests that this is because women's bodies have become an extension of the battlefield and therefore war is waged on them. Rape is also used with the intention of destabilising society and forcing citizens into exile. For example, many women in the Balkans were kept in rape camps until they became pregnant in order to interfere with the gene pool. Finally, there is a serious problem of rape in refugee camps, where women are unprotected and the incidence of rape is very high. Research has shown that rape during conflict is more brutal, often repeated and involves more than one rapist (Nikolic-Ristanovic 2000).

Although the refugee woman will not necessarily be pregnant as a result of rape, the fact of the pregnancy is likely to generate very ambivalent feelings within her. Many women never speak of their ordeals because it is so unacceptable to do so (some languages do not even have a word for rape, as they believe that a woman cannot be penetrated unless she is willing, and others punish rape victims as adulterers). On arrival in the UK there may be pressure from the woman's family to have a baby and she will be unable to explain why this may be a problem for her. Some women who have previously become pregnant as a result of rape may have had a late termination or they may have had the baby and given it away. Nikolic-Ristanovic (2000) describes as 'one of the cruellest forms of torture' the conflict of knowing that one is carrying one's rapist's child, which is also one's own child. The children born of these unions are viewed as 'monstrous' and 'evil'. For these women, pregnancy will be a major memory trigger, and together with the concerns about internal spoiling it may result in significant trau-matisation. Labour will inevitably bring back the memories of the previous experience. Zelina, a 13-year-old refugee who had been raped, had given birth to a child and had given it away, described her greatest fear as follows: 'that she would never be able to physically enjoy a man's company or love a baby' (Hinshelwood 1996: 195).

Therefore for these women, having a baby will be a pivotal moment in their lives, which may be a new beginning, but which will also be a painful reminder of what has happened. They will have fears about the baby and whether it will be deformed or evil because their internal reproductive organs have become a bad and unsafe place. Finally, many of these women will be terrified that they bear some kind of visible sign of their experiences, which will be discovered during an examination. To end this section, a vignette is taken from a speech by Gill Hinshelwood. We can assess torture, rape and torment in cool clinical language, but the cost to an individual can only be quantified in human terms. Asha's story brings to life the suffering and shame that is experienced by these women after being abused.

> Asha arrived in England in 1994 when she was 18 years old. She knew no one. Once in England, she was sent to a bed-and-breakfast hostel, where she stayed in her room, locked away from noise and danger, and only emerged to find help when she could not control her vomiting. She was pregnant. She had an abortion and went back to her miserable room. When she was referred to me some seven months later, her presenting symptom was a carrier bag of medicines – some of which she had tried to take as an overdose. Asha had 22 different medicines in her bag for complaints of aches and pains ranging from head to foot. She sat strained and rigid, her face never lightening and never making eye contact . . . The past history that Asha slowly allowed us to hear was one of violence and brutality, beginning with threats and abuse directed at those entering the Kingdom Hall and abuse hurled at her in the street, and culminating in brutal rape by five policemen in a cell leaving her unconscious, bleeding and, as it later turned out, pregnant. She had been a virgin. Asha had very few words at her disposal to describe what had happened. Many of the words we use are felt to defile the person by the very utterance of them . . . She had coped over the last seven months by her disconnectedness, by being 'a backache', 'a sore throat', 'a painful knee'. This consultation with me was the first exposure she had allowed since that day when her clothes were torn off, a rag was stuffed into her mouth and five policemen took over her body, penetrated her, cursed her . . . Asha was a walking picture of shame. (Hinshelwood 1997)

Other types of violence

Most refugees are subjected to terror prior to flight. Awareness of the destabilisation of a regime and the increased unpopularity of one's ethnic group will be frightening. During these periods, stories of rape and torture abound, and there will be much agonising over the decision of whether to leave. The ongoing threat of violence will be present. There will also be terror of being returned; as only 20–25% of applications are upheld, the great majority of refugees will be sent back home.

Disappearance of relatives

This can be extremely painful for the woman. Her relatives may have disappeared years previously, but the lack of closure will keep the pain fresh. Allodi and Rojas (1985) suggest that there is a higher incidence of mental health problems among refugees who have experienced the disappearance of a family member.

Separation and loss

All refugees will experience separation and loss. The woman will have been forcibly separated from her home, and she will have lost her belongings and status. She will no longer have a social structure around her to help her through her pregnancy. She will also have lost all of the frames of reference that contextualised her as a person, both internally and externally. Afkhami (1999: 214) described this as a 'loss of who I was.'

Coehlo (1982) describes this loss as a form of culture shock, which is particularly pertinent with regard to the pregnant woman, as childbirth is an event imbued with cultural and traditional meanings that will not be relevant in the new social culture. The woman may have lost members of her immediate family, and she will also have lost her social group who would have welcomed the baby into the world. Eisenbruch (1984) suggested that these losses are a form of cultural bereavement, and that they require adaptation that could result in denial, anger and finally depression.

Many women will also have been bereaved in the literal sense, having lost husband, relatives, friends and children in the conflict. They may be recently bereaved, and they could be experiencing feelings of guilt both about surviving and about having a new baby.

There is also loss of the woman's cultural life; in the host nation there is little interest in or respect for a refugee's homeland. This lack of knowledge and desire to learn is profoundly depressing and deeply insulting for many refugees (Van der Veer 1998). There will be cultural confusion, particularly in relation to gender, and the woman will often feel isolated and cut off from the female support networks in her own society. The rules that governed her in her homeland may not exist in a Western society where there are few limitations for women, and this can result in a loss of stability and balance in the woman's family relationships. Groenenburg (1992) has noted that this leads to conflict and ultimately a higher divorce rate within these families.

Hardship

Mrvic-Petrovic and Stevanovic (2000) stated that there is a widespread impoverishment of women refugees. This impoverishment often begins before the woman becomes a refugee, within her home country. Living in a repressive regime or an area of conflict inevitably leads to hardship of various kinds. There are frequently food and power shortages, and if the refugee is from a minority group, there could be poverty and hunger imposed by the regime itself.

During flight, refugees often experience the most gruelling physical hardship – they may walk through storms, over mountains or through deserts to escape. Some will bribe their way into lorries run by criminals, paying a terrible price to escape, as these criminals often force the women to have sex with them, rape them, rob them, and often do not give them food or water for days at a time. At the borders, guards exact a price as well, often in the form of the belongings of and sexual intercourse with the women.

A huge number of refugees will begin exile in a refugee camp. These again are places of immense poverty and hardship. There are frequently food shortages, and women receive the smallest share of what is available (Marshall 2000). As aid agencies struggle to manage the vast needs created by these camps, many residents are left without heating, water or shelter for long periods of time (Kett 2005).

Finally, having arrived in the UK, these women will again face hardship. The life of asylum seekers is not an easy one. They are often housed in the least desirable properties in the least desirable areas and are forced to live below the poverty line with no access to money, paying for goods with vouchers. Single women are placed in hostels, which are often mixed and which charge fees that use up all of the asylum seeker's allowance. Asylum-seeking mothers do not even have the right to free milk and vitamins for their babies.

McLeish (2002) published a report on the plight of pregnant asylum seekers for Maternity Alliance. It paints a depressing picture of how these women, once in the UK, continue to suffer from loneliness, depression, separation from family members and sometimes violence, and they suffer poor physical and mental health as a result. Black African women, including asylum seekers and newly arrived refugees have a maternal mortality rate nearly six times higher than white women (Lewis 2007). Special emphasis is given to migrant women in the Confidential Enquiries into Maternal Deaths recognising that their particular experiences render them vulnerable during pregnancy and childbirth. These experiences include female genital cutting and, also, the need for translators to aid effective communication (Lewis 2007).

In times of extreme hardship, the woman will be more concerned about survival than anything else. The pregnant asylum seeker will be likely to have this mind set. She may seem more preoccupied and concerned about housing or her application for refugee status than she is about the baby or attending antenatal clinics at the right time. This is not an indication of lack of interest, but rather it is simply her way of coping with the enormous hurdles that lie in front of her. She will need flexibility and understanding from the midwives, and even help with organising her time so that she can attend her appointments and receive the support she needs (Lockey and Hart 2004, Harris, Humphreys and Nabb 2006, Ukoko 2005).

Exile

All refugees, for whatever reason, have been exiled. They have been exiled from the smell, the feel and the sights of home, and this sense of not belonging often remains with refugees for the rest of their lives. Many of them will be concerned with events at home, and will be disturbed if there is news coverage of a particular event. The pregnant woman will be adapting simultaneously to her new social setting and her pregnant state. She will be aware that her child will be born into exile and may never know its country of origin. She will also be coming to terms with the fact that she has become a refugee and her child will be born with this identity and denied his or her birthright. This can cause overwhelming feelings of guilt and sadness. In exile, the woman may also have a great deal more responsibility than she had before. She may suddenly be the head of the household and be faced with decision making for the first time in her life.

REMEMBERING

People who have been through significant trauma will have a different way of remembering events. In fact, it is probably misleading to use the term 'memory' in this context, as it implies a sense of an event being viewed in the past, whereas for the traumatised refugee quite the opposite will be the case. Langer (1991) identified a concept of durational memory in Holocaust victims. This is a form of remembering that does not age or fade with time. Durational memories are fresh and are described as being 'like yesterday'. They are also physical or sensory, involving smell, sensations and emotions rather than details and overviews. This means that the woman can be remarkably vague (to the point of being difficult to believe) about details, but will nevertheless remember and feel the event as if it were yesterday. Seifert and Hoffnung (1987) suggest that this is due to an overload of information in the long-term memory causing spillage into the short-term memory, which results in flashbacks and nightmares. They also suggest that the short-term memory is then filled up inappropriately, resulting in problems with regard to memory and concentration.

This is a crucial factor to consider when caring for the refugee woman. Her pregnancy, the examinations and the birth may all trigger durational memories that could be very damaging and frightening. She needs to be treated as if her experiences had happened yesterday, as chronological time has no relevance in this situation. She should not be expected to remember things easily, so information that is given to her should be repeated and written down.

CONCLUSIONS

Faced with this list of appalling experiences and tragedy, it seems difficult to envisage that anything more than understanding can be offered to the refugee woman who is facing childbirth in the UK. However, this is not the case; as with resourcefulness and knowledge healthcare professionals can adapt their approach to the needs of the woman and greatly improve her care.

One of the most difficult problems for these women is lack of knowledge – of who they are, where they are from, what they have been through and what is important in their lives. In the busy world of the NHS these issues are rarely addressed, but they are vital to the person who has lost most of this knowledge (O'Donnell, et al. 2007, Coker 2004). We need to be able to show interest, learn a little about the countries they come from and acquaint ourselves with some of the major cultural features (particularly birthing rituals) of our refugee patients. The ability to discuss refugee topics with these women will be a step towards reducing the stigma attached to their position. It is also vital for the carer to understand the importance of survival issues to the refugee. It is pointless to assume that they feel safe now and therefore there is no longer a problem. They will *not* feel safe – they will fear strangers, fellow nationals, people in uniform, and of course the Home Office, which may send them back to their homeland. Instead of fighting this, and trying to impose the healthcare professional's own set of values on these women, it would be more productive to help them work through the survival issues or to direct them towards someone who can do this (Derluyn and Broekaert 2007, Feldman, *et al.* 2007).

For any woman, bearing a child in the UK can represent a loss of control over one's body, particularly in the hospital setting. This can be very challenging for the refugee patient, who has seen all control removed from her life in previous years. In particular, victims of torture need to have control over their bodies, as they have been subject to a total loss of autonomy during the torture. The loss of control over one's body, associated with pain such as labour, may trigger durational memories, flashbacks and terror. Because of this, the healthcare professional should ensure that any decision – even simply touching the woman – is made by the woman herself without pressure or coercion. Any refusal of an examination or treatment must be regarded as an informed choice. For example, some survivors of torture have said that they would prefer to die rather than undergo a procedure that triggered a flashback (Matthews 1997).

This chapter has provided a snapshot of the refugee woman and her life. We can see that the effects of experiences such as rape and torture are overt and numerous. Basic functions such as eating and sleeping are disrupted, as are mechanisms for communication, due to fear and lack of language. The woman's body has acquired a new set of meanings through her experiences, and these make it a dangerous place for her. We can also see how the violation of boundaries during rape and torture leads to a sense of social pollution. It is hardly surprising that many women refugees struggle to come to terms with their lives in the UK. There is a high rate of suicide and depression among refugees in this country (Aldous, *et al.* 1999). However, most refugees will carry on, despite feelings of desperation and severe traumatisation. They are survivors and that is what they do, often at immense personal cost. Importantly, Amen (1985) suggests that refugees often cope well until they are faced with something unexpected, or until physical illness undermines their ability to cope, and then they collapse. This is why pregnancy and childbirth represent such a dangerous time for the refugee woman, as it is a time of emotional significance and great vulnerability, when the woman will miss her home, her family and her loved ones more than ever and require greater support than before. Mrvic–Petrovic (2000) supports this view, stating that women refugees are especially vulnerable to new stressors when pregnant.

This chapter has focused more on what *makes* refugee women than on what *happens* to them in the UK, because if we are to understand the context of their lives, it is necessary to look back to the start of the fear and repression and how the process of becoming a refugee has affected these women. During pregnancy and childbirth they require knowledge, sensitivity and understanding. The midwife should be alert to signs of trauma and be aware of the complex issues in the refugee woman's life.

KEY POINTS

- ✑ Women seek asylum for a variety of different reasons.
- ✑ Refugee women are stigmatised, and experience poverty and hardship in their host country.
- ✑ They will be diverse will and have had widely different experiences, but certain common factors will be present.
- ✑ Many will have endured physical and mental abuse, which they will be reluctant to discuss. This could have profound psychological effects.
- ✑ Apparent lack of interest and apathy may be misleading and require the carer to consider the possible causes, such as trauma and a preoccupation with survival.
- ✑ The rape and torture of refugee women is common.
- ✑ Traumatic memories remain recent and painful.
- ✑ Pregnant refugees are particularly vulnerable and require special care and consideration. The midwife needs to understand and anticipate the difficulties that may arise.

USEFUL ADDRESSES

Medical Foundation for the Care of Victims of Torture
111 Isledon Rd
London N7 7JW
Tel: 0207 697 7777 www.torturecare.org.uk
Provides medical consultations and treatment, medical documentation of torture, practical help and advice, marital, family and child therapies, and a range of complementary therapies.

Refugee Council
240–50 Ferndale Rd
Brixton SW9 8BB
Tel: 0207 346 6700 www.refugecouncil.org.uk
Campaigns for refugee rights, provides direct services such as day care, housing advice, etc. and produces information on refugee issues.

Liberty
21 Tabard Street
London SE1 1LA
Tel: 0207 403 3888/0207 374 8659 www.liberty-human-rights.org.uk
Offers legal advice and assistance on all areas that affect asylum seekers and refugees.

REFERENCES

Afkhami M. (1999) A woman in exile. In: Agosin M, editor. *A Map of Hope*. Harmondsworth: Penguin Books.

Agger I, Jenson S. (1993) The psychosexual trauma of torture. In: Wilson J, Raphael B, editors. *International Handbook of Trauma Stress Syndromes*. New York: Plenum Press.

Aldous J, Bardsley M, Daniell R, *et al.* (1999) *Refugee Health in London: key issues for public health*. The Health of Londoners Project. London: Directorate of Public Health.

Allodi F, Rojas A. (1985) The health and adaptation of victims of political violence in Latin America. In: Pichot P, editor. *Psychiatry: the state of the art*. New York: Plenum Press.

Amen DG. (1985) Post-Vietnam stress disorder: a metaphor for current and past life events. *Am J Psychiatry*. **39**: 580–6.

Bashir H. (2008) *I was raped and taunted in a 'ghost house': a woman doctor from Darfur tells of her abuse at the hands of the Sudanese regime*. London: The Times; 14 July 2008.

Bennett K, Heath T, Jeffries R. (2007) *Home Office Statistical Bulletin: asylum statistics United Kingdom 2006: explanatory notes*. London. Available at: www.homeoffice.gov.uk/rds/immigration1.html (accessed 26 Dec 2008).

Brownmiller S. (1993) Making female bodies the battlefield. In: Stiglmayer A, editor. *Mass Rape: the war against women in Bosnia–Herzegovina*. Lincoln, NE: University of Nebraska Press.

Burnett A, Fassil Y. (2004) *Meeting the Health Needs of Refugee and Asylum Seekers in the UK: an information and resource pack for health workers*. London: National Health Service.

Chinkin CM. (1993) Peace and force in international law. In: Dallmeyer DG, editor. *Reality, Women and International Law*. New York: Asil.

Coehlo GV. (1982) The foreign student's sojourn as a high-risk situation: the culture-shock phenomenon re-examined. In: Nann RC, editor. *Uprooting and Surviving*. Dordrecht: D Reidel Publishing Company.

Coker N. (2004) Asylum seekers and refugees in the United Kingdom. In: Healy J, McKee M, editors. *Accessing Healthcare: responding to diversity*. Oxford: Oxford University Press; Chapter 11.

Derluyn I, Broekaert E. (2007) Different perspectives on emotional and behavioural problems in unaccompanied refugee children and adolescents. *Ethn Health*. **12**(2): 141–62.

Douglas M. (1966) *Purity and Danger*. London: Routledge.

Dumper H. (2005) *Making Women Visible: strategies for a more woman-centred asylum and refugee support system*. London: Refugee Council.

Eisenbruch M. (1984) Cross-cultural aspects of bereavement: a conceptual framework for comparative analysis. *Culture Med Psychiatry*. **8**: 283–309.

Feldman CT, Bensing JM, de Ruijter A, *et al.* (2007) Afghan refugees and their general practitioners in the Netherlands: to trust or not to trust? *Sociol Health Illn*. **29**(4): 515–35.

Gielis A. (1982) Geleerde hulpeloosheid all depressiemodel, Een literatuurstudie. *Gedragstherapie*. **15**: 3–31.

Groenenburg M. (1992) Female victims. In: Van der Veer G, editor. *Counselling and Therapy with Refugees*. New York: John Wiley & Sons.

Harris M, Humphreys K, Nabb J. (2006) Developing services for women seeking refuge. *RCM Midwives*. **9**(6): 226–8.

Hinshelwood G. (1996) Women, children and the family. In: Forrest D, editor. *A Glimpse of Hell*. London: Cassell.

Hinshelwood G. (1997) *Gender-Based Persecution*. Transcript of unpublished paper given to United Nations Medical Foundation Library.

Kett M. (2005) Displaced populations and long-term humanitarian assistance. *BMJ*. **331**(7508): 98–100.

Langer L. (1991) *Holocaust Testimonies*. New Haven, CT: Yale University Press.

Lewis G, editor. (2007) *Saving Mothers' Lives: reviewing maternal deaths to make motherhood safer – 2004-2005*. The Seventh Report of the Confidential Enquiries into Maternal Deaths in the

United Kingdom. Confidential Enquiry into Maternal and Child Health (CEMACH). London: CEMACH.

Lockey R, Hart A. (2004) Improving consultation with disadvantaged service users. *Br J Midwif.* 12(12): 784–9.

Marshall R. (2000) Refugee women. *Refugees Magazine.* **100**: 78–89.

Matthews J. (1997) *After the Pain: the body of the torture survivor.* Brunel: Brunel University. Unpublished research paper.

McLeish J. (2002) *Mothers in exile: maternity experiences of asylum seekers in England.* London: Maternity Alliance.

Morris T. (2000) Disguise and deny. *New Internationalist.* **327**: 28.

Mrvic-Petrovic N, editor. (2000) Social acceptance and the difficulty adapting to a new environment. In: Nikolic-Ristanovic V, editor. *Women, Violence and War: wartime victimisation of refugees in the Balkans.* Budapest: Central European Press.

Mrvic-Petrovic N, Stevanovic I. (2000) Life in refuge: changes in socio-economic and familial status. In: Nikolic-Ristanovic V, editor. *Women, Violence and War: wartime victimisation of refugees in the Balkans.* Budapest: Central European Press.

Nikolic-Ristanovic V, editor. (2000) *Women, Violence and War: wartime victimisation of refugees in the Balkans.* Budapest: Central European Press.

O'Donnell CA, Higgins M, Chauhan R, *et al.* (2007) 'They think we're OK and we know we're not': a qualitative study of asylum seekers' access, knowledge and views to healthcare in the UK. *BMC Health Services Research.* **7**: 75. Available at: www.biomedcentral.com/1472–6963/7/75 (accessed 26 Dec 2008).

Palmer D, Ward K. (2007) 'Lost': listening to the voices and mental health needs of forced migrants in London. *Medicine, Conflict and Survival.* **23**(3): 198–212.

Paulson DS. (2003) War and refugee suffering. In: Krippner S, McIntyre TM, editors. *The Psychological Impact of War Trauma on Civilians: an international perspective.* London: Praeger.

Seifert K, Hoffnung RJ. (1987) *Child and Adolescent Development.* Boston, MA: Houghton Mifflin.

Seifert R. (1991) War and rape – a preliminary analysis. In: Stiglmayer A, editor. *Mass Rape: the war against women in Bosnia-Herzegovina.* Lincoln, NE: University of Nebraska Press.

Seligman M. (1975) *Helplessness: on depression, development and death.* San Francisco, CA: Freeman.

Ukoko F. (2005) Sure Start midwife: giving a voice to the voiceless. *Br J Midwif.* 13(12): 776–80.

United Nations High Commission for Refugees. (1998) *Basic Obligations: refugee rights and the State.* Unpublished guidance document.

United Nations High Commission for Refugees. (2000) *The State of the World's Refugees.* Oxford: Oxford University Press.

Van der Veer G. (1998) *Counselling and Therapy with Refugees and Victims of Trauma.* Chichester: John Wiley & Sons.

Wali S. (1995) Muslim refugee, returnee and displaced women: challenges and dilemmas. In: Afkhami M, editor. *Faith and Freedom.* Syracuse, NY: Syracuse University Press.

Yates T, Crane R, Burnett A. (2007) Rights and the reality of healthcare charging in the United Kingdom. *Med, Conflict Surviv.* 23(4): 297–304.

CHAPTER 7

Domestic violence in pregnancy

Sally Cottrell

This chapter discusses domestic violence experienced by women in pregnancy. It explores the social context of domestic violence in the UK, from both an historical and present day perspective, and the effects it has on women and their experience of pregnancy. The impact that health professionals and the maternity services can have on women's experience is also discussed, with some suggestions of how health professionals can help to ensure women who experience violence receive appropriate support.

WHAT IS DOMESTIC VIOLENCE?

The most widely accepted definition of domestic violence is 'any incident of threatening behaviour, violence or abuse (psychological, physical, sexual, financial or emotional), between adults who are or have been intimate partners or family members, regardless of gender or sexuality' (Department of Health 2005). The abusive behaviour is frequently used by one person to control and dominate another (Hester, Pearson, and Harwin 1998), and it may include various forms of coercion and intimidation such as degradation, humiliation, deprivation, systematic criticism and belittling (Home Office 1995).

It is widely accepted that the vast majority of violence in a domestic relationship is perpetrated by men against women and their children, although it is acknowledged that abuse may occur in same-sex relationships and be committed by women against men (Department of Health 2005). Women are much more likely to be victims of multiple incidents of abuse and to experience sexual violence (Walby and Allen 2004). It is also important to acknowledge that the issue of domestic violence perpetrated against women by their male partners is not the same violence towards children or older people. Failure to do so would ignore or minimise the gender implications that are central to this issue.

The language used to describe domestic violence and the women who experience it can be problematic. Terms such as 'victim' and 'battered wife' are frequently applied to women who experience domestic violence, implying weakness and passivity. This denies women's resistance and coping strategies, and encourages victim blaming (Hester, Kelly and Radford 1996). A more appropriate descriptor might be 'survivor' to emphasise the determination, action and bravery shown by women (Dobash and Dobash 1992), and reflect the complexity of responses to the experience of domestic violence.

WHO EXPERIENCES DOMESTIC VIOLENCE?

Domestic violence is often secret, hidden and undisclosed, with only one in three incidents that result in injury being reported to the police (Home Office 1996). However, a self-reporting questionnaire used in the British Crime Survey indicates that domestic violence is a common experience, with nearly one in four women being assaulted by their partner at some point in their lives, and one in eight repeatedly so (Women's Aid 2008). Domestic violence is rarely an isolated incident; an escalating spiral of abuse is commonplace, sometimes resulting in death. The criminal statistics for England and Wales demonstrate that a present or former partner is responsible for killing almost half of all female murder victims, with an average of two women being murdered each week by a current or previous male partner (Povey 2004, Home Office 2008).

Women of all ages, classes and ethnic groups are known to experience abuse in the home (Radford 1987), although recently some differences related to age have been noted, with young women aged 16–24 years most at risk (Mirrlees-Black 1996). However, there appears to be a common view that violence is more prevalent or somehow different among those from the lower socio-economic groups. This is exemplified by the writings of Frances Cobbe (1878), who described domestic violence as:

> . . . the blow or two delivered occasionally in the gentlemen's drawing room, through thrashings with a fist in London, to its climax in the overcrowded centres of manufacturing, trade, and mining in the north, where tramplings and purrings with hobnailed boots are common. (Cobbe 1878, cited in Stark and Flitcraft 1996: 43)

Most of the research into domestic violence has been conducted amongst the lower socio-economic group, adding to the myth that it is a disorder of the poor. It is true that this group has the highest level of reporting of domestic violence; however, no differences have been found in the actual incidence of domestic abuse within different social groups in Britain. It could be suggested that middle class women might be more able to deal with the challenges of addressing domestic violence. They are more likely to be financially able to leave, and to receive respect and be taken seriously by professional support services. However, if they are married to middle class men, it may be more difficult to enlist the support of agencies such as the police, with stereotypical assumptions that middle class men do not beat their wives (Hester, Kelly and Radford 1996).

Pregnancy, a time when women are making physical, emotional and social preparations for motherhood, offers no protection from abuse. For some women pregnancy is a result of their male partner's violence towards them, conception being the result of rape. During pregnancy, the abuse may simply be 'business as usual', but for some women, the pregnancy may act as the trigger for domestic violence, with male jealousy or anger directed towards the unborn baby (Campbell, *et al.* 1993). For almost 30% of women who experience domestic violence in their lifetime, the first incident occurs during pregnancy (Helton, *et al.* 1987). Others experience an increase in the extent and nature of violence, with injuries to the breasts, abdomen and genital area more common (Hillard 1985). As part of a cycle of escalating violence, pregnant women are also murdered by their male partner/relative, with 19 cases being reported in the Confidential Enquiries into Maternal Deaths in the United Kingdom (Lewis 2007). On the other hand, pregnancy may offer some women a respite from abuse, often resulting in repeated pregnancies in a short space of time, to afford some self-protection (Mezey and Bewley 1997). However, other research has demonstrated that *postnatal* women are most at risk for moderate to severe injury (Hedin 2000).

HISTORICAL PERSPECTIVE

For many centuries women have experienced violence at the hands of men they are intimately involved with. The abusive nature of this relationship has been well documented since Roman times, with the patriarchal society being seen as the root cause of male violence towards women. There seems no doubt that the origins and perpetuation of domestic violence are a product of male authority and control and the associated subordination of women. For example, in the eighteenth century, a married woman was subject to whatever violence her husband felt was reasonably required to correct her (Blackstone 1765, cited in Dobash and Dobash 1979). This 'domestic chastisement' was thought necessary since husbands were legally answerable for their wives' misbehaviour, although there was no legal recourse for women whose chastisement was excessive or unreasonable.

Throughout the nineteenth century various Acts of Parliament were passed that made small improvements to the position of women in relation to their position as wives, and through the 1878 Matrimonial Causes Act women were finally afforded the same protection against beatings and ill-treatment that animals already had. However, these improvements made little impact on the daily lives of women living in abusive relationships. The private institution of the family, upheld by the Church and the State as sacred, maintained and promoted the subordinated position of women, and their economic dependence on their male partners. Every 20 years or so during the twentieth century, a surge of protests has occurred about the issue of domestic violence, perhaps most notably during the 1970s with the emergence of the women's movement against domestic violence. National Women's Aid organisations, working to end violence against women and children, have been a powerful force for social change, supporting individual women, providing accommodation in shelters and generally raising the profile of domestic violence, ensuring its place on the national agenda. Their work and that of others has led to a huge increase in social and political awareness of domestic violence, the experience of women who live in abusive relationships, and the impact this has on their health.

By the end of the twentieth century, Government policy began to take a strong line, promoting an interagency approach to tackling domestic violence, and encouraging the police to be proactive in the enforcement of relevant legislation. Having previously viewed domestic violence as being in the private domain of the family, the police moved from a position of largely ignoring the problem to taking a more positive stance; for example, setting up domestic violence units within each locality. However, within any institution that is inherently patriarchal, such as the police force, it is difficult not to be critical of their approach. It would seem that police discretion in dealing with the abuse of women allows an enormous number of domestic violence crimes against women to be ignored (Wright 1995). Little wonder then that women are reluctant to involve the police; the average victim has been assaulted 35 times before reporting the abuse (Bewley, Friend and Mezey 1997).

THE CONTEXT OF DOMESTIC VIOLENCE

To understand the context of domestic violence it is important to first comprehend the context of men and women's lives within society and accept the roles they play to fulfil society's expectations. Hoff (1990) asserts that violence against women occurs in a climate of socially structured inequalities for women, exemplified not only by the concept of patriarchy, but also sexism. In a social system where women's subordination to men is defined as natural, violence continues to be seen as a necessary and acceptable means of controlling women. Alternatively, women are viewed as willing participants, thriving and enjoying an abusive relationship, with frequently heard comments such as, 'If it is so bad, why doesn't she leave?' This approach typifies the ideology of women as victims, putting the onus for ending the violence on them rather than on the perpetrator who is actually responsible.

Dobash and Dobash (1979, 1998) and Dobash, *et al.* (1996) have demonstrated how violence can be seen as a result of a conflict of interests within a domestic relationship, based on the status and position of men in a patriarchal society. Four themes have been identified that exemplify conflict leading to domestic violence: men's possessiveness and jealousy, disagreements and expectations concerning domestic work and resources, men's sense of the right to punish 'their' women for perceived wrongdoing, and the importance to men of maintaining or exercising their power and authority. Their research has highlighted the specific issues that may be a source of conflict and act as a trigger for violence to occur (*see* Box 7.1).

BOX 7.1 SOURCES OF DOMESTIC CONFLICT (DOBASH AND DOBASH 1998)

- domestic work
- money
- children
- alcohol
- possessiveness and jealousy
- isolation and restriction of mobility and social life
- sex

Pregnancy and the birth of a baby could also be seen as additional sources of conflict exacerbating those highlighted above. Consider the impact of pregnancy on women's domestic work. Household chores such as cleaning, washing, ironing, shopping and food preparation are essentially the responsibility of women and may be combined with paid employment outside the home and care of other children. During early pregnancy many women experience extreme tiredness, nausea and vomiting, and in the later stages backache and tiredness are common place. In the early postnatal period women will need personal time to establish breastfeeding and recover from the physical effects of labour and birth. It is likely that domestic responsibilities will be low on their list of priorities, although the same demands will be ever present if not increased. Combine this with an existing male expectation that his needs for food, clothing and a clean house will be met and it is not hard to see how this could be an increased source of conflict.

Gelles (1975) investigated reasons why pregnant women might be abused, and suggested that the normal physiological traits of pregnant women, such as mood swings and a reduction in libido, were credible reasons for male violence towards pregnant women. Pregnancy can be seen as interfering with the woman's ability to perform the roles and duties that the male partner sees as necessary, thus justifying a violent response. Cultural beliefs about domestic violence reinforce the notion that women are somehow deserving of abuse. However, it is only within the context of a society that perpetuates women's subordination to men, that this could be viewed as such.

Domestic violence as a *women's* issue may be culturally denied; when discussing domestic violence it is common to hear of women who perpetrate violence against their male partners. Domestic violence against women is a crime where people instinctively leap to the defence of the perpetrator (Horley 1991). One of the easiest ways of avoiding the realities of domestic violence is to turn it around, and insist that it is a two-sided issue with women being seen as the abusers as well as the abused. However, there is no doubt that the overwhelming majority of adults who experience domestic violence are women, and the extent of the injuries and trauma they experience is far in excess of anything experienced by men (Dobash, Dobash and Noaks 1995). In cases of extreme domestic violence that result in death, female victims far outweigh male victims, and there is a significant difference in the way the violence is perpetrated. Women who kill their male partners typically do so as a single act of violence after many years of experiencing abuse themselves, compared to men who kill their female partners as a final act after a long series of attacks (Lloyd 1995). However, within the male-dominated criminal justice system, violence against women is yet again viewed as justified, provoked or deserved, with women who kill after experiencing years of abuse being discriminated against, and often receiving harsher sentences than men who commit similar or lesser crimes.

EFFECTS OF DOMESTIC VIOLENCE

The effect that living with violence has on women is wide and varied, from physical injury, poor mental health, social isolation, and overuse of drugs of comfort. The abuse may be apparent in a variety of ways, such as bruises, bites, cuts, grazes, broken bones, depression, suicide attempts, loneliness, alcoholism and drug abuse. On the other hand there may be no obvious outward signs.

In keeping with the secret, covert nature of the perpetration of the abuse, women may become skilled at hiding the signs and symptoms because of shame, embarrassment, or fear of retribution should anyone outside the family become aware of the abusive relationship. Women living with violence may also have a sense of personal responsibility for their partner's actions. Guilt may be a significant factor in a woman's silence; she may regard the experience of violence as a signal that she has somehow failed, and be concerned that public knowledge may be associated with social stigmatisation (Dobash and Dobash 1998). If others do become aware of the abuse, women may minimise or deny the violent incidents. When women say 'nothing really happened', perhaps what they are really implying is how much worse it could have been (Hester, Kelly and Radford 1996).

SPECIFIC EFFECTS OF DOMESTIC VIOLENCE ON PREGNANCY

Pregnant women experience domestic violence in the same ways as those who are not pregnant. However, the consequences may include some that are specific to pregnancy, including miscarriage, placental abruption, antepartum haemorrhage, premature labour, stillbirth and low-birth-weight babies (Lewis 2007, Hillard 1985, McWilliams and McKeirnan 1993, Mooney 1993, Saltzman 1990). In-utero injuries also occur, with abdominal trauma to the mother resulting in fractures to the fetus (Mezey and Bewley 1997). These effects are often not attributed to domestic violence by health professionals, and may partially account for the frequency with which many negative outcomes of pregnancy and birth remain unexplained.

For women who experience 'moderate to severe' violence in pregnancy the risk of preterm labour has been found to be up to four times greater than in women who experience no abuse (Shumway, et al. 1999). A high incidence of miscarriage has also been found. A survey of women living in refuges in Northern Ireland found that 60% had experienced violence during a pregnancy, with 13% having subsequent miscarriages (McWilliams and McKiernan 1993). Within health services considerable emphasis is placed on physiological causes of miscarriage and preterm labour. Women may be diagnosed with an 'incompetent cervix' and offered cervical cerclage, or repeated transvaginal ultrasound scans to detect changes in the cervix that may result in preterm delivery. Huge resources are poured into offering these services yet little is given to the exploration of social causes such as domestic violence.

Research has shown that 'mild and moderately' abused women are more frequently admitted to hospital during their pregnancy (Webster, Chandler and Battistutta 1996). However, it is likely that for many of these women the true cause of their need for their admission is never identified. It is apparent to anyone working within the maternity services in the UK today, that a considerable number of antenatal admissions are for symptoms that are never adequately diagnosed or explained through traditional medical approaches to care. A woman who has vague abdominal pain at 24 weeks with no specific diagnosis made, or frequent admissions for reduced fetal movements, may simply be seeking a place of refuge from an abusive relationship for a few hours or days. For other women their physical illness, caused by domestic abuse, such as a urinary tract infection, is physiologically investigated, diagnosed and treated. If the infection is severe, recurrent, or resistant to treatment, a range of further investigative tests may be performed. However, it is likely that no one will stop to consider whether the actual cause of the symptoms or the reason for the woman's self-referral could be related to an abusive relationship.

Abused women are more likely to use a range of coping strategies that have associated health risks, for both themselves and the fetus. An increased incidence of overuse of alcohol, abuse of prescribed and illegal drugs and cigarette smoking is evident (Grimstad, et al. 1998, Curry 1998, Martin, et al. 1996), with an associated impact on low birthweight (McFarlane, Parker and Soeken 1996). Strategies to support smoking cessation are becoming widespread to meet the Government's target of significantly reducing the incidence of smoking in pregnancy (Department of Health 2000a). However, in seeking to promote smoking cessation, it is uncommon for health professionals to address the social causes of women's smoking behaviour, such as domestic violence. In failing to do so, not only are health professionals facing a monumental challenge in meeting this target, they are also failing women who experience violence in their lives, and use cigarettes as a means of support easily available to them.

Violence directed at the unborn child may be apparent, with abdominal injuries more common in pregnancy (Hillard 1985). One-third of domestic violence in pregnancy is thought to be associated with jealousy or anger towards the unborn child (Campbell 1989, 1998). The welfare of children in households affected by domestic violence also causes concern, with children known to be at great risk of physical harm if their mother is abused (Mullender and Debbonaire 2000). Over half of all child protection cases involve domestic violence (Department of Health 2002).

Social isolation may be an intrinsic aspect of domestic abuse as part of the male strategy to control and dominate his partner (Stark and Flitcraft 1996). Women may be emotionally unable or physically prevented from accessing support, either from family and friends or statutory and voluntary agencies. During pregnancy women may be late bookers, unable to attend for antenatal care, and miss planned appointments. Women may be labelled by health professionals as a nuisance, deviant or uncaring of the outcome of their pregnancy, with little insight into the difficulties they face in engaging in normal social interactions.

Not surprisingly, women who experience domestic violence are known to experience mental health problems, for example, depression, anxiety, and suicide – actual or considered (Helton, MacFarlane, Anderson 1987). However, domestic violence as a cause of perinatal mental illness is largely unrecognised. In recent years, considerable emphasis has been placed upon the risks and impact of postnatal depression on new mothers, with hormonal changes proposed as the main determinant (Dalton and Holton 2001). This physiological approach denies the social context of birth, offering medical explanations and solutions for depressive illnesses that may have roots in relationship strife and domestic violence. Post-traumatic stress disorder has also been found amongst women who experience domestic violence (BMA 1998), and parallels between the effects of domestic violence on women and the impact of torture and imprisonment on hostages are apparent (Graham, *et al.* 1988). The impact of these effects includes low self-esteem, dependence on the perpetrator, and feelings of hopelessness and despair (Kirkwood 1993).

Women experience a high risk of 'moderate to severe' violence in the postnatal period (Hedin 2000). The birth of a baby, and the transition to parenthood is a time of major upheaval, stress and lifestyle changes. An increase in social status for the woman as mother is also evident, along with a need for the man to redefine his role as father, and assert his associated power and authority. If violence already exists within a relationship, this period of social role adjustment may be a time when it flourishes. It is not uncommon to find sexual assault as part of an abusive relationship, with pregnancy often the result. The early postnatal period may also be a time of vulnerability. It is not hard to empathise with the postnatal woman who has a painful swollen perineum following an episiotomy. She takes regular analgesia and frequent baths to alleviate her pain. She moves awkwardly, easing herself slowly from standing to sitting or vice versa, using every possible means to minimise her discomfort. It might be surprising therefore to discover that some midwives have found women who have had their perineal sutures removed by their partner (Hunt and Martin 2001, Steene 2001, personal communication). Imagine the power, coercion or force that must be involved, and the physical and psychological trauma women experience, in order for the partner to take his conjugal rights; although spoken about within professional circles, no documentary evidence existed until recently.

WHAT CAN HEALTH PROFESSIONALS DO?

Until recent times the NHS has largely ignored the problem of domestic violence. Given the incidence, the identification of women who access health services for injuries caused by domestic violence seems staggeringly poor. A woman may have attended for care on many occasions before her injuries became viewed as anything other than accidental. However, the advent of the new millennium saw a change in approach with domestic abuse becoming a priority throughout Government (Department of Health 2005). The Department of Health supports a joined-up approach of interagency working, and has issued clear guidance for health professionals on their role and responsibilities, with this proposal:

> It is essential that public agencies take every opportunity to identify those who may be subject to violence, and by offering practical and emotional support, help prevent the situation deteriorating. (Department of Health 2000b: iii)

The Crime and Disorder Act 1998 has placed a statutory duty upon health services to work collaboratively with others to reduce crime, including domestic violence. Primary Care Trusts must engage with local agencies to develop strategies to address domestic violence (Department of Health 2005). It is no longer considered acceptable to simply treat the consequential injuries of domestic violence. Health professionals are expected to work with the survivors of abuse, providing support, advice and appropriate referrals to other agencies empowering women to retake control of their lives. To do this they must first acknowledge domestic violence as a women's health issue and then identify those who are experiencing abuse, by being alert for possible indicators (*see* Box 7.2).

BOX 7.2 INDICATORS OF DOMESTIC VIOLENCE IN PREGNANCY (LEWIS 2007).

- late booking and/or poor or non-attendance at antenatal clinics
- repeated attendance at antenatal clinics, GP's surgery or Emergency Department for minor or trivial or non-existent complaints
- unexplained admissions
- non-compliance with treatment regimes/early self-discharge from hospital
- repeat presentation with depression, anxiety, self-harm and psychosomatic symptoms
- untreated injuries of several different ages, especially to the neck, head, breasts, abdomen and genitals

- minimisation of signs of abuse on the body
- sexually transmitted diseases, frequent vaginal and urinary tract infections and pelvic pain
- poor obstetric history including repeated miscarriage or terminations of pregnancy, stillbirth or preterm labour, preterm birth, intrauterine growth retardation/low birthweight, unwanted or unplanned pregnancy
- constant presence of the partner at examinations – may be domineering, answers all the questions for her and be unwilling to leave the room
- the woman seems evasive or reluctant to speak or disagree in front of her partner.

These indicators may alert health professionals of the possibility of domestic abuse, although the most important factor appears to be a relationship under social or financial strain. Key signs include marital separation, young children, financial pressures, drug/alcohol abuse and disability and ill health (Mirrlees-Black 1996). Great caution should be exercised before midwives, health visitors, general practitioners and others commence a 'search and rescue' mission to save these seemingly helpless, vulnerable women (Dobash and Dobash 1998). Hunt and Martin (2001) have highlighted the anger that midwives may feel when confronted with women who are experiencing violence during pregnancy, leading to a directive approach and strongly worded advice to leave the perpetrator. This, however, merely serves to reinforce the notion that women who experience domestic violence are weak, and in need of direction and control. By exercising professional power in this way, although rooted in the caring aspects of the role, health professionals may perpetuate the disempowerment of women in controlling their own lives and experiences.

Searching for indicators of abuse might not be particularly fruitful due to the covert nature of domestic violence. An alternative approach would be for health professionals to ask appropriate and timely questions of all women they come into contact with. The Royal College of Midwives advocates routine enquiry into domestic abuse throughout pregnancy and the postnatal period, with the proviso that it must be accompanied by a package of measures that includes a systematic and structured framework for referral and support of women who disclose domestic abuse (Royal College of Midwives 2006).

The form the questions take must depend upon the individual practitioner, the women, and the circumstances in which they find themselves. For example, introduce the subject to women as a routine enquiry that all pregnant women are asked about because of the greater risk during pregnancy. It is also recommended that general questions such as 'How are you feeling?' or 'How are things at home?' should be followed up with more specific questions related to abuse (Salmon, et al. 2004). Fears that women will be offended by health professionals' questions are largely unfounded; research demonstrates that a vast majority of women have no objections to being asked about domestic violence (Bradley, et al. 2002). No differences in levels of acceptability have been found between those who experience violence and those who do not (Stenson, et al. 2001). To women, what appears central to the acceptability of screening is that it is conducted in a safe, confidential environment, by a trained health professional who is empathetic and non-judgemental (Bacchus, Mezey and Bewley 2002).

Some women may voluntarily choose to disclose their experience of violence to a health professional, although this may be fraught with difficulties, not least finding the opportunity. Mezey and Bewley (1997) highlight the paradox now facing pregnant women. In the move to empower women, to promote informed choice, and make birth a social experience, the maternity services have opened doors previously closed to men, and welcomed them in with open arms. Gone is the antenatal clinic or delivery room as a sacred, female-only domain. Men are positively encouraged to attend every antenatal clinic appointment with their partner, to participate in birth preparation or 'parentcraft' classes, and stand vigil while their partner is in labour, soothing, massaging, and whispering words of encouragement. A man who is not present at his baby's birth is often viewed as somehow slightly deviant in today's post Changing Childbirth era (Department of Health 1993). The result of this is that, for pregnant women who live with domestic violence, there is no longer a place of safety, a respite from the abuse, or a confidential space in which to disclose their experience.

In this changed environment, health professionals may be reluctant to ask a woman about the cause of her injuries or symptoms, for fear of offending or upsetting her partner, although direct questioning should never occur in the presence of another person. Research has found that concerns about their own and the woman's subsequent safety may also discourage midwives from active questioning (Salmon, *et al.* 2004). Overcoming the barriers to enquiring about domestic violence require well thought out and supportive strategies that provide a structured and systematic response.

It is vital that when women do disclose an experience of domestic violence, health professionals respond sensitively, and provide ongoing support and information about other services available to assist women experiencing violence. Encouraging or cajoling a woman into leaving her abuser may not necessarily have the desired effect of protecting her from further violence. The most risky time for violence, particularly fatal injury, is when a woman leaves or attempts to leave the perpetrator (Daly and Wilson 1988, Binney, Harknell and Nixon 1988). What is essential is that women are supported to make their own decisions, and if they choose to leave, that they are well informed about support services they can use, such as a refuge or local authority accommodation to ensure their safety. If women choose not to leave, health professionals can help by offering an open door to provide ongoing support and appropriate information. This is not because women are helpless victims, but because an individual's personal coping mechanisms, on their own, may not be sufficient to counteract the social structure, cultural values and actions of perpetrators that combine to create and perpetuate the domestic abuse of women.

If health professionals are to be effective in identifying and supporting women who experience violence in pregnancy, a joined-up approach is required that has adequate resources and the support of health service managers. Close interagency liaison is required, with health professionals not afraid to challenge historical working practices, and willing to work across traditional boundaries. To promote this, staff development programmes should include training in domestic violence issues, and support mechanisms for health professionals who are themselves survivors of abuse. Particular attention should be paid to attitudes and beliefs about abuse that happens within the private domain of the family, for if health professionals are to be effective they must acknowledge domestic violence as an issue that is everybody's business.

CONCLUSION

Whilst much has changed in society's attitudes towards domestic violence, and recognition of the need for a coherent strategy to address this issue exists, there is still a long way to go before every woman living with violence receives the support and assistance she requires. For many women who live with abuse in the home, little has changed. Male violence continues to be perpetuated within a patriarchal society as a means of controlling women to assume their socially ascribed place in the natural order. It is vital that health professionals recognise domestic violence as an issue that potentially affects all women they encounter, regardless of social class, ethnicity and age. Pregnancy may be a particularly vulnerable time, with serious consequences for both maternal and fetal health. It is essential that health professionals provide sensitive, timely advice and support that empowers women to survive domestic violence.

KEY POINTS

- ∽ Domestic violence is a common experience, with nearly one in four women being assaulted by their partner at some point in their lives, and one in eight repeatedly so.
- ∽ The origins and perpetuation of domestic violence lie within male authority and control. In a social system where women's subordination to men is defined as natural, violence can be seen as a necessary and acceptable means of controlling women.
- ∽ Domestic violence may be the result of conflict of interests within a domestic relationship. The most important factor appears to be a relationship under social or financial strain. Key signs include marital separation, young children, financial pressures, drug/alcohol abuse, disability and ill health.
- ∽ Pregnancy may offer no protection from abuse. For many women the first incident of domestic violence may occur during pregnancy, although postnatal women are most at risk for moderate to severe injury.
- ∽ The physical and psychological effects of abuse are often not attributed to domestic violence by health professionals, and may partially account for the frequency with which many negative outcomes of pregnancy and birth remain unexplained.
- ∽ All pregnant women should be routinely asked about domestic violence by well-trained midwives, who have a variety of support mechanisms in place for both the women and themselves.
- ∽ It is vital that when women do disclose an experience of domestic violence, health professionals respond sensitively, providing ongoing support and information of other services available to assist women experiencing abuse in the home.

USEFUL ADDRESSES
Women's Aid Federation of England
PO Box 391
Bristol
BS99 7WS
National Domestic Violence Helpline Tel: 0808 200 0247
www.womensaid.org.uk

REFERENCES
Bacchus L, Mezey G, Bewley S. (2002) Women's perceptions of routine enquiry for domestic violence in a maternity service. *Br J Obstet Gynaecol.* **109**: 9–16.
Bewley S, Friend J, Mezey G, editors. (1997) *Violence Against Women.* London: Royal College of Obstetricians and Gynaecologists.
Binney V, Harkell G, Nixon J. (1988) *Leaving Violent Men: a study of refuges and housing for battered women.* London: Women's Aid Federation England.
Bradley F, Smith M, Long J, et al. (2002) Reported frequency of domestic violence: cross sectional survey of women attending general practice. *BMJ.* **324**: 271–4.
British Medical Association. (1998) *Domestic Violence: a healthcare issue?* London: British Medical Association.
Campbell J, Oliver C, Bullock L. (1993) Why battering during pregnancy? *Clin Issues Perinat Women Health Nurs.* **4**: 343–9.
Campbell J. (1989) A test of two explanatory models of women's responses to battering. *Nurs Res.* **38**: 18–24.
Campbell J. (1998) *Empowering Survivors of Abuse: healthcare for battered women and their children.* London: Sage.
Curry M. (1998) The interrelationships between abuse, substance use and psychosocial stress during pregnancy. *J Obstet Gynecol Neonatal Nurs.* **27**(6): 692–9.
Dalton K, Holton W. (2001) *Depression After Childbirth: how to recognise, treat and prevent postnatal depression.* Oxford: Oxford University Press.
Daly M, Wilson M. (1988) *Homicide.* New York: Aldine de Gruyter.
Department of Health. (1993) *Changing Childbirth.* London: HMSO.
Department of Health. (2000a) *The National Plan for the New NHS: the need for change.* Leeds: Department of Health NHS Executive. Available at: www.dh.gov.uk/en/Publicationsandstatistics/Publications/PublicationsPolicyAndGuidance/DH_4009362 (accessed 6 Jan 2009).
Department of Health. (2000b) *Domestic Violence: a resource manual for healthcare professionals.* London: Department of Health.
Department of Health. (2002) *Secure Futures for Women: making a difference.* London: Department of Health.
Department of Health. (2005) *Responding to Domestic Abuse: a handbook for health professionals.* London: Department of Health.
Dobash RE, Dobash RP. (1977) Love, honour and obey: institutional ideologies and the struggle for battered women. *Contemporary Crises.* **1**(4): 403–15.
Dobash RE, Dobash RP. (1979) *Violence Against Wives: a case against patriarchy.* New York: The Free Press.
Dobash RE, Dobash RP. (1992) *Women, Violence and Social Change.* London: Routledge.
Dobash RE, Dobash RP, editors. (1998) *Rethinking Violence Against Women.* London: Sage.
Dobash RE, Dobash RP, Cavanagh K, et al. (1996) *Research Evaluation of Programmes for Violent Men.* Edinburgh: Scottish Office Central Research Unit.
Dobash RE, Dobash RP, Noaks L, editors. (1995) *Gender and Crime.* Cardiff: University of Wales Press.

Gelles R. (1975) Violence and pregnancy: a note on the extent of the problem and needed services. *Family Coordinator*. **24**: 81–6.

Graham P, Rawlings E, Rimini W. (1988) Survivors of terror: battered women, hostages and the Stockholm syndrome. In: Yllo K, Bograd M, editors. *Feminist Perspectives on Wife Abuse*. London: Sage.

Grimstad H, Backe B, Jacobsen G, *et al.* (1998) Abuse history and health risk behaviours in pregnancy. *Acta Obstet Gynecol Scand*. **77**(9): 893–7.

Hedin L. (2000) Postpartum, also a risk period for domestic violence. *Eur J Obstet Gynaecol Reprod Biol*. **89**(1): 41–5.

Helton AS, McFarlane J, Anderson ET. (1987) Battered and pregnant: a prevalence study. *Am J Public Health*. **77**(10): 1337–9.

Hester M, Kelly L, Radford J, editors. (1996) *Women, Violence and Male Power*. Buckingham: Open University Press.

Hester M, Pearson C, Harwin N. (1998) *Making an Impact: children and domestic violence*. Bristol: Department of Health, School for Policy Studies, University of Bristol, NSPCC, Barnardos.

Hillard P. (1985) Physical abuse in pregnancy. *Obstetrician and Gynaecologist*. **66**: 185–90.

Hoff L. (1990) *Battered Women as Survivors*. London: Routledge.

Home Office. (1995) *Interagency Circular*. London: Home Office.

Home Office. (1996) *British Crime Survey*. London: Home Office.

Home Office. (2008) *Break the Chain: multi-agency guidance for addressing domestic violence*. London: Home Office. Available at: www.crimereduction.homeoffice.gov.uk/dv/dv08.htm#2 (accessed 11 Mar 2009).

Horley S. (1991) *The Charm Syndrome: why charming men can make dangerous lovers*. London: PaperMac.

Hunt S, Martin A. (2001) *Pregnant Women, Violent Men: what midwives need to know*. Oxford: Books for Midwives Press.

Kirkwood C. (1993) *Leaving Abusive Partners*. London: Sage.

Lewis G, editor. (2007) *Saving Mothers' Lives: reviewing maternal deaths to make motherhood safer – 2004–2005*. The Seventh Report of the Confidential Enquiries into Maternal Deaths in the United Kingdom. Confidential Enquiry into Maternal and Child Health (CEMACH). London: CEMACH.

Lloyd A. (1995) *Doubly Deviant, Doubly Damned: society's treatment of violent women*. London: Penguin Books.

Martin S, English K, Andersen K. (1996) Violence and substance abuse among North Carolina pregnant women. *Am J Public Health*. **86**(7): 991–8.

McFarlane J, Parker B, Soeken K. (1996) Abuse during pregnancy: associations with maternal health and infant birthweight. *Nurs Res*. **45**(1): 27–41.

McWilliams M, McKieran J. (1993) *Bringing it Out into the Open*. Belfast: HMSO.

Mezey G, Bewley S. (1997) Domestic violence and pregnancy. *Br J Obstet Gynaecol*. **104**. 528–31.

Mirrlees–Black C. (1996) Domestic violence: findings from a new British crime survey self completion questionnaire. *Home Office Research Study 191*. London: Home Office.

Mooney J. (1993) *The Hidden Figures: the North London domestic violence survey*. Middlesex: Middlesex University Centre for Criminology.

Mullender A, Debbonaire T. (2000) *Child Protection and Domestic Violence*. Birmingham: Venture Press.

Povey D, editor. (2004) *Crime in England and Wales 2002/3: Supplementary Volume 1 – Homicide and gun crime*. London: Home Office.

Radford J. (1987) Policing male violence, policing women. In: Hanmer J, Maynard M, editors. *Women Violence and Social Control*. Basingstoke: Macmillan.

Royal College of Midwives. (2006) *Domestic Abuse in Pregnancy*. Position paper. London: Royal College of Midwives.

Salmon D, Baird K, Price S, *et al.* (2004) *Bristol Pregnancy and Domestic Violence Programme*. Bristol: University of the West of England.

Saltzman L. (1990) Battering during pregnancy: a role for physicians. *Atlanta Medicine*. **64**(3): 45–8.

Shumway J, O'Campo P, Gielen A, *et al.* (1999) Preterm labour, placental abruption, and premature rupture of membranes in relation to maternal violence or verbal abuse. *J Matern Fetal Med*. **8**(3): 76–80.

Stark E, Flitcraft A. (1996) *Women at Risk: domestic violence and women's health*. London: Sage.

Steene M. (2001) Personal communications. Research Fellow in Midwifery. Leeds: St James University Hospital; 3 May 2001.

Stenson K, Saarinen H, Heimer G, *et al.* (2001) Women's attitudes to being asked about exposure to violence. *Midwifery*. **17**: 2–10.

Walby S, Allen J. (2004) *Domestic Violence, Sexual Assault and Stalking: findings from the British crime survey*. London: Home Office Research, Development and Statistics Directorate.

Webster J, Chandler J, Battisutta D. (1996) Pregnancy outcomes and healthcare use: effects of abuse. *Am J Obstet Gynecol*. **174**: 760–4.

Women's Aid. (2008) *Statistics: domestic violence*. Available at: www.womensaid.org. (accessed 26 Dec 2008).

Wright S. (1995) The role of the police in combating domestic violence. In: Dobash RE, Dobash RP, Noaks L, editors. *Gender and Crime*. Cardiff: University of Wales Press.

CHAPTER 8

Female genital mutilation

Comfort Momoh

Female Genital Mutilation (FGM) is a violation of the rights of women and children. It denies women and children security, personal liberty and the right to health. This chapter discusses the historical and social context of FGM, types of FGM, why it is practised and its prevalence. The effect on women's physical, sexual and psychological health is discussed, as well as issues related to childbirth and the law. The power of older women, as key decision makers in perpetuating FGM, is a further point of focus. Child protection issues and what professionals should do when a child is at risk of FGM are addressed along with the role of the midwife as advocate and carer.

INTRODUCTION

> All societies have norms of care and behaviour based on age, life stages, sex, gender and social class. These 'norms', often referred to as traditional practices, originate either from social, or cultural objectives, or from empirical observations related to the well-being of individuals or the society. Traditional practices may be beneficial, harmful or harmless. Traditional practices may have a harmful effect on health and this is often the case in those relating to female children, relations between men and women, marriage and sexuality. (World Health Organization [WHO] 1997: 1)

Female Genital Mutilation (FGM), also known as Female Circumcision, is considered to be a violation of women and children's rights. A human rights perspective sets FGM in the context of women's social and economic powerlessness. FGM has no health benefit; it is a deeply rooted, cultural, traditional, and largely African practice, which affects the short- and long-term physical and psychological health of women and girls.

The practice of FGM dates as far back as fifth century BC (El Dareer 1983, Eke 2000) and today transcends all religious, racial and social boundaries (Webb 1995). FGM is supported by centuries of tradition, culture and false beliefs and is perpetuated by poverty, illiteracy, low status of women and inadequate healthcare facilities (Dorkenoo 1995, Allam, *et al.* 1999, Eke 2000).

It is estimated that more than 130 million girls and women worldwide have undergone FGM (WHO 1997); FGM is now a growing problem in Western countries due to the increasing number of immigrants and the practice has become an issue for health and social care practitioners who may be unfamiliar with the problem and its complexities. The influx of immigrants to the UK has presented challenges for midwives who must, therefore, develop knowledge and understanding of FGM.

Approximately 10 000 girls and young women are at risk of FGM in the UK and Boot (1994) is of the view that there are 3000–4000 new cases each year. In this country FGM is seen mainly among women from Somalia, Eritrea, Ethiopia, Sudan, Sierra Leone and the Yemen. In Britain, despite the Female Genital Mutilation Act (House of Commons 2003), women were still taking their children to other countries in the holidays for circumcision and it was impossible to prevent this happening since it was not illegal at that time.

The age at which FGM is performed depends on the country, tribe and circumstances, and varies from a few days old to adolescence, adulthood, just before marriage or after the first pregnancy. For example, Somalis tend to perform FGM on girls aged from four to nine years while the Ethiopian Fallashas perform the operation when the baby is a few days old (Ng 2000). In Eastern Ethiopia, the Adere and the Oromo groups carry out FGM from four years to puberty, while the Amhara perform FGM on the eighth day of birth (Missailidis and Gebre-Medhin 2000).

Due to lack of systematic data collection real numbers of affected women and girls with FGM are unknown. However, according to WHO (1997) the prevalence of FGM is still high in 28–30 countries in Africa (Table 8.1) and the Middle East; it can also be traced to Latin America, India, Malaysia and Indonesia and is estimated to range from 50–98% (Dorkenoo 1995, Toubia 1999).

TABLE 8.1 Estimated prevalence of FGM by country (Hosken 1993, Toubia 1995, WHO 1998)

Country	% of women affected	Number of women affected
Benin	50	1 365 000
Burkino Faso	70	3 656 800
Cameroon	20	1 336 800
Central African Republic	43	759 810
Chad	60	1 932 000
Djibouti	98	248 920
Egypt	97	27 905 930
Eritrea and Ethiopia	90	26 323 250
Gambia	80	396 800
Ghana	30	2 635 200
Guinea	60	1 999 800
Guinea Bissau	50	272 500

(cont.)

Country	% of women affected	Number of women affected
Ivory Coast	60	3 750 000
Kenya	50	6 967 5000
Liberia	60	902 400
Mali	99	5 155 900
Mauritania	25	295 250
Niger	20	921 200
Nigeria	40	25 601 200
Senegal	20	838 000
Sierra Leone	90	2 167 200
Somalia	98–100	5 034 260
Sudan	89	12 816 000
Tanzania	10	1 552 000
Togo	50	1 044 500
Uganda	5	513 050
Zaire	5	945 000

DEFINITION

The WHO (2008) defines FGM as, 'all procedures involving partial or total removal of the external female genitalia or other injury to the female genital organs whether for cultural or other non-therapeutic reasons'. The WHO also classified FGM into four types (Figures 8.1 and 8.2):

Type 1 – excision of the prepuce, with or without excision of part or all of the clitoris. When it is required to differentiate between the variations of type 1 FGM, the following subtypes are suggested: (WHO 2008)
- **Type 1a** – removal of the prepuce only
- **Type 1b** – removal of the prepuce and the clitoris

Type 2 – excision of the clitoris with partial or total excision of the labia minora
- **Type 2a** – removal of the labia minora only
- **Type 2b** – partial or total removal of the clitoris and the labia minora
- **Type 2c** – partial or total removal of the clitoris, the labia minora and the labia majora

Type 3 – excision of part or all the external genitalia and stitching/narrowing of the vaginal opening (also known as infibulation)

Type 4 – unclassified: this includes pricking, piercing or incising of the clitoris and/or labia, stretching of the clitoris and/or labia, cauterisation by burning of the clitoris and surrounding tissue.

FIGURE 8.1 WHO (1997) Classification of Female Genital Mutilation

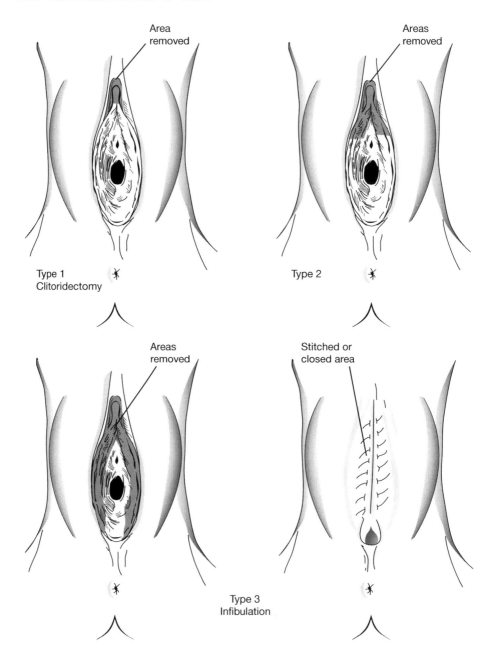

FIGURE 8.2 Some of the different types of female genital mutilation. (Reproduced from Momoh 2000)

Most procedures are irreversible and their effects last a lifetime (WHO 1997). Ten per cent of girls and women die from the short-term complications of FGM, for example, haemorrhage, shock and infection. Another 25% die in the long-term, as a result of recurrent urinary and vaginal infections and complications during childbirth, such as severe bleeding and obstructed labour; however, such tragedies do not occur here in Britain or in other Western countries.

FGM PROCEDURE

The procedure is sometimes carried out using crude tools and instruments such as razors, knives and scissors. Anaesthetics or antiseptics are not generally used; however, in urban areas FGM is being performed more frequently in hospitals by trained doctors and midwives. Girls may be circumcised alone or with a group of peers from their community (Dorkenoo 1995). With Type 3 excision or infibulation, elderly women, relatives and friends secure the girl in the lithotomy position. A deep incision is made rapidly on either side from the root of the clitoris to the fourchette. A single cut of the razor excises the clitoris, labia majora and minora. Bleeding is profuse but application of various poultices, threading of the edges of the skin with thorns, or clasping them between the edges of a split cane, usually controls it. A piece of twig is inserted between the edges of the skin to ensure a patent foramen for urinary and menstrual flow. The lower limbs are then bound together for two to six weeks to promote haemostasis and to encourage union of the two sides (McCaffrey, *et al.* 1995).

Healing takes place by primary intention and, as a result, except for a small hole, the introitus is obliterated by a drum of skin extending across the orifice (WHO 1996, Momoh 1999, Toubia 1999). Much, however, will depend on the circumstances at the time. The girl may struggle so vigorously that incisions may become uncontrolled and haphazard. The girl may be held so tightly that she suffers bone fractures.

This procedure still continues in some villages and rural areas in some African countries, but can be done in hospitals and cities with sterile equipment and under general or local anaesthesia to reduce the pain (Bridgehouse 1992, Baker, *et al.* 1993). However, having the procedure done in hospital makes no difference in terms of short- and long-term complications; it violates the injunction 'to do no harm' and is unethical by any standards (Eke 2000, WHO 2001).

CONSEQUENCES AND COMPLICATIONS OF FGM

Women who have had FGM present with very specific medical, gynaecological, obstetric and psychosexual problems, which doctors, midwives and/or other professionals are not usually trained to recognise or treat (Gordon 1998, Morris 1999), *see* Table 8.2.

TABLE 8.2 Complications of FGM

Immediate	Haemorrhage from the dorsal artery, shock, pain, retention of urine, and infection/tetanus that could lead to death
Intermediate and long-term	Cysts and abscesses, keloid scar formation, damage to the urethra resulting in urinary incontinence, dyspareunia, neuromata (trapped clitoral nerve), haematocolpos and sexual dysfunction

From Momoh (2005)

In most cases women do not link the problems they are experiencing to FGM because they have, in many instances, been told that pain is part of growing and is, therefore, normal. Such women accept problems as being part of the natural order of things (Cameron and Rawlings-Anderson 2001). Furthermore, it needs to be remembered that FGM, for many women, is a part of the struggle for everyday survival in areas of war and famine, where women are not well educated and there is a lack of healthcare provision (Scherf 2000).

FGM is unnecessary and is damaging to girls' and women's physical and emotional well-being. It can also have lifetime effects, such as psychological trauma and flashbacks. Girls are usually conscious when FGM is performed with no anaesthesia and it is not surprising that the experience lasts for a lifetime. This can lead to feelings of deep anger, fear, bitterness and betrayal at having been subjected to such pain (FORWARD 2000).

The effects of FGM on women and girls greatly depend on a number of factors: severity and type of FGM, competence of the person performing FGM, the un/sanitary conditions under which it is performed, 'cooperation' and health of the child at the time of FGM. The treatment or its complications may contribute to a wide range of psychological effects including chronic irritability, depression and anxiety, which may in some cases lead to suicide (Dorkenoo 1995, Allam, *et al.* 1999, Ciment 1999, Eke 2000, Weir 2000).

In relation to sexual and psychological problems, anxieties due to anticipation of pain at menarche, intercourse, childbirth and medical vaginal examination have also been reported (Lightfoot-Klein 1998). Rushwan (2000) reports that intercourse and conception may not be achieved in women with Type 3 FGM, as the tough fibrotic skin closing the vaginal introitus could hinder penetration. He also suggests that intercourse may take place in some women through the small opening (false vagina) and this may induce detrimental effects on women such as severe pain during intercourse, and infertility.

WHO (1996) and Gibeau (1998) believe that many women who have had FGM experience various degrees of sexual dysfunction, including the inability to achieve orgasm, as the clitoris is believed to be key to the normal functioning and mental and physical development of female sexuality. FGM interferes with sexual feelings and pleasure because the clitoris contains a large number of receptor nerve endings and its removal may affect the physical receptivity of sexual stimulation (Hopkins 1999). FGM may also result in damage to the concentrated nerve complex responsible for clitoral erection, pelvic muscular and secretory activity and the transmission of sensory information to the central nervous system (Bridgehouse 1992).

It is difficult to generalise about what form of sexual dysfunction occurs. Rawlings-Anderson and Cameron (2000) published a study of 97 circumcised Sudanese women and found that 90% of these women had experienced orgasm after FGM. However, many of these women said that orgasms were weak, infrequent or hard to achieve. Some women may also experience marital conflicts or disharmony due to some of the above sequelae (Wright 1996).

RATIONALES GIVEN FOR PERFORMING FGM

Historical background

The history of FGM is not well known but theories and suppositions date it as far back as the fifth century BC (Koso-Thomas 1987). Some believe it was practised in ancient Egypt as a sign of distinction amongst the aristocracy and affirm that trace evidence of infibulation can still be found on Egyptian mummies (Izett and Toubia 1999). Many believe that the practice evolved from early times in primitive communities desirous of establishing control over the sexual behaviour of women.

The concern over women's sexual and moral behaviour does not seem to have been confined to Africa, neither is the ingenuity to curb or conceal female sexuality displayed only on that continent (WHO 1996). The early Roman technique of slipping rings through the labia majora of their female slaves to prevent them becoming pregnant is an indication that FGM has been practised outside the African continent for a long time, (Bridgehouse 1992). The Scoptsi sect of Russia performed FGM to ensure virginity (Eke 2000).

History also traces FGM to the UK and USA and evidence suggests that it was performed in the nineteenth century by gynaecologists to cure so-called 'female weaknesses' such as nymphomania, aberrant behaviour such as reaching orgasm, insanity, masturbation, hysteria, epilepsy and other female disorders (Koso-Thomas 1987, Eke 2000).

Explanations for FGM are complex, multifactorial, interrelated, and woven into beliefs and values that communities uphold; hence it is extremely difficult to isolate why the practice occurs (Rahman and Toubia 2000). Reasons can be classified as follows: myths, social pressure, religious teaching, sex, hygiene and tradition/culture. It is important to realise that parents and/or relatives do not decide to circumcise their daughters with malicious intent, but see it as an act of love and part of their culture, and consider it neither unethical nor immoral (Momoh 1999, Toubia 1999).

Socio-cultural reasons for FGM

FGM has formed part of the cultural identity of many groups; it is embedded in social values, beliefs and culturally defined norms and is linked to strongly held ideas about identity, sexuality, gender and power (Rahman and Toubia 2000). FGM may be seen as an act of love to be celebrated with ceremonial events and embraced with excitement and anticipation. It may be seen as a rite of passage to womanhood ensuring that daughters, as virgins, are marriage worthy and virtuous (Momoh 2000).

Traditionally, women who have undergone the procedure are said to be highly regarded within practising societies, since the belief is that unless a girl is circumcised, she will not become a mature woman and will lose the right to marry and bear children commensurate with others of her age group and her ancestors. This fear of social ostracism and being considered deviant in the community is a powerful motivator that ensures the continuation of the practice.

Peers and family reject girls who are not circumcised, which is disastrous since they have no means of security or support (Gibeau 1998, Momoh 1999). Furthermore, in some societies, circumcision is not only positively reinforced through the social benefits described above, but also negatively reinforced. For example, within certain groups, the greatest insult is to be referred to as 'son of an uncircumcised woman' (Lightfoot-Klein 1989).

Wright (1996) and FORWARD (2000) argue that for women living in a patriarchal society with no land, no education and no effective power base, marriage is their main means of survival and access to resources. In this context one can understand why FGM continues. WHO (1996) also argues that social reasons for FGM are centred on the dominant role of the male within the family and society, as men in most African countries are the head of the family.

Interestingly, Savane (1984) complicates the picture further by describing how university-educated women occupying administrative posts are still victims of traditional models of behaviour. She suggests that they are pulled each way by the traditional and the modern in that they aspire to the freer Western philosophies but also need the traditional structures and roles, which offer psychological security. It may be argued that even if they felt they needed the 'traditional structures and roles', it would be reasonable to assume that they would also be subjected to strong peer and family pressure to conform.

It is always very difficult to be the first to deviate from the norm; however, Missailidis and Gebre-Medhin (2000) paint a conflicting picture. In their study of three ethnic groups in Eastern Ethiopia, they found that some women felt that it made little difference to a man whether a woman was circumcised or not, as long as she was a virgin. Other women felt that men did prefer circumcised women. It seems here that society acts as a mechanism supporting the roles of men and women in a vicious circle that perpetuates FGM.

Religion

FGM is not associated with any one religion. Some practising communities make claim to its existence in the Koran or the Hadith but it predates Islam (Gibeau 1998). Although FGM is not cited in the Koran, Muslim principles are derived not only from the Koran but also from the anthology of 'Sunna' – a term that represents words and actions attributed to the Prophet Mohammed. It is within Sunna that one finds opinion regarding FGM. Despite this, leading Islamic theologians refute the argument that the practice is based on religious doctrine (Khaled and Vause 1996).

There is evidence that Jews, Christians, Muslims and indigenous religious groups practice FGM in Africa. However, despite the fact that FGM is not known in a lot of Muslim countries, for example, Saudi Arabia, which is the locus of Islam (Wright 1996), it is strongly identified with Islam in several African nations. Furthermore, many members of the Muslim community believe that it is a religious obligation as it ensures 'spiritual purity' (Bridgehouse 1992). It may be then that religion here is being used to legitimise FGM as a means of female social control (Lightfoot-Klein 1989, Brooks 1995).

Sexual reasons

There are many strange, and often inaccurate, reasons given for the perpetuation of FGM. Some believe that FGM reduces sexual desire and, therefore, preserves virginity or that the uncut clitoris will grow big and pressure on this organ will arouse intense desire (WHO 2001). Uncircumcised girls are perceived to have an overactive and uncontrollable sex drive, which will lead to the premature loss of their virginity and this will bring disgrace to her family and damage her chances of marriage. Some nomadic tribes circumcise their daughters to prevent them from being raped in the desert while they are left alone to care for the animals.

Some socio-political theories state that FGM is perpetuated to oppress women and girls and control their sexuality (Lightfoot-Klein and Shaw 1990, Boot 1994, Khaled and Vause 1996, WHO 1996). It is likely that FGM (as well as the use of chastity belts or the closing of the external organs with steel pins or iron tacks) is undertaken in order to control female sexuality and to cause women to be more submissive to moral, social, legal and religious constraints, especially the constraints of monogamy. Only by restricting female sexuality can the man be sure that the children are his own (El Saadawi 1980).

A narrow vaginal opening is believed by both Somalis and Sudanese to heighten male sexual pleasure. Unfortunately, following marriage, penetration can take up to three months to achieve and, in some cases, opening up is necessary before intercourse can take place. However, Shandall (1967, cited in Dorkenoo 1995) surveyed 300 Sudanese husbands who had one infibulated wife and one non-infibulated wife; 266 of the husbands stated categorically that they preferred non-excised or Sunna-circumcised women, sexually.

El Saadawi (1980) adds that men are not alone in promoting FGM to protect their economy and that of the family. There are many traditional birth attendants, nurses, paramedical staff, doctors, midwives and laywomen who make their living from FGM. They may derive much social standing and status within their community because they are upholding traditional, cultural practices, which are seen as vital in maintaining the social fabric of groups who may perceive themselves to be under threat from Western ideals.

Myths

Mythical reasons for FGM include the promotion of fertility, the notion that the clitoris poses danger and will grow and harm the baby, and the idea that FGM assists in the health and survival of the child. Protagonists argue that, like male circumcision, FGM promotes cleanliness but there is no supporting evidence for this argument (Koso-Thomas 1987). In Sierra Leone, women were interviewed who believed the clitoris to be a source of disease and that failure to excise it would result in infertility (WHO 1996). Village communities will testify to the validity of such assumptions.

Custom and power

In many countries, FGM is an accepted and expected part of their custom and for many women FGM is a fact of life, a pain that must be borne because they must conform to social expectation in order to survive. Toubia (1999) considers that traditional values and methods of relating to each other in many African cultures are hierarchical and therefore favour respect for authority figures and elders. Because of this social power and hierarchy most women do not question FGM.

Women have been socially conditioned to accept FGM within social definitions of womanhood and identity and this encourages older women to perpetuate the practice; they play a strong role in FGM and its continuation because in most cases they are the key decision-makers. They see it as an important component in the socialisation process of girls into the social, familial, sexual and reproductive roles of women and they strongly oppose sex before marriage. They believe that circumcision increases the chances of achieving a favourable marriage and the family's chances of obtaining a high price for the bride (Dorkenoo 1995). The concept of marriage in most cultures where FGM is practised is viewed as security for life for the woman and her family.

Older women often see FGM as a very beneficial custom and an integral part of the social and cultural heritage with the community. The degree of power held by older women within practising societies enables them to reinforce and pass on cultural norms from one generation to the next. They have the ability to influence members of the social network and even override other decision-makers. They are the custodians of family traditions and an authoritative influence. FGM gives them the chance to exercise real command in a patriarchal culture, where before they were powerless and, as such, could be seen to be unwittingly colluding with their own oppression.

For older women to accept that FGM is a harmful practice means having to psychologically face the fact that their mother/grandmother did something harmful to them and this may cause a fragmentation of their psyche. There is also the fear of leaving their daughters uncircumcised, as this may lead to social ostracism from the tribe or clan upon which they rely for their food, shelter and well-being. The communities, and especially the female elders, therefore, see FGM as an act of love and a rite of passage to womanhood. FGM is not seen as violation of human rights or child abuse, as perceived by the Western world.

FGM: THE LEGAL POSITION

Is has been the goal of many governments throughout the world, including those in Africa, to eradicate the practice of FGM. Strategies to accomplish this have included awareness raising, education, incentives to discourage practitioners, and laws making FGM illegal. African nations include Benin, Burkina Faso, Central African Republic, Chad, Ivory Coast, Djibouti, Eritrea, Ethiopia, Ghana, Guinea, Kenya, Niger, Senegal, South Africa, Tanzania, and Togo; they have enacted laws and introduced penalties that include fines and varying terms of imprisonment. Industrialised nations (Australia, Belgium, Canada, Cyprus, Denmark, Italy, New Zealand, Norway, Spain, Sweden, United Kingdom, and United States) have introduced legislation in the light of rising immigration of people from countries that still practice FGM. Legislation has been deemed necessary to support the commonly held view that FGM is a violation of universally recognised human rights, which include the right to integrity of the person and the highest attainable level of physical and mental health (WHO 1997, Chelala 1998, Ciment 1999).

In 2000, the All Party Parliamentary Group on Population, Development and Reproductive Health aimed to raise awareness of FGM in the UK and abroad and to generate support for a prevention and eradication programme (Kmietowicz 2000). Some recommendations made following the hearing were that:

- the UK Government should undertake a full assessment of local authority provision and guidance of FGM, particularly with reference to child protection
- the UK law be amended to ensure that UK residents who take girls abroad to have them circumcised can be prosecuted under the UK law on their return, regardless of the status of FGM in the country where the circumcision takes place
- funds should be available for non-government organisations and for research into the prevalence of FGM in Britain
- it should be a legal requirement for health professionals and other relevant authorities to report all incidents of FGM
- the Act should be publicised in a media campaign.

Whilst FGM has been illegal in the UK since 1985, a loophole – whereby people were taking their daughters abroad to undergo FGM – was not closed until 2004 with passage of the Female Genital Mutilation Act that reinforced previous legislation. The UK Government also funded an information campaign amongst practising communities, and those breaking the law now face up to 14 years in jail whereas previously maximum sentence was 5 years. In 2001, a general practitioner was struck off the General Medical Council register for agreeing to perform FGM (Dyer 2001) but prosecution has proved difficult and rates are very disappointing.

NATIONAL POLICY

The UK Government's Every Child Matters: Change for Children Programme (which includes the National Service Framework for Children, Young People and Maternity Services [Department of Health 2004], and is supported by the Children Act), requires all agencies to take responsibility for safeguarding and promoting the welfare of every child to enable them to be healthy, stay safe. Many professional bodies in the UK have now created, or are in the process of creating, guidelines on FGM. The Royal College of Midwives (1998) published a position paper on FGM, the British Medical Association (2001) has revised its guidelines, and the latest guidelines from the Royal College of Obstetricians and Gynaecologists were published in 2003.

THE MIDWIFE'S ROLE

Midwives need to have better knowledge, effective communication, and understanding of the cultural factors influencing FGM in order to understand the reasons for its occurrence and provide insightful support for women and girls. Midwives should be advocates for women and girls and possess up-to-date clinical expertise in order to help these women give birth (McCaffrey, *et al.* 1995, Momoh 2000, Chalmers and Kowser 2000). Counselling can be provided and women given the option of defibulation where the aim is to restore normal anatomy as far as possible. Dunkley (2000) suggests that strategies to ensure that all members of society have an equal right to health and health-care may seem utopian, but continued efforts toward meeting this standard should be adopted and remain high on the agendas of health professionals.

CONCLUSION

As midwives are now caring for many pregnant refugees and immigrant women who are circumcised and from different socio-cultural backgrounds, they need to be aware of issues relating to FGM in the UK. The African Well Woman Clinic is an excellent example of how the needs of the community have been addressed. As we now live in a multicultural society, FGM is becoming increasingly challenging for midwives and this requires great sensitivity and awareness. A sensitive and caring approach by midwives is essential in order to gain the trust of women so that they will seek help if and when required. This, in turn, should open up opportunities for midwives to empower the women with the education, advice and support they require in order to help them give birth and, hopefully, assist in the abolition of an age-old harmful practice. Working within policies and FGM framework is essential for all professionals, as we all have a statutory responsibility to safeguard children from being abused through FGM.

KEY POINTS

- ∽ FGM is a deeply rooted cultural practice and a violation of human rights.
- ∽ FGM continues to be a major problem in the UK despite laws prohibiting the practice.
- ∽ FGM has no health or medical benefit for women and girls.
- ∽ Midwives need to gain knowledge and understanding of FGM in order to act as advocates and carers.

USEFUL ADDRESSES

The African Well Woman's Clinic
St Thomas' Hospital Trust
C/o Admin Office
10th Floor North-Wing
London SE1 7EH
Tel: 0207 188 6872/0795 654 2576
Pager: 087 0055 5500 (code 881018)
Email: cmomoh@hotmail.com or comfort.momoh@hotmail.com

African Well Woman's Health Clinic
Whittington Hospital
Level 5 Highgate Hill
London N19 5NF
Tel: 0207 288 3482

Multicultural Antenatal Clinic
Liverpool Women's Hospital
Crown Street
Liverpool L8 7SS

Birmingham Heartlands Hospital
Princess of Wales Women's Unit
Labour Ward, Bordesley Green East
Birmingham
Tel: 0121 424 3514
Contact: Alison Hughes or Teresa Ball

African Well Woman's Clinic
Antenatal Clinic
Central Middlesex Hospital
Acton Lane, Park Royal
London NW10 7NS
Tel: 0208 965 5733

African Women's Clinic
The Elizabeth Garret Anderson and Obstetric Hospital
Huntley Street
London WC1E 6DH
Tel: 0207 380 9773
Email: egappts@uclh.nhs.uk

African Well Woman's Clinic
Northwick Park and St Marks Hospitals
Watford Road
Harrow
Middlesex HA1 3UJ
Tel: 0208 869 2880

Black Women's Health and Family Support
82 Russell Lane
Bethnal Green
London E2 9LU
Tel: 0208 980 3503

Foundation for Women's Health
Research & Development (FORWARD)
765–767 Harrow Road
London NW10 5NY
Tel: 0208 960 4000

Midlands Refugee Council
5th Floor
Smithfield House
Digbeth B5 6BS
Tel: 0121 242 2200

Agency for Culture and Change Management
The Old Coroners Court
14–38 Nursery Street
Sheffield S3 8GG
Tel: 0114 275 0193/0123 435 6910
Email: info@accmsheffield.org

Rainbo
Queens Studios
121 Salisbury Road
London NW6 6RG
Tel 0207 625 3400

WoMan Being Concern International
31 Ispden House
Windmill Walk
London SE1 8LU
Contact: Dr Rahmat Mohammed
Tel: 0777 594 4805

REFERENCES

Allam MF, de Irala-Estevez J, Navajas RF, *et al.* (1999) Student's knowledge of and attitudes about female circumcision in Egypt. *N Engl J Med.* **341**: 1552–3.

Baker CA, Gilson GJ, Vill MD, *et al.* (1993) Female circumcision: obstetric issues. *Am J Obstet Gynecol.* **169**: 1616–8.

Boot J. (1994) *Female Genital Mutilation.* London: Borough of Waltham Forest.

Bridgehouse R. (1992) Ritual female circumcision and its effects on female sexual function. *Can J Hum Sexuality.* **1**: 3–10.

British Medical Association. (2001) *Female Genital Mutilation: caring for patient and child protection.* London: BMA.

Brooks G. (1995) *The verses.* Manchester: Guardian Weekend; 11 March 1995; pp. 12–19.

Cameron J, Rawlings-Anderson K. (2001) Genital mutilation: human rights and cultural imperialism. *Br J Midwif.* **9**(4): 231–5.

Chalmers B, Kowser OH. (2000) 432 Somali women's birth experiences in Canada after earlier female genital mutilation. *Birth.* **27**(4): 227–34.

Chelala C. (1998) An alternative way to stop female genital mutilation. *Lancet.* **352**: 126.

Ciment J. (1999) Senegal outlaws female genital mutilation. *BMJ.* **318**(7180): 348.

Dorkenoo E. (1995) *Cutting the Rose: Female Genital Mutilation: the practice and its prevention.* London: Minority Rights Publications.

Dunkley J. (2000) *Health Promotion in Midwifery Practice: a resource for health professionals.* London: Balliere Tindall.

Dyer O. (2001) GP struck off for agreeing to perform female circumcision. *BMJ.* **322**(7277): 9.

Eke N. (2000) Female genital mutilation: what can be done? *Lancet.* **356**(Suppl.): S57.

El Dareer A. (1983) Epidemiology of female circumcision in the Sudan. *Trop Doct.* **13**: 41–5.

El Saadawi N. (1980) *The Hidden Face of Eve.* London: Zed Press.

FORWARD. (2000) *Female Genital Mutilation Fact Sheet.* London: FORWARD. Available at: www. forwarduk.org.uk/download/11 (accessed 27 Dec 2008).

Gibeau AM. (1998) Female genital mutilation: when a cultural practice generates clinical and ethical dilemmas. *J Obstet Gynecol Neonat Nurs.* **27**(1): 85–91.

Gordon H. (1998) Female genital mutilation: female circumcision. *The Diplomate.* **5**(2): 86–90.

Hopkins S. (1999) A discussion of the legal aspects of female genital mutilation. *J Adv Nurs.* **30**(4): 926–33.

Hosken FP. (1993) *The Hosken Report: genital and sexual mutilation of females.* Revised ed. Lexington, MA: Women's International Network News.

House of Commons. (1985) *Prohibition of Female Circumcision Act.* London: HMSO; Chapter 33: 217.

Izett S, Toubia N. (1999) *A Research and Evaluation Guidebook Using Female Circumcision as a Case Study: learning about social changes.* New York: Rainbo.

Khaled K, Vause S. (1996) Genital mutilation: a continued abuse. *Br J Obstet Gynaecol.* **103**: 86–7.

Kmietowicz Z. (2000) MPs recommend tightening the law on female circumcision. *BMJ.* **321**(7273): 1365.

Koso-Thomas O. (1987) *The Circumcision of Women: a strategy for eradication.* London: Zed Press.

Lightfoot-Klein H, Shaw E. (1990) Special needs of ritually circumcised women patients. *J Obstet Gynecol Neonatal Nurs.* **20**:(2): 102–7.

Lightfoot-Klein H. (1989) *Prisoners of Ritual: an odyssey into female genital mutilation in Africa.* New York: The Haworth Press.

Lightfoot-Klein H. (1998) The sexual experience and marital adjustment of circumcised and infibulated females in the Sudan. *J Sex Reprod.* **26**(3): 375–92.

McCaffrey M, Jankowska A, Gordon H. (1995) Management of female genital mutilation: Northwick Park Hospital experience. *Br J Obstet Gynaecol.* **102**(10): 787–90.

Missailidis K, Gebre-Medhin M. (2000) Female genital mutilation declines in eastern Ethiopia. *Lancet.* **356**: 137–8.

Momoh C. (1999) Female genital mutilation: the struggle continues. *Pract Nurs.* **10**(2): 31–3.

Momoh C. (2000) *Female Genital Mutilation: information for healthcare professionals.* London: King's Fund.

Momoh C. (2005) *Female Genital Mutilation.* Oxford: Radcliffe Publishing.

Morris R. (1999) Female genital mutilation: perspectives risks and complications. *Urol Nurs.* **19**(1): 13–19.

Department of Health. (2004) *National Service Framework for Children, Young People and Maternity Services.* London: Department of Health. www.dh.gov.uk/PolicyAndGuidance/HealthAndSocialCareTopics/ChildrenServices/ChildrenServicesInformation/fs/en (accessed 27 Dec 2008).

Ng F. (2000) Female genital mutilation: its implication for reproductive health: an overview. *Brit J Fam Plan.* **26**(1): 47–51.

Rahman A, Toubia N. (2000) *Female Genital Mutilation: a guide to laws and policies.* London: Worldwide Zed Books.

Rawlings-Anderson K, Cameron J. (2000) Female genital mutilation: a global perspective. *Br J Midwifery.* **8**(12): 754–60.

Royal College of Midwives. (1998) *Female Genital Mutilation (Female Circumcision) Position Paper 21.* London: RCM. Available at: www.rcm.org.uk (accessed 6 Mar 2009).

Royal College of Obstetricians and Gynaecologists. (2003) *Female Genital Mutilation Statement No.3.* London: RCOG. Available at: www.rcog.org.uk (accessed 6 Mar 2009).

Rushwan H. (2000) Female genital mutilation: management during pregnancy, childbirth and the postpartum period. *Int J Obstet.* **70**: 99–104.

Savane MA. (1984) Elegance amid the phallocracy. In: Morgan R, editor. *Sisterhood is Global.* Harmondsworth: Penguin.

Scherf C. (2000) Ending genital mutilation: women in Africa have many other problems besides genital mutilation. *BMJ.* **321**(7260): 570–1.

Toubia N. (1995) *Female Genital Mutilation: a call for global action.* New York: Rainbo.

Toubia N. (1999) *A Technical Manual for Healthcare Providers Caring for Women with Circumcision.* New York: Rainbo.

Webb E. (1995) Cultural knowledge is the key to understanding. *BMJ.* **70**: 441–4.

Weir E. (2000) Female genital mutilation. *CMAJ.* **162**(9): 1344–5.

World Health Organization. (1996) *Female Genital Mutilation: a report of WHO technical working group.* Geneva: World Health Organization.

World Health Organization. (1997) *FGM: a joint WHO/UNICEF/UNFPA statement.* Geneva: World Health Organization.

World Health Organization. (1998) *Female Genital Mutilation: an overview.* Geneva: World Health Organization.

World Health Organization. (2001) *A Teacher's Guide.* Geneva: World Health Organization.

World Health Organization. (2008) *Eliminating Female Genital Mutilation: an interagency statement.* Geneva: World Health Organization.

Wright J. (1996) Female genital mutilation: an overview. *J Adv Nurs.* **24**: 251–9.

CHAPTER 9

Transition to motherhood

Nicola Winson

This chapter compares some definitions of motherhood, but focuses on the transition to the state of motherhood. Three theorists have described the process from different perspectives at different times so that a behaviourist model and a social model of feelings involved in the process can be presented. The experience of giving birth is thought to influence a woman's transition to the state of motherhood. Postnatal events, mood and personality type can influence the woman's adaptation to the state, as (it is thought) can her age, although this is not yet proven in the literature. Finally, the need for social change, as a means of facilitating acceptance of the status of mother, is explored.

INTRODUCTION

Childbirth is portrayed in the media as a happy and joyous event (Paradice 1995, Gibson 2001), and society maintains and feeds the myth that mothering is both easy and natural. These sentiments do not reflect the enormous psychological adjustment that a woman undergoes to make it appear easy and natural. She has completed a complex and demanding task (Paradice 1995). She has possibly been financially independent, professionally competent, socially in demand and emotionally balanced with broad horizons, and she may now change into someone who is physically tired (Larkin and Butler 2000), scarred, bruised (Ockenden 2000), nervous, socially isolated, intellectually under-stimulated, unable to participate rationally in or digest a discussion, financially dependent, professionally non-existent, emotionally labile and hypersensitive.

The processes that occur during this transition are poorly understood, but some research has been done. This chapter will sample the antenatal literature that considers women's views about their future role change during pregnancy. The work of three major theorists will be examined as they state how these changes in role identification occur.

The birthing experience is also a major influence on the transition to motherhood; in the recent past it has been regarded as less traumatic only because women now rarely die from it. Recent research demonstrates that birthing is mentally traumatic and possibly injurious both to the transition to motherhood and to the woman's mental health. Postnatally, a woman's mental health is valued less than her caring for the baby. This chapter will examine some postnatal issues, including role conflict and the effects that occur when the transition to motherhood appears to be incomplete. As the average age at which women are having children is rising, the transition to motherhood among older women will also be addressed. This social phenomenon is not the only one referred to here. Society's expectations of women, the influence of the media on women, and the control of women by society are subtle issues that will thread through this chapter.

WHY STUDY THE TRANSITION PROCESS?

Why study the transition process at all when it is viewed by the media as easy and as a normal stage in family development (Morse, *et al*. 2000)? The literature answers this question by revealing that for some it is a serious challenge or even a crisis (Underdown 1998, Morse, *et al*. 2000). Becoming a parent involves labour-intensive activity that absorbs enormous amounts of time, energy and effort almost continuously every day of the week for up to two decades (Fedele, *et al*. 1988), and it has a psychological, physiological and relational impact, which will test the resources of each individual in a partnership (Goldberg 1988). It seems that the 'normative' transition has very extensive and profound dimensions.

Rubin (1984) looked at areas of the transition process where nurses could provide help. She did this because it had been established that should the mother not make the transition, it would be noticed and she would be considered an inadequate mother. No definition of inadequate or its consequences was offered. As little help with this transition seems to be available in society, clearly there is a need for healthcare professionals and midwives to understand it.

Millar (2002) suggested that there is a gap or even a gulf between social expectations and reality. Culture, as represented in part by the newspapers, tells surprising stories. The volume of personal stories that appear at least weekly in each journal is significant. 'She once confessed to being terrified of becoming a parent . . . but yesterday any fear had vanished as *Big Brother* presenter Davina McCall described her joy at becoming a mother for the first time' (Bonnici 2001). It seems that the transition to motherhood has taken place, but why do so many personal testimonies of it appear? If it is easy and normal, why should it be reported? If it is a trouble-free process, why should people write about it? The article quoted suggests that the public need to be told that the process of becoming a parent can be achieved by celebrities (i.e. people whom the rest of the population may regard as role models). The picture is very glamorous, suggesting the subtle message that the transition to motherhood is easy, natural and does not detract from one's public or personal appeal. This is a different idea to that offered above by Morse, *et al*. (2000).

SOME DEFINITIONS

Transition is defined as the process of changing from one state to another (Rooney 1999). Life is full of change – from baby to infant to child to adolescent to parent to old person. Most of these stages are marked culturally by events, celebrations and certain rituals, even if only birthday parties. They are considered to be achievements.

Vehviläinen-Julkunen (1995) described transitions as forming an integral part of human development. Profound change with dramatic effects on the lives of significant others and major significance for health and welfare, are other aspects of the definition of transition.

The dictionary definition (Rooney 1999) of a *mother* as producing young emphasises her role as a parent, originator and protector. On chicken farms, the apparatus used for generating warmth so that eggs can be hatched and chicks reared without a hen is called a mother! The characteristic that is required in order to mother is the ability to give physical warmth so that the development occurs. Perhaps this lighthearted view has hidden depth if warmth is defined as having physical, psychological, social and emotional aspects. Schmied and Lupton (2001) consider that breastfeeding forms a major part of the definition of motherhood, and that it is central to women's experience of motherhood. Some women have portrayed breastfeeding as a crucial part of maternal identity and as being representative of good mothering. However, this perspective is not universally shared. The idea of including breastfeeding in the definition of motherhood will seem strange and inaccurate, if not oppressive, to some people. The debate about breastfeeding involving more than merely ensuring the physical survival of the infant is beyond the scope of this chapter. It could be argued that breastfeeding focuses the woman's mind more acutely on the issues and transitional processes that she is undergoing, but to suggest that it is integral to the concept of motherhood when the processes involved in the transition to motherhood are still poorly understood or researched, would seem presumptuous.

Chick and Meleis (1986, cited in Pridham and Chang 1992), define the *transition to motherhood* as a process of personal and interpersonal change that occurs as a woman assumes maternal tasks and appraises herself as a mother. Pridham and Chang (1992) point out that the previous definitions have been limited to problem solving with regard to infant care and parenting issues, and mothers have focused on assessment of their problem-solving competence, their relationship with the infant, and their attention to the infant's development and individual characteristics. This definition relates to behaviour rather than to psychological attitudes, mental processes, emotional development or change. It moves current thinking beyond psychomotor skills and towards the psychological, but it still lacks information about the processes and strength of feeling that are associated with motherhood.

MATERNAL PERCEPTIONS OF THE FETUS BEFORE BIRTH

Before discussing the major theorists' research on the transition process undergone by the mother during pregnancy, it is useful to consider other aspects of this transition. For example, does the ultrasound scan (USS) affect attachment? How does it affect the psychological processes of transition? During early pregnancy, few women are aware of more than the fact that they are feeling very sick and tired. The fetus is not a person for whom they want to care. Before USS was available, the fetus became a person only when their movements could be felt (quickening). At that point, realisation of the reality of motherhood dawned. Ram and Lerman (1993) wanted to determine whether this realisation (which they referred to as maternal-fetal attachment in the psychological sense rather than the physiological one) is affected by the early USS. From the sample of 139 women who completed questionnaires, it was found that the early USS before or after quickening made no difference to the maternal–fetal attachment.

Verny (1988) wrote extensively about the fetal life and what the fetus remembers. He stated that interactions between the parents and the unborn child have consequences for personality development of the child. Verny (1988) quotes research by DeCasper, who demonstrated that fetuses recognise their own mother's voice, or pieces of music that are played during uterine life.

Sorenson and Schuelke (1999) wanted to know how women fantasised about their unborn child, and whether these fantasies differed accordingly to gestational age and multiparity. A total of 184 completed questionnaires (to the open-ended question that was asked) were returned. Some women wrote full-page descriptions. No definitive pattern emerged from the study to indicate normality or abnormality. The researchers decided that the only aspect of note was that women had started the process of transition to motherhood. When these fantasies start, and what they mean with regard to women's psychological transition to the role of mother, is still unknown.

MAJOR THEORIES

Three theories will be discussed here. Van Gennep (1960) considered transition to be a rite of passage, and proposed a simple model. Reva Rubin (1967a) conducted qualitative research into certain behaviours and the mental processes underpinning them. Rogan, *et al.* (1997) investigated the transition to motherhood with focus groups using a grounded theory approach, and they developed a model describing 'change', which has much in common with the models proposed by Rubin (1967a) and Van Gennep (1960).

Van Gennep (1960) describes how a woman exchanges one social status for another. The value of each social status will be debated later in the chapter. The woman starts as an independent person, so the first phase of the process involves separation from her former social status. She is viewed by society as different. The next phase is marginality, when the woman is between socially recognised states. This phase occurs during pregnancy. The woman starts to look different and to behave differently (perhaps with regard to her diet, alcohol consumption, energy levels and sporting activities). The third stage is that of reincorporation of the woman back into society with an altered social status. She is now a mother and has different responsibilities and priorities. Previously, society regarded her as a wife or as a single person, but after the process of transition she is seen as neither of these. Society recognises that her responsibilities have changed, and now changes its view of her value in terms of whether she is employable, intelligent or dependent.

Van Gennep's (1960) 'marginality' phase is considered by Western society to be indicative of sexual activity, and as such has great curiosity value and is even a cause of envy for some people. In some societies pregnancy is regarded as shameful and defiling because it demonstrates that the woman has been sexually active. These contrasting views are dependent on the social values of the culture in which they live. In one culture, men may regard women as available (or as having been so if they are pregnant) to gratify their sexual drive, whereas in another culture men may regard the sexual drive in women (as demonstrated by pregnancy) as something that needs to be guarded against because it might lead to all kinds of undesirable behaviour. It could be said that men have a poor understanding of women's sexuality, and that therefore the idea of women having a libido can be frightening. In order to control this sexual drive and avoid possibly inexplicable behaviour, men in some cultures try to suppress it or even demonise it. This attitude may be manifested by the practice of female genital mutilation to make women submissive and controllable.

Rubin (1967a) followed five primiparous and four multiparous women through their pregnancies and the first month after birth. She interviewed them on average 12 times during pregnancy and 11 times during the first month after birth, so that the process of transition could be analysed in depth. Three main topic areas emerged, namely, the 'taking in' process, the self-system, and operations.

The 'taking in' process (Rubin 1967b) is a description of how earnestly and sensitively the woman tries to understand the meaning of becoming a mother. Nothing – be it her husband's job, her sister's wedding or medical opinion – is considered relevant to her unless she can link it in some way to her maternal role. The self-system theory suggests concern for the body image, the self-image and the ideal image. The ideal image is not so much concerned with morals but with the capacity to suffer/endure out of love for another, with gifts and giving, and so on. The self-image sees self as 'here and now' rather than in relation to the previous experiences that constituted the self-image. The body image theory focuses not on the physical changes but on the body's ability to accommodate and function. Self-esteem and role achievement or failure are linked

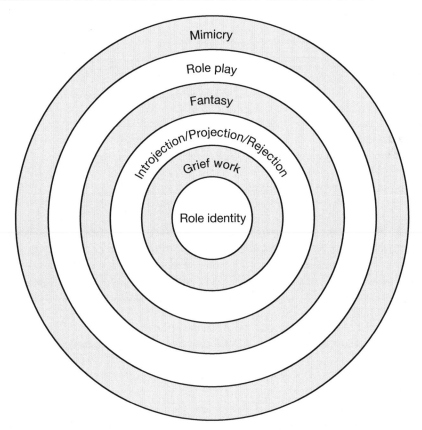

FIGURE 9.1 Operational level from superficial to deep psychological change (Rubin, 1967b)

to this ability. 'Operations' are the active processes. There are five operational levels, which from the outside inward are mimicry, role play, fantasy, introjection/projection and grief work (*see* Figure 9.1). Finally, after all of these processes have been worked through, role identity is achieved.

Mimicry is the adoption of simple behaviours, from dressing the part to following a myriad of taboos on lifting, eating, buying, and so on. Thus one sees women who have only just become pregnant wearing a maternity dress or bending backwards to see what it feels like before they have to. Role play is less symbolic and more concerned with 'acting out' situations and new role relationships. The woman searches for a young child with whom to establish a friendship, to help, to play 'hide and seek', to babysit, or even to feed. In a given situation, fantasy is concerned with the question 'how will it be for me?' The woman asks other mothers what their labour pains were like; what they really want to know is whether they will be able to cope or whether they will humiliate them-selves by shouting or swearing. Wishes, fears and dreams indicate a deeper involvement in the forthcoming role. Information is gathered in relation to the fantasies. There may be negative fantasies as well as positive ones, and silences, loneliness and darkness may exacerbate these fantasies.

Introjection/projection/rejection refers to the manner in which the mimicry and role playing are internalised to see whether they 'fit' the woman's personality and experience. This is the most important aspect of the model. The woman has been pre-tending to change nappies according to the way her friends do it. At this stage she must decide for herself whether she will do things the same way. She may reject the way her friend changes nappies because she feels that disposable nappies are environmentally unfriendly. Her experience and personal philosophy have been applied to the mimicry she has been practising. If she decides to follow her role model's way of changing nappies, and considers that her friend's barrier cream is the most effective type available, then the mimicry and role play are reinforced. Some issues may be talked through in face-to-face conversations with a role model, but the final decision is made silently. When these decisions have been made, the woman can be said to have identified with the role that she had previously been mimicking. She no longer thinks that motherhood is something that happens to other people, but rather that it is something which is going to happen to her, and she will use the present and future tense when speaking about herself.

Grief work involves 'letting go' of former identity. It is a review of previous attach-ments and associated events in the former role. Relying on work colleagues as friends, and going to the pub at lunchtime, need to stop and be grieved for because they are no longer compatible with the woman's new role. Although it is not final, some degree of resolution of the two lifestyles (i.e. that of a paid worker and that of a mother) occurs, and if it does not, there is a marked depression in role taking.

Rubin then discusses the relationship of significant others (e.g. partner and par-ents) to the above processes. All of the study subjects began the process by using their own mothers as models. Their peers then replaced them. Fantasies were experienced in relation to significant others at home. Husbands and partners were regarded as just that – husbands and partners – rather than as fathers. They were sometimes used not as a reference, but as a support or reinforcement.

A new theory has recently been described by Rogan, *et al.* (1997) on the basis of research conducted by Barclay, *et al.* (1997). They used nine antenatal focus groups with a total of 55 women to discuss the experience of becoming a mother. They concentrated on the process and after coding and categorising, they described six stages in the process. 'Realising' occurs when the impact of the life changes that are required becomes fully apparent. Women found reality to be different from their expectation and reported that being able to narrate their birth experiences repeatedly, allowed them to move into the reality. The enormity of the impact caused women to feel unready and unprepared. Being 'drained' refers to the enormous physical, mental and emotional demands that the experience of childbirth makes upon mothers. Change is fundamentally tiring, and sleep is normally used to compensate for and adapt to it, but that is not possible for new mothers. Their lack of confidence and their awareness of the amount that they have to learn, leads to the third stage, termed 'alone'. Partners are not always supportive, and new mothers are awake at unsociable hours, so the loneliness is not easily alleviated. 'Unreality' is experienced by many women, and is unaffected by attendance at antenatal classes. 'Loss' in many areas of life is also difficult to rectify. This 'loss' relates to time for a partner, friends and oneself, freedom and independent control over one's own life, and the loss of a sense of self. These losses are not reversed until the baby grows older. The final stage, namely 'working it out', seems to have been experienced by most of the women in the study, after a period of time. They felt that they needed resources of personal resilience and assertiveness, and to start to trust their own judgements and feelings rather than expert opinion. This final stage of the process is not reached by all women, and some reasons for and consequences of this will be explored later in the chapter.

This social process, which is experienced by so many women, occurs as the mother undergoes a major reconstruction of self without being prepared, supported or recognised by society. It is increasingly challenging in contemporary Western society (Rogan, *et al.* 1997). According to one feminist writer (Rich 1976), the absence of social recognition is deliberate and aims to ensure that women remain under male control. The process of transition has been considered to be problematic, and easy transition is unusual (Oakley 1980, Rogan, *et al.* 1997). Nuclear households that reduce women's contact with the outside world have been blamed for the difficulties in transition, which can result in 'disorientation, depression and despair' (Oakley 1980, Rubin 1984).

Dysphoria refers to distressed mood, and is not as serious as 'disorientation, depression and despair'. Dysphoria has been measured by Morse, *et al.* (2000) at four stages during the transition process, namely 24 weeks' gestation, 36 weeks' gestation and 1 and 4 months postnatally. The number of women who experienced dysphoria (measured with a variety of psychological tests) was 19.5% at 24 weeks, rising to 21.6% at 36 weeks before dropping to 14.9% by 4 months postnatally. This rise and fall is the only evidence in the literature of the timescale of the transition process, and the only serious evidence of the number of mothers for whom it may be a 'normative stage' in family development. It may well be that if future studies replicate these data, the term 'normative' will need to be redefined and the transition issue addressed more seriously within society.

A recent qualitative study by Schneider (2002) has offered an easy to understand model of the process of transition.

First trimester	Second trimester	Third trimester
'A world turned upside down'	'Getting back on track'	'Feeling a little better but when will it end?'
Dis-ease – physical	Well-being – physical	

(*continued*)

First trimester	Second trimester	Third trimester
Ambivalence – emotional	Feeling better – emotional	Discomfort – physical
Disorientation – cognitive	Forgetful – cognitive	Stable – emotional
Support – family and friends	Comfort – friends and family	Normalcy – cognitive
Seeking information	Acceptance of the pregnancy	Needing assurance, interaction with family
Healthcare system	Healthcare system familiarisation	Teamwork – healthcare system
Control	Control	

There are many quotes in the study to support the categories above.

Many studies have identified the amount of emotional work the woman needs to do. Nelson (2003) identifies this in her meta-synthesis but called it 'being actively involved', and suggests that without active engagement the woman cannot grow and be transformed. Other studies quoted by Nelson express the same concepts in terms like engrossed, engaged and giving of self. This idea of growing personally is not new but has not been emphasised before.

THE EXPERIENCE OF GIVING BIRTH

The physical process of giving birth affects the above psychological and sociological process. The fact that a woman's emotional reaction to motherhood is affected by her delivery and care has been documented (Ball 1987). Many women consider labour to be a challenge they are uncertain they can meet at the end of their first pregnancy. They have preconceived ideas, which they have acquired from their mothers and friends, and from reading. Emotionally, relief that labour has started is mixed with fear of the unknown and their reaction to it, and with anticipation of seeing the child. There are insufficient words in the language to describe the psychological depth referred to earlier. In the following scenario, emotional elation and euphoria are poor descriptive words in the writer's experience. 'Within minutes a woman who has experienced natural birth is extremely engaged with her baby, talks to the baby, tries to make eye contact, and feels a happiness that she has not experienced before. What emotional elation and euphoria . . .' (Righard 2001: 2). As far as Western cultural values are concerned, staying in control is very important, which may explain why there are no accurate words for the 'euphoria'. They may be emotions that are out of control, but whose control? Women may be afraid of 'losing control and making a fool of themselves' (Burke 1985: 23) by shouting, screaming and swearing. It is thought by this author and others (Burke 1985) that the current practice of offering epidural analgesia to women who shout adds to the woman's sense of failure if she does 'lose control'. Oakley (1980) found that the women who had experienced 'loss of control' were depressed after childbirth.

Another dimension of the 'control' aspect of labour has been described by Righard (2001). She believes that doctors attend normal births because they want to be in control of what is happening. They have the power to prescribe 'lying in bed', induction, caesarean sections and electronic monitoring. By using these tools they can stay in control. If this is true, it is unlikely that many women will either be or feel in control. Most women will avoid a power struggle in the delivery suite. Righard's (2001) observations in practice led her to point out that, according to the doctors and some midwives, it is 'easier to have her under control'. Thus it is the emotions of anxiety, fear and intimidation that cause the woman to submit to the doctor's authority. A woman has much debriefing (i.e. telling her story) to do after birth before she can carry on the process of transition to motherhood at the same time as meeting the demands of her infant.

Receiving appropriate support in labour is known to result in a positive experience (Sosa, *et al.* 1980, Klaus, *et al.* 1986, Hofmeyr, *et al.* 1991). Both emotional well-being and the way in which women relate to their babies, are affected (Gottlieb 1978). This researcher found that positive maternal health facilitates attachment. Otamiri, *et al.* (1992) looked at the effect of the type of delivery on mother-infant relationships. Women who underwent elective caesarean sections had more doubts about their ability to care for their babies during the first few days after birth than did the mothers who had experienced vaginal deliveries. After one month the elective caesarean section mothers were much more 'care-taking' towards their babies than the control group. It may be that the one-month measurement was made when the mothers had physical problems, and that once these were resolved they attempted to compensate for their earlier incapacity. Thanks to the work of Britton, Gronwaldt and Britton (2001) some measurements of the mother-infant relationship can be made following birth: close physical contact, eye contact, loving touch, examination of the infant, loving talk, positive comments, and appearance of happiness despite the exhaustion associated with labour. These authors suggest that the level of attachment observed in the hour after birth is likely to predict the success of the mother's transition to the mothering relationship her infant requires 6 and 12 months later. The midwife will be aware of some of the above behaviours, but as yet there is no process for documenting the observations or for using them as a means of encouraging the woman in her role as mother.

How traumatic birth may be perceived has not been clearly defined because it relates to how individual women feel. In the past, women not uncommonly died in childbirth, but today it is (according to the media) a healthy and joyous experience. Post-traumatic stress disorder (PTSD) is a condition associated with national catastrophes rather than with childbirth! Three studies have looked at childbirth and the potential stress syndrome associated with it. In one study, 6% of women were found to have the condition (Menage 1993). In a UK study (Ayers and Pickering 2001), it was found that 2% of women had the disorder at six weeks and 1% had it at six months. It was felt that after six months the incidence was unlikely to decrease further.

In an Australian study (Creedy, *et al.* 2000), one in three women reported a stressful birthing event with three or more post-traumatic symptoms such as flashbacks, re-experiencing the birth, avoidance and autonomic arousal. In that study, the level of intervention was a strong predictor of traumatic symptoms; a forceps delivery being as traumatic as an emergency caesarean section. It is felt that after this degree of psychological morbidity, it will take the mother a long time to come to terms with her feelings, and this will need to happen before she can focus her mind on caring for herself and her baby. The transition to motherhood may thus be temporarily, but hopefully not permanently, suspended.

POSTNATAL CONSIDERATIONS: FEELINGS AFTER CHILDBIRTH

Anderson, *et al.* (1994) measured mood antenatally and postnatally and found a correlation. They measured the desire to seek information about childcare, body image, perception of pain, tolerance and social boredom. These parameters could be used to indicate how far the mother has moved in the transition process. They suggested that if there is a negative response to these variables, then there will be a negative mood postnatally, which may give rise to clinical depression or unhappiness. The mood swings were found to be more labile in pregnancy and did not improve until day 28 postnatally. Happiness in the parental relationship was associated with positive mood during pregnancy. Women who were dissatisfied with the appearance of their bodies had a lower tolerance of pain. Added to this psychological stress is cultural stress caused by the media stereotype of what is considered to be an attractive female body, namely a very slender one, which not many healthy pregnant woman can achieve. Another cultural image that women are expected to emulate is that of a fun-filled mother. Anderson, *et al.* (1994) did not explore this image. It may be achievable by women who have domestic help and much free time, but not by those who return to paid employment and juggle it with childcare, as the economic climate suggests should be done.

Paradice (1995) points out that postnatal depression is not clearly understood despite being extensively studied, and that it could be a condition that arises in response to the complex life changes and demands that motherhood brings. The claim that it is a *normal* response is justified by hearing women's observations such as, 'a completely new situation', 'never fully prepared', 'not fully aware of the impact on their life', 'exhausted', 'life has changed for ever' and 'no break, even for illness'. Paradice (1995) considers that a *pathological* condition has been created by perceiving childbirth as a happy and joyous event. This myth that is propagated by society makes it difficult for new mothers to admit they are unhappy. Thus a pathological condition seems to have been caused by a myth. Paradice (1995) does not suggest who is responsible for generating and maintaining the myth, but the media should be named and shamed for imposing this misconception on women. Paradice does not want the 'condition' to be regarded as normal; rather, that women's experiences will not continue to be trivialised and mothering will be acknowledged as the complex and demanding task that it really is. The clinical symptoms of depression may be slight, but the woman feels dysfunctional. As yet there is no satisfactory terminology to describe the condition, apart from a medical one which Paradice suggests is inaccurate. Medical treatment may or may not be used. Alternatively, a social management programme may be appropriate, thus taking the problem out of the clinical realm of influence into the social realm where it truly belongs.

On a more practical level, Ockenden (2000) urges us to respect the postnatal period as an essential interval of time when the new mother needs to recover, rest and come to terms with her new life. In some Moslem, Arabic and African societies, women rest in near isolation for 40 days, during which time they receive special foods and help. In eighteenth-century England, women stayed in bed for 28 days after childbirth, but in twenty-first-century England, the market economy drives women to return to work. Ockenden also points out that 'Western imagery surrounding motherhood does not match reality' (Ockenden 2000: 11). Women need realistic care for themselves, partnership with the professional, and above all for motherhood to be regarded as special. Western society is lacking in rituals that promote mothers' mental health. In cultures that do not celebrate the post-partum period, a high incidence of postnatal depression is reported.

Herbert's (1994) research reinforced the work of Rubin (1967a, b), as it found that after birth the transition to motherhood took three months. The problems of being tired, visitors outstaying their welcome, and the need to develop a new support network took at least three months to work through. Pridham and Change (1992) used questionnaires to explore the transition to being a parent and carer. They noticed how the mothers developed and used problem solving to obtain emotional support, feedback on their performance, and information. She found that better-educated mothers had to be more proactive in their problem solving. They and older women reported less satisfaction with the maternal role.

One could be justified in assuming from the above that mothers' mental health may be impaired. It would be helpful to know whether or not an incomplete process of transition to motherhood has long-term effects. There is very limited literature available in the form of follow-up studies. Walker (1994) conducted a study after 8–10 years on 124 mothers (only 77 of whom were available), using a postal survey to assess children's social competence and behavioural problems. When compared with the maternal role indicators measured during the puerperium, there was no strong or clear prediction of the children's competence or behaviour. This finding has not been verified in other studies.

OLDER WOMEN

Various researchers have investigated whether age is relevant or affects the process of transition to motherhood. Few researchers have studied older women in their own right, yet the average age at which women start a family is rising. Randell (1993) interviewed 18 married Caucasian women at an average of 13 weeks' gestation. The average age of the women was 34 years (which might not be classed as 'older women' by some authorities). It seems that these women were experiencing problems reconciling their ideal image with their real self. They were uncertain about the way in which work colleagues would view them. Their previous identity as non-pregnant seemed to remain with them, suggesting that for them the pregnancy was not real. Other conflicts were between the need to be responsible and the urge to remain self-centred, and between having a child and being that child's mother. It may be concluded that women in Western society are saying that they love their children but they find motherhood difficult. Although this research was informative, because there was no control the question arises as to whether the results would be the same or different if the average age of the women had been 24 years.

The research of Morse, *et al.* (2000) into dysphoric moods (distress in antenatal women) showed that women's distressed moods in mid-pregnancy were strongly correlated with younger age and low levels of instrumental (physical) and emotional support from their partners. This suggests that younger women find the transition to motherhood more difficult. Older women's distress levels decreased more quickly during the early postnatal period, suggesting that they managed better than expected. These findings are supported by other research (Gottesman 1992), which suggests that older women are at lower risk of postnatal depression than younger ones.

A Study by Welles-Nystrom and de Chateau (1987) found older women to be more anxious than a group of younger women in their first pregnancy. This could be due to their greater experience of life, known medical conditions, or just having had time to hear other women's accounts of raising children and their uncertainty as to whether they are up to the challenge. Before drawing conclusions it should be noted that this was a very small study.

There is evidence that older women require more medical intervention during their pregnancy (Gilbert, *et al.* 1999). Certainly they are at greater risk of having a child with Down's syndrome, but the idea that they will require more intervention gives rise to much debate. There is no doubt that pregnancy for older women is likely to be more stressful. Berryman and Windridge (1993) studied 40 nulliparous pregnant women aged 35 years or over, and asked them to complete a Maternal-Fetal Attachment Scale. Each woman was matched with a multiparous woman over 35 years of age. The unstated question related to whether their self-image was that of a woman having a baby or that of being the child's mother, and whether age made any difference. Was the transition process happening? Berryman and Windridge (1993) found that, for the multiparous mother, age had no effect. For the older nulliparous pregnant woman, there was a decreased level of attachment, but it was not statistically significant. If this is true, it may be due to the failure of Western capitalist society to value the woman as a mother as highly as it did the woman as a wage earner. This would make the transition to motherhood very difficult to achieve. Western society still needs to grapple with this.

Windridge and Berryman (1999) conducted a longitudinal study on 107 women to compare the birth experience and postnatal depression across age bands. The study found no age-related difference with regard to obstetric outcome. The older women were more anxious about their baby's safety, but were not more likely to develop postnatal depression.

Welles-Nyström (1997) undertook research to examine how influential feminist thought had been with regard to women's perceptions of having children after the age of 35 years. Not all of her findings are relevant to the current topic. However, one minor finding of the study was that American women had a more symptomatic transition to motherhood than did Swedish women. The term 'symptomatic' was not defined, but seemed to be related to 'off-line transition' behaviour, and it was found that American women over 35 years of age viewed their body changes negatively compared with Swedish women of the same age. The explanation for this was that because these women had timed their reproduction at an abnormal time in their culture, it was inevitable that the transition itself would be unusual. Welles-Nyström (1997) postulated that the postponement of motherhood results from latent immaturity, a disturbed mother-daughter relationship or rejection of one's feminine identity. The questionnaire that was used in the research indicated that all mothers became attached to their infants with little anxiety (despite antenatal 'off-line' transition behaviour).

THE ROLE OF THE MIDWIFE

A research-orientated, evidence-based practice environment may be responsible for midwives focusing on the physiology and patho-physiological aspects of pregnancy and childbirth. Midwives may need to revise their vision of childbirth as an emotional and social event. Most midwives work within the institutions of the NHS. The culture of the institution favours care based on the greatest good for the greatest number. Against this background the midwife needs to remember; 'The woman must be the focus of maternity care. She should be able to feel that she is in control of what is happening to her and able to make decisions about her care based on her needs' (Department of Health

1993: 9) This statement suggests that individualised care is required from the midwife. Each pregnancy occurs in a different set of circumstances. An aspect of the midwife's role in the transition process is to engage fully with the notion that each pregnancy is unique and allow the woman to develop her own frame of reference for care.

The midwife needs to be aware that many women are experiencing grief and loss and need support. For some women it is a heavy work load as they may feel they are losing their identity, financial independence, career progression, body image, perceived sexual attractiveness, social stamina and status. They may not be aware of their new identity, family standing, sense of achievement, perceived proof of womanhood and fertility (highly valued in some cultures).

It may be useful, as a means of empowering her, to remind the woman of what she has already achieved. The list should be individually constructed but is likely to include: changes in behaviour such as stopping smoking, overcoming minor disorders such as nausea and vomiting, making decisions, returning to work or not, and acquiring information about labour.

The midwife must not forget the power of antenatal classes. If she/he is able to understand group dynamics, she/he will enable women to openly discuss the changes they have experienced. This has the effect of validating and normalising their changes and experiences and developing new social networks within the group.

CONCLUSION

Change is a part of our lives as a consequence of physical, chronological and professional development. Many girls grow up expecting to become mothers, but they do not understand how much their lives will be affected and the adaptation that they will have to experience (Gibson 2001). 'New mothers are expected to continue with life as usual – as well as coping with the baby' (Ockenden 2000: 10). The media dramatically misrepresent women's lives in this area. Why does Western culture not recognise that motherhood can be one of the most stressful occupations? Two explanations can be offered for this. The first is that men – who are not usually the main caregivers in early infant life – control the media and cultural practices; even the most sensitive man cannot understand the intensity of a concept for which language does not have words. For example, there is only one word for pain, yet pain due to contractions of labour, pain due to a dental abscess, emotional pain, pain due to terminal illness, pain due to sleep deprivation and the pain of grieving are all different, though this is not apparent in the terminology. However, this view is not well supported.

The second explanation is that the media are controlled. Women rarely exercise this control. There are few rituals and celebrations in Western culture that recognise changes in women's lives. This is more of a problem in Western society, because other cultures have rituals involving social recognition of women after childbirth. In Britain there used to be 'Churching of Women' after childbirth, but this is no longer practised. In other cultures, women's lives are conducted in less isolation from other women (Yearley 1997). Understanding and support are often non-verbal, but Western society communicates through newspapers, computers and mobile telephones, all means by which non-verbal communication, empathy and support are difficult to express. These means of communication are highly valued in Western culture, and were developed by and are controlled by men.

The lack of recognition of the transition to motherhood means that there is no channel by which women can express themselves. In these circumstances, postnatal depression could be interpreted as a normal response (Paradice 1995) to the buildup of fear, anxiety, responsibility, discomfort, exhilaration and guilt (Burke 1985). It seems that the lip-service that is currently paid to motherhood must turn into reality before the role conflicts that women experience are to be resolved.

The midwife has an active role in the transition to motherhood for women. Above all she/he must listen and reflect on her/his role within the NHS, on her/his personal philosophy and on the ideas women present. She/he must listen to women and sometimes reflect back to them their ideas or those of others, including researchers, with a view to empowering them.

KEY POINTS

- The transition to motherhood requires psychological adjustment.
- This transition is hindered by the media's idealistic portrayal of the process of becoming a mother.
- Western capitalist society values women as earners and taxpayers rather than as mothers.
- Women are left to work through the conflict of ideas (*mother* versus *wage earner*) on their own.
- In Western society, motherhood is isolating and conflict can lead to women experiencing poor mental health.

REFERENCES

Anderson VN, Fleming AS, Steiner M. (1994) Mood and transition to motherhood. *J Reprod Infant Psychol.* **12**: 69–77.

Ayers S, Pickering AD. (2001) Do women get post-traumatic stress disorder as a result of childbirth? A prospective study of incidence. *Birth.* **28**: 111–18.

Ball J. (1987) *Reactions to Motherhood: the role of postnatal care.* Cambridge: Cambridge University Press.

Barclay L, Everitt L, Rogan F, *et al.* (1997) Becoming a mother: an analysis of women's experience of early motherhood. *J Adv Nurs.* **25**(4): 719–28.

Berryman JC, Windridge KC. (1993) Pregnancy after 35: a preliminary report on maternal–infant attachment. *J Reprod Infant Psychol.* **11**: 169–74.

Bonnici T. (2001) *Davina's darling.* London: Daily Mail; 26 September 2001. p. 23.

Britton HL, Gronwaldt V, Britton JR. (2001) Maternal postpartum behaviours and mother–infant relationship during the first year of life. *J Pediatr.* **138**: 905–9.

Burke B. (1985) The transition to motherhood. *Nurs Mirror.* **161**: 22–4.

Creedy DK, Shochet IM, Horsfall J. (2000) Childbirth and the development of acute trauma symptoms: incidence and contributing factors. *Birth.* **27**(2): 104–11.

Department of Health (1993) Changing childbirth (the Cumberledge Report). *The Report of the Expert Maternity Group.* London: HMSO.

Fedele NM, Godling ER, Grossman FK, *et al.* (1988) Psychological issues in adjustment to first parenthood. In: Michaels GY, Goldberg WA, editors. *Transition to Parenthood: current theory and research*. New York: Cambridge University Press.

Gibson J. (2001) Motherhood: unrealistic expectations? *Pract Midwife*. 4: 32–4.

Gilbert WM, Nesbitt TS, Danielsen B. (1999) Childbearing beyond age 40: pregnancy outcome in 24 032 cases. *Obstet Gynecol*. 93(1): 9–14.

Goldberg WA. (1988) Perspective on the transition to parenthood. In: Michaels GY, Goldberg WA, editors. *Transitions to Parenthood: current theory and research*. New York: Cambridge University Press.

Gottesman MM. (1992) Maternal adaptation during pregnancy among adult early, middle and late childbearers: similarities and differences. *Matern Child Nurs J*. 20: 93–110.

Gottlieb L. (1978) Maternal attachment in primiparas. *J Obstet Gynecol Nurs*. 7(1): 39–44.

Herbert P. (1994) Support of first-time mothers in the three months after birth. *Nurs Times*. 90: 36–7.

Hofmeyr GJ, Nikodem VC, Wolman C, *et al.* (1991) Companionship to modify the clinical birth environment: effects on progress and perceptions of labour and breastfeeding. *Br J Obstet Gynaecol*. 98(8): 756–64.

Klaus MH, Kennell JH, Robertson SS, *et al.* (1986) Effects of social support during parturition on maternal and infant morbidity. *BMJ*. 293: 585–7.

Larkin V, Butler M. (2000) The implications of rest and sleep following childbirth. *Br J Midwif*. 8: 438–42.

Menage J. (1993) Post-traumatic stress disorder in women who have undergone obstetric and/or gynaecological procedures: a consecutive series of 30 cases of post-traumatic stress disorder. *J Reprod Infant Psychol*. 11: 221–8.

Millar T. (2002) Adapting to motherhood: care in the postnatal period. *Community Pract*. 75(1): 16–18.

Morse CA, Buist A, Durkin S. (2000) First-time parenthood: influences on pre- and postnatal adjustment in fathers and mothers. *J Psychosom Obstet Gynecol*. 21: 109–20.

Nelson AM. (2003) Transition to motherhood. *J Obstet Gynecol Neonatal Nurs*. 32: 465–77.

Oakley A. (1980) *Women Confined: towards a sociology of childbirth*. Oxford: Martin Robertson.

Ockenden J. (2000) After the birth is over . . . rest and support for new mothers. *Pract Midwife*. 3: 10–13.

Otamiri G, Berg G, Lcijon I, *et al.* (1992) Mother-infant relationship: effect of mode of delivery. *J Psychosom Obstet Gynecol*. 13: 209–22.

Paradice K. (1995) Postnatal depression: a normal response to motherhood? *Br J Midwif*. 3: 632–5.

Pridham KF, Chang AS. (1992) Transition to being the mother of a new infant in the first 3 months: maternal problem solving and self-appraisal. *J Adv Nurs*. 17(2): 204–16.

Ram A, Lerman M. (1993) Ultrasound, mother-attachment and the quickening fetus. *Int J Prenatal Psychol Med*. 5: 127–35.

Randell BP. (1993) Growth versus stability: older primiparous women as a paradigmatic case for persistence. *J Adv Nurs*. 18: 518–25.

Rich A. (1967) *Of Woman Born*. New York: Bantam Books.

Righard L. (2001) Making childbirth a normal process (guest editorial). *Birth*. 28(1): 1–4.

Rogan F, Shmied V, Barclay L, *et al.* (1997) 'Becoming a mother': developing a new theory of early motherhood. *J Adv Nurs*. 25(5): 877–85.

Rooney K. (1999) *Encarta World English Dictionary*. London: Bloomsbury Publishing.

Rubin R. (1967a) Attainment of the maternal role, Part I: processes. *Nurs Res*. 16: 237–45.

Rubin R. (1967b) Attainment of the maternal role, Part II: models and referrants. *Nurs Res*. 16: 342–6.

Rubin R. (1984) *Maternal Identity and Maternal Experience*. New York: Springer.

Schmeid V, Lupton D. (2001) Blurring the boundaries: breastfeeding and maternal subjectivity. *Sociol Health Illn*. 23(2): 234–50.

Schneider Z. (2002) An Australian study of women's experiences of their first pregnancy. *Midwifery.* **18**(3): 238–49.

Sorenson DS, Schuelke P. (1999) Fantasies of the unborn among pregnant women. *Am J Matern Child Nurs.* **24**(2): 92–7.

Sosa R, Kennell J, Klaus M, *et al.* (1980) The effects of a supportive companion on perinatal problems, length of labour and mother-infant interaction. *NEJM.* **303**(11): 597–600.

Underdown A. (1998) The transition to parenthood. *Br J Midwif.* **6**: 508–11.

van Gennep A. (1960) *The Rites of Passage.* London: Routledge and Kegan Paul.

Vehviläinen-Julkunen K. (1995) Family training: supporting mothers and fathers in the transition to parenthood. *J Adv Nurs.* **22**: 731–7.

Verny TR. (1998) Some aspects of prenatal parenting. *Int J Childbirth Educ.* **3**: 19–20.

Walker LO. (1994) Maternal identity and role attainment: long-term relations to children's development. *Nurs Res.* **43**: 105–10.

Welles-Nyström B. (1997) The meaning of postponed motherhood for women in the United States and Sweden: aspects of feminism and radial timing strategies. *Healthcare Women Int.* **18**(3): 279–99.

Welles-Nyström BL, de Château P. (1987) Maternal age and transition to motherhood: prenatal and perinatal assessments. *Acta Psychiatr Scand.* **76**(6): 719–25.

Windridge KC, Berryman JC. (1999) Women's experiences of giving birth after 35. *Birth.* **26**: 16–23.

Yearley C. (1997) Motherhood as a rite of passage: an anthropological perspective. In: Alexander J, Levy V, Roth C, editors. *Midwifery Practice: core topics 2.* Basingstoke: Macmillan.

CHAPTER 10

Maternal–infant attachment

Cathy Rowan

The way you treat your child before birth and after is the way the child will treat the world. This is the whole truth about primary prevention.

(Professor Fedor Freybergh, cited in Lee 2000: 5)

This chapter explores some of the theories and characteristics of the nature of the early relationship between a mother and her baby in relation to attachment behaviour. Some of the implications for midwifery practice are discussed, including the possible effects of antenatal screening tests, the type of birth and the effects of early separation if the baby requires special care. The implications for babies whose mothers are depressed are considered, and although no firm conclusions can be drawn, a baby whose mother is depressed may be affected by his or her mother's mood. Early detection and appropriate care for these women may be important in helping to facilitate the relationship and enable the mother to understand her baby's behaviour. The woman's own experience of mothering may affect the way in which she relates to her baby, and in cases where difficulties are evident specialist support may be beneficial.

INTRODUCTION

The attachment relationship between mother and baby is important not only for the physical survival of the baby in terms of the provision of food, warmth and shelter, but also for his or her psychological well-being and development. Several attachment theories have been suggested that have different implications for mothers and babies. Most would agree that the relationship a child forms with its primary caregiver in the first year of life is a key part of the infant's psychological development and has implications for their future relationships, affecting their responsiveness to others and to their own children if they become parents. Adams and Cotgrove (1995) suggest that these patterns are established by one year of age. Attachment between the mother and baby may begin prior to conception when the mother is contemplating pregnancy, and it develops during pregnancy, when the woman is coming to terms with being a mother.

Midwives and healthcare professionals are in a prime position to facilitate the development of a positive relationship between the mother and her baby, and to identify and support those women who may be at risk of developing difficulties in the relationship with their baby. This chapter will examine current understanding of maternal–infant attachment and the factors that may affect this, and will discuss the implications for midwifery practice.

MOTHER–INFANT ATTACHMENT: SOME THEORETICAL APPROACHES

Much has been written about the significance of early attachment between a mother and her baby, although there is not always a clear consensus. Rousseau, an eighteenth-century French writer and philosopher, was the first to use the concept of attachment in relation to the mother–infant relationship. Bowlby (1969) defined attachment as a strong affectional tie between two people, usually an infant and their mother, which develops during the first 18 months of life. Later, in 1988, Bowlby identified the first nine months of life as significant. Klaus and Kennell (1982) stated that the first few moments after birth are an important 'sensitive period' during which a woman is hormonally primed to accept her infant. Their focus was on the mother's perspective of the attachment relationship. They found that mothers who had an extra 16 hours of contact with the baby after birth showed better mothering skills, and their infant performed better on developmental skills than others who did not have this extra contact. Brazelton (1963) and Gay (1981) proposed that attachment is a mutual relationship in which both mother and child contribute, and that it takes time to develop. It is characterised by a strong orientation to each other, discriminative abilities and a desire or need to maintain proximity and contact. The pleasure and synchrony in the interaction serve as catalysts for further exploration of the relationship and its evolution towards a durable attachment (Brazelton and Cramer 1991).

The original idea of maternal–fetal attachment in humans developed from ethnological data from a variety of animal observations, which suggested that there is a species-specific maternal behaviour prior to, during and immediately after birth that leads to the mother's attachment to her offspring. In animals, early removal of the offspring after parturition results in a loss of maternal behaviour. For example, a mother goat will not accept her kid if it is removed from her for more than two hours, before it is one hour old. However, if five minutes of contact are allowed after birth, virtually all young are reaccepted even after three hours (Klopfer 1971). It has been demonstrated in sheep that the longer the period of 'togetherness' before separation, the more likely it is that the mother will continue to display maternal behaviour towards her offspring after reintroduction. Poindron and Le Neindre (1979) found among sheep that when separation begins at birth and lasts for 12–24 hours, 25% of lambs are accepted by their mothers. In contrast, if a 24-hour separation begins two to four days after parturition, all ewes will reaccept their lambs. Klaus and Kennell (1982) postulated that human mothers may also perhaps show species-specific behaviours that facilitate attachment to the infant, but it is uncertain whether observations from animal behaviour can be extrapolated to humans. In an Israeli hospital, after two mothers had accidentally taken home each other's babies they were reluctant to give them up when the error was discovered at the two-week check (Klaus and Kennell 1982).

However, the significance of the early period after birth in humans has been debated. In the 1980s, the findings of Klaus and Kennell were met with considerable criticism to the effect that the research methods were flawed, having been inspired by work with animals (Eyer 1992). However, Korsch (1983) suggested that the critics of the bonding research were reacting as much to the exaggerated practices that had been triggered by Klaus and Kennell's work as to the research ideas. Klaus and Kennell later adapted their views, making it clear that the human experience is much less influential, and that although the early postpartum experience is significant, it is not nearly such a critical period as in animals.

CHARACTERISTICS

The basis of the infant–mother attachment is thought to be biological, in that biologically determined behaviour is triggered by danger or anticipated danger to the infant, to which the infant responds by seeking greater proximity to its primary caregiver (Adams and Cotgrove 1995). This elicits care. When the threat is resolved, the infant returns to exploration. The process is geared towards saving and maintaining life and enhancing the survival of the species. As a result of these early interactions, the child predicts and anticipates responses and develops internalised representations of these key relationships, behaving towards others in a way that has been learned. Depending on the way in which a mother responds when her infant is frightened or needs to be comforted, and how consistently she is sensitive or insensitive to her infant's needs, the infant will learn what to expect from her and other people (Gutbrod 1999).

The maintenance of proximity between mother and baby is considered to be a requirement for the development of attachment. Early and extensive contact enables the parents to become acquainted with their infant. Feeding, embracing, rocking and maintaining prolonged visual contact foster the development of an affective tie. Seeking and maintaining proximity arouses feelings of love, security and joy (Karen 1994). Parents who develop sensitivity in recognising the particular ways in which the infant communicates will respond appropriately by smiling, vocalising, touching and kissing until the infant signals the need to end it. By learning to decode the infant's language the parents can synchronise themselves with their baby so as to maintain certain states for longer periods of time (Brazelton and Cramer 1991). After birth, newborns will synchronise their movements to the rhythm of a mother's voice, who in turn adapts her speech to the response that she perceives from the baby. Parents learn to rely on these responses from the infant as guides to their own behaviour. This interaction enables the infant to develop a sense of him- or herself as a separate person. Thus this sense of identity is developed from the way in which the child perceives him- or herself as a result of the mother's interactions with him or her.

A mother who has sufficient capacity for reflection is able to think about the infant's internal state as separate from her own. When the infant is distressed, she will be able to respond with understanding. A mother may mirror or reflect the child's anxiety. This perception organises the child's experience and they begin to know what they are feeling. Thus the infant learns that their internal feelings are understandable and tolerable (Fonagy and Target 1997). A mother who is unable to reflect on the infant's mind as independent from her own will be unable to provide containment when the infant is distressed, thus increasing his or her anxiety. This can lead to psychological difficulties for the child later.

Klein, a psychoanalyst, stated that infants are capable of relating to figures that are identified as separate from the self at birth, and that psychological development involves the taking into the mind from outside to create 'internal objects'. This view is supported by the work of infant researchers such as Stern (1985). Each individual lives with their own version of the world coloured by models or representations that they carry in their own mind from parental figures. Klein describes the baby's experiences as 'good' (e.g. being fed and nourished) or 'bad' (e.g. being hungry or upset). During the early months the boundaries between the baby and the mother become clearer, and by about six months the child begins to suspect that these good and bad experiences are caused by the same person. The baby needs to integrate these feelings and find a balance where the mother can be both loved and hated. The infant requires a sensitive and emotionally containing caregiver if they are to develop their own capacities to contain and assimilate experiences and feelings (Bion 1967). If this does not occur, defence mechanisms may begin to operate, disrupting the experience of self. Subsequently, the mother and later the world may be experienced as either ideal or malign.

For mother–infant attachment to be facilitated, there needs to be emotional availability of the caregiver, emotional warmth, support-sensitive responses, appropriate stimulation, prompt responsiveness to stress, consistency over time and synchrony and mutuality in the interaction (Belsky, *et al.* 1995). Sufficient space and the ability to detach at the appropriate stage of development of the infant constitute an authentic sign of a secure attachment. A mother's most effective technique for maintaining an interaction seems to be sensitivity to her infant's capacity for attention and need for withdrawal. Infants also differ from each other. Some babies may be difficult to understand, some may take a long time to respond, and some may overreact to stimuli and react negatively with relentless crying. Parents may feel shut out or ineffective, which may have the effect of increasing their anxiety. Parents and babies need to develop an understanding of each other, and some parents may need help to understand their baby and his or her responses (Brazelton and Cramer 1991). It may be helpful if the midwife points out to the mother the ways in which the baby is demonstrating his or her ability to communicate with the mother by highlighting his or her body language.

In 1978, Ainsworth, *et al.* developed what became known as the 'strange situation' for assessing attachment security in 12- to 18-month-old children. Parents, their infants and an experimenter were involved in separation and reunion episodes in order to cultivate attachment behaviours. Infants were classified according to how they responded to their parents during separation and especially upon reunion. Infants who showed separation anxiety but were happy to be reunited with their parents were termed secure. Insecure infants were those who showed distress during separation and ignored their parent upon reunion, and those who were extremely distressed during separation and were unable to be comforted (Gutbrod, 1999). However, such strategies of emotional regulation may make the adult or child very vulnerable and lead to psychological difficulties later. Moreover, focusing on the strange situation as a measure of attachment behaviour ignores the possible influence of temperament and the child's familiarity with separations.

There are four types of parent–infant attachment, three organised types (secure, avoidant and resistant) and one disorganised type. Infants whose caregivers respond in a reassuring way learn to feel secure. Infants whose caregivers respond in insensitive or rejecting ways may demonstrate avoidant or inconsistent behaviour, such as angry displays of distress or resistance. Infants exposed to disorganised forms of parenting may display bizarre or contradictory behaviour (Benoit 2004). It is as if children evolve attachment patterns that are optimal for ensuring their survival in that environment (Thompson and Calkins 1996). Analysis of play using different observations showed a significant difference in the quality of play and quantity of aggression between dyads of securely and insecurely attached children. The presence of an insecurely attached child in a group was associated with more victimisation behaviour, which was shown to continue during childhood (Egeland, *et al.*1990).

Within the scientific literature pertaining to attachment, very few factors have been singled out as being significantly associated with the development of a strong link between parents and their baby. Much that has been written adopts a largely white, middle-class view of motherhood. However, regardless of different parenting styles, which may vary according to historical period and culture, children have grown and developed normally. Tizard (1991) states that a child's relationship with his or her mother is only one of a number of significant relationships that are established in child-hood. He also argues that children are resilient and have the ability to overcome the ill effects of negative periods in their development.

It may be that the infant has the capacity to interact and form bonds with more than one person (Bowlby 1969; Brazelton and Cramer 1991). Families, too, share working models of how to behave, and Byng-Hall (1991) terms these 'family scripts'. Children may therefore be able to view their whole family (rather than just their mother or father) as a secure base from which to explore their environment, secure in the knowledge that they can seek proximity and reassurance at times of stress.

ATTACHMENT IN PREGNANCY

The relationship between the mother and her baby begins in pregnancy or even before the child is conceived, when the woman has ideas of what her child may be like. During the first stage of pregnancy, the woman is coming to terms with becoming a mother, and parents usually look forward to developing the relationship with their baby. Some of the mother's feelings about the baby will depend on her individual situation and whether she has the support of her partner. Cranley, *et al.* (1983) found an association between maternal attachment scores and level of social support. There is a growing awareness of the baby in the uterus as a separate individual, which usually starts with quickening. From the baby's point of view, he or she may become aware of the sounds, activities and rhythms of the mother's world prior to birth.

The experience of screening and diagnostic tests for fetal abnormalities may have a complex effect on the woman's feelings about her baby. A positive association between attachment during pregnancy, and the presence of fetal activity and ultrasound move-ments has been demonstrated by Heidrich and Cranley (1989). Lumley (1990) suggests that scans performed early in pregnancy may slightly improve maternal–fetal bonding, but those performed after quickening are not associated with attachment. Short-term positive effects on maternal health behaviour, such as a reduction in smoking, have been detected when detailed information was given during the scan. Lumley (1990) sug-gested that maternal anxiety may be increased by scanning and then allayed by positive feedback. Hyde (1986) confirmed the anxiety–allaying effect of ultrasound scans, but reported that not all women found them reassuring. A trial by Kemp and Page (1987) found a significant association between ultrasound scans and attachment, although this was much smaller than the association of attachment with the presence of fetal movement. The study did not specify the timing of the ultrasound scans. Some parents may be disappointed when they discover the sex of the baby. The work of attachment takes time, and early attempts to consolidate it may be rejected (Brazelton and Cramer 1991). Kemp and Page (1987) concluded that ultrasound scans may hasten, but do not substantially alter, the development of attachment in the long term, although the skill and communication of the operator may affect the mother's perceptions.

The midwifery literature reflects an increasing awareness of the psychological costs of screening (Grayson 1996, Massey-Davis 1998). Although screening tests for fetal abnormalities may be reassuring for some women, the resultant anxieties may postpone the maternal–fetal attachment process during the antenatal period. Care that focuses on potential abnormalities may undermine a woman's knowledge and her confidence in her ability to produce a fit and healthy baby. Statham and Green (1993) described the psychological effects, such as increased anxiety, experienced by women who receive a result that indicates increased risk. In the study by Fairgreave (1997) of women at greater risk of having a baby with an abnormality, 89.4% of women expressed worry or apprehension prior to the results of amniocentesis. For the remainder of the pregnancy, 14% of the women constantly worried and 44.7% occasionally worried. Farrant (1980) commented that while they were waiting for the results, women smoked more and took tranquillisers. Green, *et al.* (1996) found that women who received a false-positive result continued to show raised anxiety levels during pregnancy, even when subsequent diagnostic tests showed that there was no problem. A lack of privacy, confidentiality or sensitivity in relaying test results can also cause distress.

Concern has now been expressed about the possible psychological, emotional and physical effects of prenatal experiences on postnatal life (Lee 2000). Some degree of anxiety may be a normal part of pregnancy, but increased anxiety levels may be harmful. Teixeira, *et al.* (1999) showed an association between maternal anxiety in pregnancy and increased uterine artery resistance index, suggesting a mechanism whereby the psychological state of the mother may affect fetal growth and development. Hall, *et al.* (2000) found that mothers who were given a false-negative result had higher parenting stress levels and more negative attitudes towards their children, and had a greater tendency to blame others, than those who declined the test. They suggested that a false-negative result seems to have a small adverse effect on parental adjustment, which is evident from two to six years. The false-positive test can make a woman detach from her baby as a means of coping should she need to terminate the pregnancy (Lawrence 1999). For example, if further tests prove that the baby does not have Down's syndrome, such mothers may have great difficulty in rebuilding an emotional attachment to their unborn baby. Robinson (2001) has postulated that the unborn child could be sensitive to the temporary rejection by its mother that is brought about by prenatal screening, and that this could have an ongoing effect. If the uterus is becoming an insecure place for the baby to be, one of the consequences could be suppressed anger in the unborn child (Lee 2000).

The offer of screening tests and their acceptance by the mother can lead to distressing adverse findings, and mothers need to be informed that the tests have limitations as well as benefits. Professionals need up-to-date information and also skills in developing a more facilitative style of counselling to improve the mother's understanding. They need to be able to recognise and refer those women who may be unsure or anxious about the test, and who need help to explore the implications for themselves in more depth.

Parent education may provide opportunities for pregnant women to share their experiences, which may help to reduce some of their anxiety. Rosser (1999) suggests that pregnant women should be offered opportunities to enjoy themselves in pregnancy, such as yoga or aquanatal classes. Michel Odent, a French obstetrician, advocated weekly singing groups!

THE EFFECT OF LABOUR

The mother's active participation during labour sets the stage for the reception of the baby at birth. Emotional support during labour, analgesia, interventions, episiotomies and instrumental delivery may all affect the mother's state postnatally as well as her opportunities to feed, feel and hold her baby (Hillan 1992b). If opiate analgesia is given to the mother during labour, this may affect both the responsiveness of the baby after birth and the ability of the mother to adjust to the baby (Belsey, *et al.* 1981). Redshaw (1982) suggests that it may be the mother's lack of participation in the care of her baby immediately after birth that contributes to the psychological separation of mother and baby that has been ascribed to analgesia given during labour.

Home birth may offer the optimal setting for early bonding to occur. The familiar, safe and relaxed environment, with little or no intervention, allows natural attachment processes to take place immediately after birth. Stevenson (1997) states that it is often at the time of the birth that the mother has a spontaneous, automatic, overwhelming feeling of love and protectiveness towards her new baby, particularly in the first hour after birth, and it is important for her to see and touch the baby. Bonding between parents and their infants can be enhanced by giving them the opportunity to feed, feel and hold their baby after birth, when the baby is often wide awake, settled, calm and interested in his or her surroundings. This quiet alert state is usually present for about 45 minutes after birth when rapid learning takes place, giving mothers and babies the opportunity to get to know each other (Klaus and Kennel 1982, Trevathan 1987). Touching and massaging the infant after birth, stimulates breathing and provides warmth, and holding the baby so he or she can hear the heartbeat may calm the baby as well as facilitate eye contact; contact with the nipple also stimulates the release of oxytocin (Trevathan 1987). A recent Cochrane review to assess the effects of early skin-to-skin contact on breastfeeding behaviour and psychological adaptation in mother and infant dyads, concluded that early skin-to-skin contact may enhance breastfeeding, early attachment, infant crying and cardiorespiratory stability (Moore, *et al.* 2007). Within minutes the baby can show his or her preference for contact with people rather than with objects. The baby will turn its head to the sound of someone's voice, and will also be attracted to faces (Murray and Andrews 2000).

The performance of caesarean section will inevitably influence the amount of contact that the mother has with her baby immediately after delivery, and reactions are likely to be affected by the stress associated with the operation. A large study (Hillan 1992a) found that morbidity among women following a caesarean birth included tiredness, backache, headaches, sleeping difficulties and depression. It is difficult to determine the effect of caesarean birth on the mother–baby relationship. Hillan (1992b) compared 50 primigravid women who gave birth by caesarean section with 50 women who delivered vaginally, by interviewing them on day three or four postnatally and again six months after the birth. She found that women who delivered by caesarean section took significantly longer than those who gave birth vaginally to feel close to their infants, and these differences persisted for several months after the birth. Only 43% of mothers stated that they felt close to the baby immediately, compared with 64% in the control group. Cranley, *et al.* (1983) found that by two months there was still a difference; those women who had had a caesarean birth did not feel as close to the baby. Among those who had had an emergency caesarean section as opposed to an elective one the problem seemed to be worse. It may be that a period of physical and emotional 'self-repair' following any traumatic birth makes the mother less available to her infant. After a long and difficult labour she may have feelings of rejection and resentment that she may find difficult to acknowledge.

However, it is difficult to draw firm conclusions from these studies, and for some mothers maternal affection may be lacking after any form of birth. Some of the effects of a caesarean section may be mitigated by preparation. A woman who has read about it, discussed it and prepared herself may feel very differently to a woman who was faced with an urgent decision after a long labour. Cranley, *et al.* (1983) suggested that women who have regional analgesia and remain conscious throughout the procedure feel more in control of their situation and benefit from early parent–infant contact. The midwife is in a key position to promote early contact between mother and baby, whatever the type of birth. It may help some women if they are given the opportunity to clarify any confusion, reconstruct their experiences and express their feelings, which may facilitate adjustment during the postnatal period.

THE INFANT WHO REQUIRES SPECIAL CARE

Early and prolonged separation of the mother from her baby may hamper the attachment process and play a part in later parenting difficulties. Many studies have highlighted the fact that a lengthy stay in the neonatal intensive-care unit denies the mother a close relationship with her infant, which may jeopardise the development of attachment (Dormire, *et al.* 1989, Coffman 1992). The mother's confidence and self-esteem may be shattered by feelings of inadequacy because she could not achieve a full-term pregnancy, and a premature infant has limited abilities to show a response to parental love. Fear of the baby dying, and the presence of incubators and other technology can have a negative effect on the bonding process. Dawson (1994) found that parents may become overwhelmed by the noise, monitors and flashing lights and be unable to focus on their infant. Hunter, *et al.* (1978) found an eight-fold increase in the incidence of maltreatment for premature and ill newborns.

If the baby has a defect or a malformation, the formation of an attachment can be difficult because the parents are going through a grieving process for their 'perfect' child, and they may also feel guilty. On the other hand, increased contact with the infant has been associated with increased attachment behaviours (Norr, *et al.* 1989). Good social support may aid positive maternal role function (Bass 1991). Providing information and helping the parents to develop caregiving skills are also important. Attempts to support parents whose baby is born prematurely, and to facilitate the development of the early attachment have been shown to produce positive results (Meyer, *et al.* 1994, Als 1997).

As mentioned previously, the evidence for an extremely short 'critical' period in human parents is inconclusive, and the guilt and anxiety generated by this belief may be an unnecessary burden on parents. Infants and their parents are considerably more resilient and flexible than they are often given credit for, as is evidenced by their ability to cope with very different experiences of birth. Although a caesarean birth or preterm delivery may cause some problems, this does not necessarily mean that the relationship between the mother and her infant is permanently affected or that the child will experience emotional difficulties later (Redshaw 1982).

INFANTS OF DEPRESSED MOTHERS

Infants are prepared for an environment of human care and are highly sensitive to the quality of their interpersonal contacts, demonstrating sensitivity to the emotional states of others (Murray 1992). They come into the world ready to respond to people. An association has been found between depression in the mother and insecure attachments (Martins and Gaffan 2000). Murray and Trevarthen (1985) demonstrated that when the mother was interacting with her infant normally, the baby responded with positive emotions, by smiling and adopting a relaxed posture. If the mother had an expressionless face, as she might do if she was feeling unhappy or depressed, the relaxed expression of the baby faded. Tronick, *et al.* (1986) asked the mothers in their sample to act as if they were depressed. The mothers still talked to their infants, but their interaction was less lively. The researchers reported that the infants also began to look depressed. Murray and Stein (1989) found that if mothers maintained a blank facial expression, the babies initially protested, then became distressed and eventually withdrew. When the babies became disappointed and withdrawn, the mothers became agitated and depressed as well (Brazelton and Cramer 1991). Thus it would seem that the emotional state of either the mother or the baby will affect the other in turn.

Mothers who are depressed may create insecure attachments to their infant (Byng-Hall 1991) because they often cause a violation of their baby's expectancy. When they are able to interact normally, they set up expectancy in the babies. Their later withdrawal leaves the baby in a state of depression and hopelessness, confused by the contradiction. Field (1984) found that the behaviour of the infant appeared to mirror that of the mother. Cohn, *et al.* (1990) studied a cohort of depressed and non-depressed mother–infant dyads and found that depression had a negative influence on the behaviour of both. Studies on the impact of postnatal depression on the mother–child relationship have shown that depressed women have difficulties in sensitively attuning their responses to the infant and in keeping their infant's experience in mind, rather than being preoccupied with their own concerns. Murray (1992) studied women with a previous history of depression and a control group for up to 18 months, and found that infants of postnatally depressed mothers performed less well on object concept tasks, and showed mild behavioural difficulties and more insecure attachments.

A number of studies have assessed the longer-term impact of maternal depression by interviewing the mother later about the child's current behaviour (Williams and Carmichael 1985, Caplan, *et al.* 1989). However, these studies have methodological limitations and yielded inconsistent findings. The balance of evidence suggests that although mild levels of difficulty may be evident, serious behavioural disturbances are not a significant consequence of postnatal depression (Murray and Stein 1989). However, in a four-year follow-up of a postpartum sample, Cogill, *et al.* (1986) found that children of postpartum depressed mothers were significantly delayed in terms of cognitive development compared with controls. Stein, *et al.* (1991) found that at 19 months, mother–infant interactions were less effectively positive and less mutually responsive in cases where the mother had suffered from depression during the postnatal period than in cases where the mother had not been depressed. Murray, *et al.* (1999) found that there were more behavioural disturbances at home and less creative play when the child was five years of age if the mother had been depressed, and there was an increase in difficulties for the child at school (Sinclair and Murray 1998). Carter, *et al.* (2001) found that boys were at greater risk of being affected by maternal depressive symptoms than girls, but they suggest that caution is needed in interpreting these findings. The results with regard to the remission from depression on interaction are inconclusive. Stein, *et al.* (1991) found that poor interaction was present at 19 months regardless of whether the depression had remitted by then. However, Campbell, *et al.* (1995) found that the characteristics in remitted mothers were better than those in still depressed mothers at six months.

Holden, *et al.* (1989) observed a considerable improvement in maternal mood in women who were treated over eight weekly sessions by health visitors trained in non-directive counselling. Seeley, *et al.* (1996) demonstrated the benefits of increased health visitor intervention following specific training in cognitive behavioural counselling skills. The difficulties experienced and relationship problems were significantly less in the group that had received additional input from the health visitor. Antidepressant medication may also be effective, but the majority of women are likely to prefer 'talking' therapy (Chilvers 2001). Murray (1992) concluded that even if postnatally depressed mothers recover from their depression within the first three months, this does not bring about an improvement in the mother–infant relationship, and that the focus on therapeutic intervention should extend beyond maternal depressive symptoms to the infant–mother relationship. However, there may be other causal factors with regard to mood disorder, such as difficult social circumstances in terms of poverty or loneliness. Maternal and infant characteristics may also interact. Maternal depressive symptoms, if combined with vulnerabilities in the baby (e.g. premature birth), may increase a child's risk of developing unfavourable patterns of attachment (Poehlmann and Fiese 2001).

Little information is available on the impact of more comprehensive treatment approaches on the longer-term outcome of mothers and babies. Psychotherapy has been shown to change a mother's depressive behaviour, with beneficial effects on the child (Teti and Gefland 1997). Cramer, *et al.* (1990) used a psychodynamic treatment to focus on the mother's internal representation of the baby in her mind, and to explore the links with the mother's unresolved conflicts in relation to her own childhood. This approach has shown promising results.

Psychiatric illness in general and suicide in particular have been identified as the leading cause of maternal death in the UK (Lewis and Drife 2004) and although the more recent report (Lewis 2007) indicates that there had been a reduction in the incidence of suicide, psychiatric illness is still an important health concern. Both reports identify the fact that many of the women who committed suicide had a previous history of psychiatric illness which had not always been identified. CEMACH (Confidential Enquiry into Maternal and Child Health) (Lewis 2007) and (NICE [National Institute for Health and Clinical Excellence] 2006) recommend that midwives ask pregnant women about their mental health and any family history of mental illness, and that specialist services are available for those women who require this.

THE RELEVANCE OF THE MOTHER'S OWN EXPERIENCE OF ATTACHMENT

It is believed that parents' own attachment experiences in childhood influence their internal model of attachment as adults, which in turn influences whether their infant develops a secure or insecure attachment relationship with them (Bowlby 1988). A study by Fonagy, *et al.* (1991) of 100 women showed that the mother's account of her childhood may be an indicator of subsequent attachment behaviour with her own children. Steele, *et al.* (1996) interviewed mothers during pregnancy about their childhood attachment and were able to predict quite accurately which mothers would have an insecurely attached child 15 months later. Brazelton and Cramer (1991) suggest that mothers can tolerate the tremendous selfishness of babies because, in caring for them, they are vicariously satisfying their own selfish needs and wishes, and that these energise a woman's capacity to mother and nurture and set the stage for attachment to the baby.

However, if the mother's dependency needs are too great (e.g. if she is very young), she may regard her baby as a rival, she may treat him or her as an envied sibling, and mothering may seem very difficult. Parents may re-establish old patterns of the past (positive or negative) through their children. Some children may be viewed as a replacement parent. Unresolved loss or mourning can be projected on to the newborn and expressed as an obsessive fear that the child will die. Family therapy may help to identify and resolve some of these issues. However, if the mother can regain or retain access to unhappy memories and reprocess them in such a way that she can come to terms with them, she will be just as able to respond to her child as a woman whose childhood was happy (Bowlby 1988). Fonagy, *et al.* (1997) concluded that individuals who have overcome adversity from their childhood have broken the intergenerational transmission of insecurity.

LIFE EVENTS

Life events and stresses will also influence the mother, and even the most securely attached mother may become highly stressed in difficult circumstances (e.g. poverty, bereavement, difficult relationships). The mother's stress levels may have a negative effect on the child's well-being and sense of security (Belsky, *et al.* 1995). There may also be a number of contextual variables that may affect the infant's emotional well-being, such as the mother's personality, the infant's temperament, the quality of the relationship with her partner and social support, as well as the relationship between work and family. However, significant characteristics of the infant's emotionality (e.g. irritability) can be substantially modified by the mother's behaviour and personality, as well as by the quality of the relationship between the mother and her partner (Nachmias, *et al.* 1996). Women who receive strong support from a partner may be more responsive to their infants.

Women from families where one or both parents had died have been shown to interact significantly less with their 20-week-old babies (Hall, *et al.* 1980). Mothers who feel unsupported and those from a difficult family background or whose pregnancy was unwanted may be particularly vulnerable. A parent who has ambivalent feelings about their child may give inconsistent messages to the infant, which may lead the child to feel that its world is unpredictable and insecure.

Vulnerable parents may also include substance abusers, teenage mothers and those with a learning disability. Insecure attachments are considered to increase internalised feelings of helplessness and low self-esteem, which are linked to depression in adults.

ATTACHMENT AND THE EFFECTS OF FERTILITY TREATMENT

Individuals who are undergoing treatment for infertility are known to experience physical pain and psychological distress, and adoption procedures can be prolonged and emotionally stressful. Holditch-Davis, *et al.* (1998) examined the early parent–infant interactions in infertile couples who became parents through pregnancy or adoption. Two groups of infertile couples (30 couples who achieved pregnancy and 21 couples who adopted) and a group of 19 couples without fertility problems were observed interacting with their babies 7 days and 21 days after the birth (or adoption) and a week later. The behaviours of the mother, father and infant were recorded. The findings suggest that neither infertility nor adoption *per se* impairs early parenting, but additional research is needed to determine whether the experience of infertility and adoption might have a greater impact as the child matures. It may also be useful to explore the effect of particular fertility treatments and the length of time spent trying for a child, and the effect of different types of adoptions. McMahon, *et al.* (1999) found that IVF mothers were more anxious and talked less to their unborn child, but also reported positive idealised attitudes to pregnancy. Previous studies did not find any difference compared with control mothers on self-reports of attachment to their unborn babies (McMahon, *et al.* 1997a), or any differences in maternal sensitivity at four months postpartum (McMahon, *et al.* 1997b). In their pilot study, Dunnington and Glazer (1991) found that previously infertile mothers had lower postpartum maternal identity scores and less self-confidence in performing mothering tasks. However, Gibson, *et al.* (2000) found no evidence that the early anxieties and concerns of IVF mothers translated into negative socio-emotional sequelae for their relationship with their infants at 12 months of age.

The issues with regard to surrogacy are more complex. Although the Surrogacy Arrangements Act (1995) makes commercial surrogacy illegal, non-commercial and privately arranged surrogacy is legal. It is speculated that surrogate mothers do have attachment feelings for their fetus, and that giving up the baby could be difficult and emotionally damaging, and for some mothers impossible (Winston 1994). However, it may be that the surrogate mother is able to dismiss her feelings of attachment (Smith 1998). Furthermore, it may be easier to hand over the child after birth because of the lack of a genetic connection (Singer and Wells 1984). A study by Snowdon (1994) found that it was more difficult for the surrogate to give up the baby if it was her own ovum, and that gestational surrogacy was less of a bond. However, other researchers suggest that many surrogate mothers deny their true feelings (Fischer and Gillman 1991). Chestler (1988) warns that surrogates tend to exhibit a high degree of dissociation from their feelings, their bodies and reality. It is clearly important that there is adequate support, counselling and monitoring of surrogacy arrangements. Midwives need to be aware both of their own feelings and of the fact that the feelings of the surrogate may be unpredictable.

With regard to the parents of children conceived as a result of surrogacy arrangements, Snowdon (1994) found that genetic and gestational connections mean different things to different women, and that it is the emotional investment a woman has in pregnancy that is of consequence. For some, the genetic link was not crucial in defining the relationship to a child. Another finding was that adoption was more balanced because the child would not be genetically linked to either partner.

PROMOTING THE MOTHER–BABY RELATIONSHIP

If a mother is finding it difficult to relate to her baby, it cannot be concluded from the available research that there will be lasting negative consequences for the child. However, it is clear that babies come into the world ready and willing to be sociable, and they seem to enjoy interacting with people. There is some evidence that the quality of early relationships may have later consequences for cognitive, emotional and social development. Helping parents to recognise the potential of their baby may help them to realise that there is a point in interacting with their baby (Paradice 1993). Promoting early contact between the mother and baby at birth by giving them time together, and keeping the baby with the mother during the postnatal period is helpful. It may also be useful to emphasise the importance of parental response to infant cues, and to highlight the infant's abilities and his or her attempts to communicate (e.g. through smiling and eye contact).

What might seem at first glance to be random and confused infant behaviour is in fact highly organised. The most dramatic of the baby's abilities, even in the first weeks of life, are his or her social responses. By watching the subtle changing pattern of a baby's expression and movement, and by appreciating the significance of these cues, parents can become aware of the richness of the baby's experience and can be guided to help their infant (Murray and Andrews 2000). Tiny babies as young as half an hour old can copy facial gestures such as tongue protrusion (Meltzoff and Moore 1977). Infants seem to quickly recognise and prefer aspects of their mother or primary caretaker, such as her voice and her face (Field and Fox 1985). Face-to-face play with babies in the second and third months can seem like a musical duet where the baby's initiative is taken up by the parent who, quite unconsciously, mirrors and develops the baby's original communication.

Babies are also attracted to particular types of visual stimulation, as well as to people's faces. They will look intently at patterns that have strong clear contrasts. The optimum distance for them to focus is 22 cm. Mothers can be made aware of the various ways in which the baby is communicating with them. Giving care that is sensitive to the baby's unique signals, reliable, and predictably structured, will help the baby to build up a sense of a familiar world where events can be anticipated, and in which minor delays and difficulties can be more easily tolerated.

CONCLUSION

It may be concluded that early contact does seem to facilitate mother–infant attachment under certain conditions with certain groups of individuals. Because of the subtleties of the behaviours involved, socio–economic status, age, feeding methods, behaviour of the baby and so on, it is not possible to make generalisations. The ability of the mother to develop a healthy relationship with her baby will be influenced by many factors, extending back to the relationship that the mother had with her own parents. Our ideas about the nature of the relationship between mother and baby are also shaped by our culture, and there are many dimensions to the nurturing of children. Focusing on the early bonding experience may over-simplify complex issues and put unnecessary blame on the mother.

However, it may be that in stressful or traumatic circumstances the child who feels insecure may be more vulnerable to emotional difficulties, have low self-esteem and find it difficult to trust others. Early interventions by healthcare professionals may help to prevent the formation of insecure attachment patterns in some women and increase the likelihood of transmission of secure attachments across the generations (Adams and Cotgrove 1995). Working in partnership with mothers, considering the way in which screening tests are presented, providing flexible and humane care during labour, and promoting early contact with the baby may be beneficial to the developing relationship between mother and baby. It may also be appropriate not to insist that there is only one way to care for the baby, in order to avoid lowering the mother's self-esteem and confidence.

It is important to acknowledge that some women themselves never experienced quality mothering or secure attachment as children. For them, the task of mothering may seem overwhelming and highly frustrating and they may need extra support. It may be possible to identify those at risk of postnatal depression before delivery (e.g. those with a poor partnership/marital relationship, social and economic stress or a previous psychiatric history). O'Hara (1997) found that mothers who are experiencing negative life events are more likely to become depressed. Paying close attention to vulnerable mothers during the postnatal period may be important. Facilitating early contact after birth and helping the mother to understand the ways in which the baby is attempting to communicate with her may promote the development of a healthy relationship. Extra support may range from increased education, extra visits, recognising and reducing stressful demands and increasing emotional support, through to individual or group counselling or psychotherapy (Raphael-Leff 1990). The midwife is in a key position to recognise the individual needs of each mother.

KEY POINTS

- ∞ Midwives should work in partnership with mothers, enabling them to make choices with regard to their care, and to increase their self-esteem and confidence.
- ∞ Midwives should identify those mothers who may require extra support during pregnancy and the postnatal period, and continuity of care for such women should be promoted.
- ∞ For women with a past history of severe mental illness, clear multidisciplinary planning should take place because of the risk of recurrence.
- ∞ Where possible, early contact between the mother and her baby after birth should be encouraged.
- ∞ Teaching the mother about the abilities of her baby and encouraging recognition of the baby's communication skills may promote healthy development of the relationship between mother and child.
- ∞ Women with a history of depression or psychiatric illness should be identified and given appropriate support.
- ∞ Women who are or who may become depressed during pregnancy or after the birth should be identified and offered appropriate support. This may include psychological treatment.
- ∞ Attention should be given to the mother's emotional well-being at the six-week check.

REFERENCES

Adams L, Cotgrove A. (1995) Promoting secure attachment patterns in infancy and beyond. *Prof Care Mother Child.* 5: 158–60.

Ainsworth MDS, Blehar MC, Waters E, *et al.* (1978) *Patterns of Attachment: a psychological study of the strange situation.* Hillsdale, NJ: Lawrence Erlbaum Associates.

Als H. (1997) *Earliest Intervention for Preterm Infants in the Newborn Intensive Care Unit.* London: Paul H Brookes Publishing Company.

Bass LS. (1991) What do parents need when their infant is a patient in the NICU? *Neonat Network.* 10: 25–34.

Belsey EM, Rosenblatt DB, Lieberman BA, *et al.* (1981) The influence of maternal analgesia on neonatal behaviour. 1. Pethidine. *Br J Obstet Gynaecol.* 88: 398–406.

Belsky J, Rosenberger K, Crnic K. (1995) The origins of attachment security: classical and contextual determinants. In: Goldberg S, Muir R, Kerr J, editors. *Attachment Theory: social, developmental and clinical perspectives.* London: Analytic Press.

Benoit D. (2004) Infant-parent attachment: definitions, types, antecedents, measurements and outcomes. *Pediatr Child Health.* 9(8): 541–5.

Bion WR. (1967) A theory of thinking. In: Bion WR, editor. *Second Thoughts: selected papers on psychoanalysis.* London: Heinemann.

Bowlby J. (1969) *Attachment and Loss, Volume 1: Attachment.* New York: Basic Books.

Bowlby JA. (1988) *A Secure Base: clinical application of attachment theory.* London: Routledge.

Brazelton TB. (1963) The early mother–infant adjustment. *Pediatrics.* 32: 931–7.

Brazelton TB, Cramer MD. (1991) *The Earliest Relationship*. New York: Karnac Books, Addison-Wesley.

Byng-Hall J. (1991) The application of attachment theory to understanding and treatment of family therapy. In: Parkes CM, Stevenson-Hinde J, Marris P, editors. *Attachment Across the Life Cycle*. London: Routledge.

Campbell SB, Cohn JF, Meyers T. (1995) Depression in first-time mothers: mother–infant interaction and depression chronicity. *Dev Psychol*. 31: 349–57.

Caplan HL, Cogill SR, Alexandra H, *et al.* (1989) Maternal depression and the emotional development of the child. *Br J Psychiatry*. 154: 818–22.

Carter A, Garrity-Rokous FE, Chazan-Cohen R, *et al.* (2001) Maternal depression and comorbidity: predicting early parenting attachment, security, and toddler socio-emotional problems and competencies. *J Am Acad Child Adolesc Psychiatry*. 40: 18–26.

Chestler P. (1988) *Sacred Bond: motherhood under siege*. London: Virago.

Chilvers C, Dewey M, Fielding K, *et al.* (2001) Antidepressant drugs and generic counselling for treatment of major depression in primary care: randomised trial with patient preference arms. *BMJ*. 322(7289): 772–5.

Coffman S. (1992) Parent and infant attachment: review of nursing research 1981–1990. *Pediatr Nurs*. 18: 421–5.

Cogill SR, Caplan HL, Alexandra H, *et al.* (1986) Impact of postnatal depression on cognitive development of young children. *BMJ*. 292: 1165–7.

Cohn JF, Campbell SB, Matias R, *et al.* (1990) Face-to-face interactions of postpartum depressed and non-depressed mother–infant pairs at 2 months. *Dev Psychol*. 26: 15–23.

Cramer B, Robert-Tissot C, Stern DN, *et al.* (1990) Outcome evaluation in brief mother–infant psychotherapy: a preliminary report. *Infant Ment Health J*. 11(3): 278–300.

Cranley MS, Hedahl KJ, Pegg SH. (1983) Women's perceptions of vaginal and caesarean deliveries. *Nurs Res*. 32: 10–15.

Dawson B. (1994) Put the parent and baby first: nurse/parent relationships in neonatal intensive care. *Prof Nurse*. 10: 30–5.

Dormire SL, Strauss SS, Clarke BA. (1989) Social support and adaptation to the parent role in first-time adolescent mothers. *J Obstet Gynecol Neonatal Nurs*. 18: 327–7.

Dunnington R, Glazer G. (1991) Maternal identity and early mothering behaviour in previously infertile and never infertile women. *J Obstet Gynecol Neonatal Nurs*. 20: 309–17.

Egeland B, Kalkoski M, Gottesman N, *et al.* (1990) Preschool behaviour problems: stability and factors accounting for change. *J Child Psychol Psychiatry*. 31(6) 891–910

Eyer DE. (1992) *Mother–Infant Bonding: a scientific fiction*. New Haven, CT: Yale University Press.

Fairgrieve S. (1997) Screening for Down's syndrome: what women think. *Br J Midwif*. 5: 148–51.

Farrant W. (1980) Stress after amniocentesis for high serum alpha-fetoprotein concentration. *BMJ*. 281: 452.

Field T. (1984) Early interactions between infants and their postpartum depressed mothers. *Infant Behav Dev*. 7: 517–22.

Field TM, Fox N. (1985) *Infant Social Perception*. Norwood, NJ: Ablex Publishing Company.

Fischer S, Gillman I. (1991) Surrogate motherhood: attachment, attitudes and social support. *Psychiatry*. 54: 13–20.

Fonagy P, Target M. (1997) Attachment and reflective function: their role in self-organisation. *Dev Psychopathol*. 9: 679–700.

Fonagy P, Steele H, Steele M. (1991) Maternal representations of attachment during pregnancy predict the organisation of infant–mother attachment at one year of age. *Child Dev*. 62: 891–905.

Fonagy P, Steele M, Steele H, *et al.* (1997) *Reflective Functioning Manual Version 4.1: for application to adult attachment interviews*. London: University College London Psychoanalysis Unit.

Gay J. (1981) A conceptual framework of bonding. *J Obstet Gynecol Neonatal Nurs*. 10: 440–4.

Gibson FL, Ungerer JA, McMahon CA, *et al.* (2000) The mother–child relationship following *in vitro* fertilisation (IVF): infant attachment, responsivity, and maternal sensitivity. *J Child Psychol Psychiatry*. **41**: 1015–23.

Grayson A. (1996) The triple test decision. *Modern Midwife*. **6**: 16–19.

Green JM, Statham H, Snowdon C. (1996) Pregnancy is a testing time. *Report of the Cambridge Prenatal Screening Study*. Cambridge: Centre for Family Research, University of Cambridge.

Gutbrod T. (1999) Mother and infant relationships. *Int J Altern Compl Med*. **17**: 18–19.

Hall F, Pawlby SJ, Wolkind S. (1980) Early life experiences and later mothering behaviour: a study of mothers and their 20-week-old babies. In: Shaffer D, Dunn J, editors. *The First Year of Life*. New York: John Wiley & Sons.

Hall S, Bobrow M, Marteau TM. (2000) Psychological consequences for parents of false-negative results on prenatal screening for Down's syndrome: retrospective interview study. *BMJ*. **320**: 407–12.

Heidrich SM, Cranley MS. (1989) Effect of fetal movement ultrasound scans and amniocentesis on maternal–fetal attachment. *Nurs Res*. **38**: 81–4.

Hillan EM. (1992a) Short-term morbidity associated with caesarean section. *Birth*. **19**: 190–4.

Hillan EM. (1992b) Maternal–infant attachment following caesarean delivery. *J Clin Nurs*. **1**: 33–7.

Holden J, Sgovsky R, Cox J. (1989) Counselling in a general practice setting: controlled study of health visitor intervention in treatment of postnatal depression. *BMJ*. **298**: 223–6.

Holditch-Davis D, Sandelowski M, Harris BG. (1998) Infertility and early parent–infant interactions. *J Adv Nurs*. **27**: 992–1001.

Hunter RS, Kilstrom N, Kraybill EN, *et al*. (1978) Antecedents of child abuse and neglect in premature infants: a prospective study in a newborn intensive care unit. *Paediatrics*. **61**: 629–35.

Hyde B. (1986) An interview study of pregnant women's attitudes to ultrasound scanning. *Soc Sci Med*. **22**: 587–92.

Karen R. (1994) *Becoming Attached: unfolding the mystery of the infant–mother bond and its impact on later life*. New York: Warner Books.

Kemp VH, Page CK. (1987) Maternal prenatal attachment in normal and high-risk pregnancies. *J Obstet Gynecol Neonatal Nurs*. **16**: 179–84.

Klaus MH, Kennell JH. (1982) The family during pregnancy. In: Klaus MH, Kennell JH, editors. *Parent Infant Bonding*. St Louis, MO: CV Mosby Company.

Klopfer PH. (1971) Mother love: what turns it on? *Am Sci*. **59**: 404–7.

Korsch BM. (1983) More on parent infant bonding (editorial). *J Pediatr*. **102**: 249–50.

Lawrence S. (1999) Counselling for Down's syndrome screening. *Br J Midwif*. **7**: 368–70.

Lee B. (2000) Attached or detached? Aspects of baby–parent attachment. *RCM Midwives J*. **3**: 158–9.

Lewis G, editor. (2007) *Saving Mothers' Lives: reviewing maternal deaths to make motherhood safer – 2004–2005*. The Seventh Report of the Confidential Enquiries into Maternal Deaths in the United Kingdom. Confidential Enquiry into Maternal and Child Health (CEMACH). London: CEMACH. Available at: www.cemach.org.uk (accessed 6 Mar 2009).

Lewis G, Drife J, editors. (2004) *Why Mothers Die: 2000–2002*. The Sixth Report on Confidential Enquiries into Maternal Deaths in the United Kingdom. CEMACH. London: RCOG Press. Available at: www.cemach.org.uk (accessed 6 Mar 2009).

Lumley J. (1990) Through a glass darkly: ultrasound and prenatal bonding. *Birth*. **17**: 214–17.

McMahon CA, Tennant C, Ungerer JA, *et al*. (1999) 'Don't count your chickens': a comparative study of the experience of pregnancy after IVF conception. *J Reprod Infant Psychol*. **17**: 345–56.

McMahon CA, Ungerer JA, Beaurepaire J, *et al*. (1997a) Anxiety during pregnancy and fetal attachment after IVF conception. *Hum Reprod*. **12**: 176–82.

McMahon CA, Ungerer JA, Tennant C, *et al*. (1997b) Psychological adjustment and the quality of the mother–child relationship at four months postpartum after conception by in vitro fertilisation. *Fertil Steril*. **68**: 492–500.

Martins C, Gaffan EA. (2000) Effects of early postnatal depression on patterns of infant–mother attachment: a meta-analytic investigation. *J Child Psychol Psychiatry*. **41**: 737–46.

Massey-Davis L. (1998) A woman's right not to choose. *Pract Midwife*. 1: 23–5.

Meltzoff AM, Moore MK. (1977) Imitation of facial and manual gestures by human neonates. *Science*. 198: 75–8.

Meyer EC, Coll CT, Lester BM, *et al.* (1994) Family-based intervention improves maternal psychological well-being and feeding interaction of preterm infants. *Pediatrics*. 93: 241–6.

Moore ER, Anderson GC, Bergman N. (2007) Early skin-to-skin contact for mothers and their healthy newborn infants. *Cochrane Database Syst Rev*. 3: CD003519.

Murray L. (1992) The impact of postnatal depression on infant development. *J Child Psychol Psychiatry*. 33: 543–61.

Murray L, Andrews L. (2000) *The Social Baby*. Richmond: CP Publishing.

Murray L, Sinclair D, Cooper P, *et al.* (1999) The socio-emotional development of 5-year-old children of postnatally depressed mothers. *J Child Psychol Psychiatry*. 40: 1259–71.

Murray L, Stein A. (1989) The effect of postnatal depression on the infant. *Baillieres Clin Obstet Gynecol*. 3: 921–33.

Murray L, Trevarthen C. (1985) Emotional regulation of interaction between two-month-olds and their mothers. In: Field T, Fox W, editors. *Social Perception in Infancy*. Norwood, NJ: Ablex Publishing Company.

Nachmias M, Gunnar M, Mangelsdorf S, *et al.* (1996) Behavioural inhibition and stress reactivity: the moderating role of attachment security. *Child Dev*. 67: 508–22.

National Institute for Health and Clinical Excellence. (2007) *Antenatal and postnatal mental health: NICE guideline 45*. London: NIHCE. www.nice.org.uk/Guidance/CG45

Norr KF, Roberts JE, Freese U. (1989) Early postpartum rooming in and maternal attachment behaviours in a group of medically indigent primiparas. *J Nurs Midwifery*. 34(2): 85–91.

O'Hara M. (1997) The nature of postpartum depressive disorders. In: Murray L, Cooper P, editors. *Postpartum Depression and Child Development*. London: Guildford Press.

Paradice R. (1993) How important are early mother–infant relationships? *Health Visit*. 66: 211–13.

Poehlmann J, Fiese BH. (2001) The interaction of maternal and infant vulnerabilities on developing attachment relationships. *Dev Psychopathol*. 13: 1–11.

Poindron P, Le Neindre P. (1979) Hormonal and behavioural basis for establishing maternal behaviour in sheep. In: Zichella L, Pancheri R, editors. *Psychoneuroendocrinology in Reproduction*. Amsterdam: Elsevier/North Holland Biomedical Press.

Raphael-Leff J. (1990) Psychotherapy and pregnancy. *J Reprod Infant Psychol*. 8: 119–35.

Redshaw M. (1982) The influence of analgesia in labour on the baby. *Midwife Health Visit Community Nurse*. 18: 126–32.

Robinson J. (2001) Does prenatal screening provoke anticipatory grief? *Br J Midwif*. 9(5): 307–11.

Rosser J. (1999) Anxiety and pregnancy: bad for women, bad for babies. *Pract Midwife*. 2: 4–5.

Seeley S, Murray L, Cooper P. (1996) The outcome for mothers and babies of health visitor interventions. *Health Visit*. 69: 134–8.

Sinclair D, Murray L. (1998) Effects of postnatal depression on children's adjustment to school. *Br J Psychiatry*. 172: 58–63.

Singer P, Wells P. (1984) *The Reproductive Revolution: new ways of making babies*. Oxford: Oxford University Press.

Smith M. (1998) Maternal–fetal attachment in surrogate mothers. *Br J Midwif*. 6: 188–92.

Snowdon C. (1994) What makes a mother? Interviews with women involved in egg donation and surrogacy. *Birth*. 21: 77–83.

Statham H, Green G. (1993) Serum screening for Down's syndrome: some women's experiences. *BMJ*. 307: 174–6.

Steele H, Steele M, Fonagy P. (1996) Associations among attachment classifications of mothers, fathers and their infants. *Child Dev*. 67: 541–5.

Stein A, Gath DH, Bucher J, *et al.* (1991) The relationship between postnatal depression and mother–child interaction. *Br J Psychiatry*. 158: 46–52.

Stern D. (1985) *The Interpersonal World of the Infant*. New York: Basic Books.

Stevenson J. (1997) Pondering about bonding. *Midwif Matters*. **74**: 20–2.

Teixeira J, Fisk N, Glover V. (1999) Association between maternal anxiety in pregnancy and increased uterine artery resistance index: cohort-based study. *BMJ*. **318**: 153–7.

Teti DM, Gelfand DM. (1997) Maternal cognitions as mediators of child outcomes in the context of postpartum depression. In: Murray L, Cooper PJ, editors. *Postpartum Depression and Child Development*. London: Guildford Press.

Thompson RA, Calkins SD. (1996) The double-edged sword: emotional regulation for children at risk. *Dev Psychopathol*. **8**: 163–82.

Tizard B. (1991) Working mothers and the care of young children. In: Lloyd E, Phoenix A, Wollett A, editors. *The Social Construction of Motherhood*. London: Sage.

Trevathan WR. (1987) *Human Birth: an evolutionary perspective*. New York: Aldine de Gruyter; 193–220.

Tronick EZ, Conn J, Shea E. (1986) The transfer of affect between mother and infants. In: Brazelton TB, Yogman MW, editors. *Affective Development in Infancy*. Norwood, NJ: Ablex Publishing Company.

Williams H, Carmichael A. (1985) Depression in mothers in a multi-ethnic urban industrial municipality in Melbourne: aetiological factors and effects on infants and preschool children. *J Child Psychol Psychiatry*. **26**: 277–88.

Winston R. (1994) *Infertility: a sympathetic approach*. London: Optima.

CHAPTER 11

The medicalisation of childbirth

Alyson Henley-Einion

Childbirth in the UK takes place within a medical context and is defined by medical norms. It is no longer a purely social or personal event, nor is it the specific province of women. This chapter explores the roots of the medicalisation of childbearing, and the underlying advances in science and medicine. The emergence of the concept of risk and risk management is considered with a particular focus on its relevance to women being given informed choice as reality or illusion. The express aim of the chapter is to deconstruct and make explicit the ways in which such processes have occurred and how they continue to affect childbearing women. Studies of the way in which women experience the maternity services have long revealed an iceberg of dissatisfaction (Kirkham 1986, Oakley 1990, Kitzinger 1992). If this iceberg is to be melted, an exploration of its structure and form is necessary, and the resulting understanding used to set up measures to redress the balance. Sociological, midwifery and feminist theory is used to explore these issues.

INTRODUCTION

Most women's experiences of childbearing in the UK today are medicalised, as birth takes place predominantly in a hospital, on a maternity ward and in the presence or under the surveillance of doctors, whether the birth is defined as 'low risk' or not. The maternity unit and the labour ward are their domain. The act of birth is surrounded by all the symbols of the medical profession and all that it stands for – science, power and authoritative knowledge, and the suggestion that control of the supposedly inherent risks of birth is possible.

The medicalisation of childbirth can essentially be viewed as a process that has resulted in childbirth being regarded as a medical event rather than a social one, an event in which human experiences are redefined as medical problems (Becker and Nachtignall 1992). The process concerns the experiences of women and their partners on becoming pregnant and giving birth. Nowadays, a pregnant woman, when asked what she anticipates in relation to labour and birth, is more likely than not to include the word 'hospital' in her reply, despite the rising profile of the homebirth movement in the UK. Part of her childbirth classes will prepare her for hospital, introducing her to the delivery room and the machinery and technology that are available to assist her to experience a safer birth. Governance procedures pertaining to the management and reduction of risk have now become embedded in all aspects of daily life. Those relating to maternity care practices, emphasise medical models of care intended to offer women safety and reassurance but are perceived as claiming the power to control natural processes of the body. Yet it is the reassurance that women yearn for that is the province of midwifery care.

There are many critiques of the medical control of childbearing. They stem from midwifery practice and theory, and feminist and social theory. The cultural and social meanings of birth and its rituals have developed in parallel with the relentless march of technological progress. In today's Western world, medical frames of reference and knowledge have been accepted and legitimated within a system of maternity care, which has brought about not only a surge in engineering obstetrics but also a steady erosion of maternal choice, control and satisfaction in relation to many aspects of pregnancy and labour, usually justified in the name of safety (Cahill 2001). Illich (1976) associates medicalisation with industrialisation, and this culture is based on the industrialisation of all areas of human experience. Risk management has come to permeate every aspect of modern society – home, school, leisure, travel, industry and professions – and its irresistible influence is particularly apparent in the fields of medicine, health and maternity care.

Feminist writing refers to the way in which women's social experiences (including their health and healthcare) are mediated by the institutions of patriarchy, usually in oppressive ways (Annandale and Clark 1996). These institutions are the focus of much of the discussion of the medicalisation of childbearing. Sociological theories, such as functionalism, relate women's experiences of childbearing to specific behavioural directives that are related to gender-specific roles and norms (Haralambos and Holborn 1995). In this chapter, some of these theories underpin the analysis of medicalisation and risk in relation to the UK maternity services.

Childbirth is in itself a natural physiological process. Prior to the advent of scientific medicine, birth was a social event, and the only 'intervention' was the presence of a midwife, who provided social support and had the experience of having attended other births, so possessed knowledge of childbirth and its processes. The social setting in which birth now occurs is one where the dominant culture is that of science, and the dominant discourse is that of risk. Midwives are part of this. Obstetrics, the dominant form of knowledge, is regarded as mainstream, *male-stream*, knowledge, whereas natural childbirth is labelled as 'alternative' and associated with greater risk. Midwives are part of this scientific movement, and are not exempt from protocols, standards and policies based upon risk assessment.

The care that is given to labouring women is prescribed by doctors, and the interventions that are used to achieve 'normal' birth are based on Western notions of time and scientific calculations, and on economic and resource-linked concerns of minimising risk. Pregnancy and birth, the latter being possibly the most potent and powerful natural event of a woman's life, are regularised and constantly scrutinised by medical professionals, acting on a definition of childbirth as inherently risk-laden. The current rhetoric of risk management is couched almost entirely in terms of obstetric management of risk. Scholefield (2005), for example, links it clearly with improving patient safety, but also with the financial implications of 'risk' where errors and negative outcomes cannot be avoided.

The dominant philosophy of modern obstetrics, particularly within the UK context, appears to be that of risk prediction (*see*, for example, Scholefield 2005, Thompson and Owen 2005, Cottee and Harding 2008). It is the inherently unpredictable nature of pregnancy and birth that seems to doom all pregnant women to increased medical surveillance. This has alienated women from a potentially empowering experience.

This chapter addresses the evolution of childbearing within the context of the science, technology and scientific/political rhetoric that now restricts women's liberties even further as they make the transition into motherhood. It draws upon feminist concerns with the social structure of science as representing an inherently sexist, classist and culturally coercive practice and hegemony (Oakley 1990). The express aim of the chapter is to deconstruct and make explicit the ways in which such processes have occurred and how they continue to affect childbearing women. Studies of the way in which women experience the maternity services have long revealed an iceberg of dissatisfaction (Kirkham 1989, Oakley 1990, Kitzinger 1992). If this iceberg is to be melted, an exploration of its structure and form is necessary, and this understanding must be used to set up measures to redress the balance.

CHILDBEARING: A HISTORY OF THE RISE OF SCIENCE, TECHNOLOGY AND OBSTETRICS, AND THE EMERGENCE OF THE CONCEPT OF RISK AND RISK MANAGEMENT

Medicalisation and control of childbirth are inextricably linked with patriarchy, which has dominated the religious, cultural and political ideologies of Western civilisation for nearly 2000 years, founded on Judaeo–Christian principles. The rise of medicine as a political and social force within the female sphere of motherhood can be traced back as far as the fourteenth century. Physicians, who had been trained at universities (which only admitted men), managed to gain approval from the Church and set out to shake the faith of the people in traditional remedies (Towler and Bramall 1986). This was the beginning of medicine's assumption of authority over the mysteries of the body, health, birth and death.

Historical analyses show that, until the seventeenth century, childbirth in Britain was firmly located within the domestic arena (Cahill 2001), with women being attended by lay midwives, family and close friends. The seventeenth and eighteenth centuries saw a rise in the power and status of the medical profession, which was achieved largely by the denigration and usurping of traditional or non-licensed practitioners, such as midwives. Since this time, medicine and religion together have systematically devalued female roles and traits and excluded women from power in society through the dissemination of patriarchal ideology (Cahill 2001).

The explosion of scientific knowledge, especially in the fields of physiology and anatomy, attracted men to the practice of midwifery. With the application of their knowledge as physicians and their skills as surgeons (using their newly-acquired forceps) these 'men-midwives' irrevocably changed the nature and pattern of midwifery practice (Towler and Bramall 1986), and seem to have introduced the concept of risk reduction through the application of superior knowledge and 'scientific practice', leading to a change in the role and function of women within the sphere of pregnancy and birth.

The popularity of 'men–midwives' and male medical practitioners among the upper classes, who set the standards for the rest of society, led to a social 'shift' in the frames of reference and behaviours surrounding birth. The use of the term 'brought to bed' in accounts of childbirth among the gentry implies that this class abandoned the traditional birth chair for the bed, and at the same time they abandoned the traditional midwife for the male attendant (Towler and Brammall 1986); the role of women as childbearers changed from active to passive.

The first 'lying-in' hospitals were established in the middle of the eighteenth century, reflecting the shift in emphasis from birth as a home-based family event to birth as a hospital-based medical event. It was only in the late nineteenth and early twentieth centuries that pregnancy on the whole became viewed as a condition that warranted some kind of supervision, stemming from the need to reduce an unacceptable level of maternal mortality (Field 1990). This was complemented by the introduction of x-rays between 1900 and 1910. Such technical developments in turn began to define the form that antenatal care would subsequently assume (Field 1990) in that surveillance of the fetus became an important factor. This is a continuing theme in the increasingly dominant risk culture of modern obstetrics.

Political moves to regularise the practice of midwifery, instigated and controlled by the medical profession, brought about legislation that established the role of the midwife as a provider of care, but within strict boundaries. As well as limiting the midwives' role to attendance only at normal births, medicine served to control the profession of midwifery through control of their education and examinations (Boyle 2000). Even the earliest midwifery textbooks were written by doctors, so it is hardly surprising that the values of the medical profession have been ingrained in midwifery (Boyle 2000). This is mirrored in the current situation, where the rhetoric of obstetrics has become the rhetoric of the maternity services, with risk the central feature of service design and delivery (Scholefield 2005).

The twentieth century saw the greatest and most rapid advances in obstetric medicine and reproductive technology, mirroring advances in science and industry in general. The formation of the National Health Service (NHS) consolidated the medical status and control of pregnancy and birth, by assuming responsibility for the health of everyone, for the treatment of their illnesses, and for ushering them to and from this world. Thus the shift from home to hospital occurred at both ends of life, and any time in between when health was less than optimal.

Advances within the pharmaceutical industry added a new twist when contraceptive drugs became available, a positive and welcome option for large numbers of women, which led to women having more control over their own reproduction, but resulted in women having less personal experience of, knowledge of, and self-confidence in, giving birth. Women were no longer witnessing births within extended families. The growing complexity of childbirth management meant that women's knowledge, gained through personal experience and passed on to others, was less applicable to the newer, more medicalised approach, and meant placing more reliance on the 'experts' in the scientific paradigms of obstetrics (Simkin 1996). This led to the ascent of obstetrics beyond the sphere of lay people and the assumption by the medical profession of a paternalistic role to ultimately define what was best for childbearing women. This is clearly linked to the current situation, where obstetrics appears to have wed itself so firmly to the risk culture, which in turn is explicitly linked to the financial side of service provision.

Not all aspects of the medical management of pregnancy and birth are negative. Biomedicine has contributed to higher maternal and fetal survival rates due to a number of factors. The availability of safe blood transfusions has redressed a major risk factor in giving birth, namely the risk of haemorrhage. Medical and surgical advances, especially the use of general and spinal/epidural anaesthesia for caesarean section, mean that women and babies with complications can be treated effectively. Antibiotics have proved invaluable for the treatment of puerperal fever. The issue is not that medicine has no place within maternity care, but that *all* pregnancies are now medically managed; *all* of them are viewed as inherently pathological or risky, and normality is only ever defined in retrospect.

Another possible benefit of the medicalisation of reproduction is that women can be freed from biological determinism. Women have achieved some control over their reproductive activities through the availability of effective contraception, and can also benefit from the exponential development of reproductive technologies that help women with fertility problems to conceive and bear children. However, the ethics and parameters of the use of assisted fertility technologies is an ongoing debate that is becoming more topical as we move through the twenty-first century. It is here, in this century, that the emerging dominance of the risk rhetoric becomes a stark warning about medical hegemony allied with the bean-counting focus of modern NHS systems. Reduction of risk is aligned with cost reduction, and quality with standards; the experience of the individual, particularly of the woman giving birth, is invisible.

MIDWIFERY OR OBSTETRICS

A clear line of demarcation appears, both within the literature and within the culture of healthcare provision, between obstetrics and midwifery. This can be viewed through a critical, feminist lens, as a gendered split. The medical profession and its scientific philosophies can be seen historically as gendered male, but despite the increasing numbers of female doctors visible within obstetrics this situation has not changed. This divide in obstetrics sees midwives standing within the domain of the 'normal', while the obstetrician stands within the domain of the 'abnormal', in the form of medical conditions or complications affecting pregnancy or arising from it. However, in order to practise, the midwife must function within the dominant paradigm, and so must straddle this divide, working within obstetric frameworks increasingly structured around terminology such as 'risk', in which all pregnancies are viewed as more or less risk laden. The obstetrician/midwife divide appears to mimic the two competing models of childbirth, namely the biomedical/technocratic model and the natural/holistic model (Viisainen 2001).

However, it is the medical model that increasingly dominates all aspects of pregnancy and birth. Not only do the majority of births in the UK take place in hospitals, but midwives are trained within hospitals, and must become as conversant with the pathology of pregnancy and birth as with its natural processes. Midwives must understand the terminology of risk management, and be skilled in the use of medical technology and with medical and surgical procedures. This is in part due to the constant struggle for professional survival that midwifery must engage in. The 'experts' in normal birth can no longer solely concern themselves with the predominantly supportive role of the 'classic' midwife. In their drive to gain recognition as both a profession and an academic discipline, midwives have adopted the common understanding that scientific knowledge, developed through research, is superior to other forms of knowledge, being objective, impersonal, value-free, theoretical, generalisable and universal (Bjornsdottir 2001). This begs the question of how much such a reorientation has changed the very nature of the profession, and affected how birth is defined even within the realms of 'normality'.

One of the effects of this process of medicalisation and 'male-streaming' of midwifery and childbearing, with its associated surveillance and regulation, has been the emergence of a demand that in order for midwives to fulfil their role they must commit to midwifery at the expense of their personal and domestic lives (Ball, *et al.* 2002). A new stressor now exists for the 'professional midwife' as it seems that she must approach her work in the same way that men are expected to – as her primary occupation. Within UK maternity care there are some midwives who do this and other midwives who do not. The midwives who conform to a capitalist patriarchal model, ordering their lives into 'work first, family later' mode, are those who advance through the ranks of seniority most rapidly, and in these positions, rather than taking advantage of their power to influence the practice of obstetrics and midwifery for the greater benefit of all women, they ally themselves to the dominant preoccupations with risk, which continue to marginalise and undermine women's choices. Those who 'opt out', putting family life before work, are left out in the cold, and experience what Kirkham and Stapleton (2000) have described as 'horizontal violence' from colleagues who regard them as not complying with expected behaviours. These may be the midwives who most readily understand the unequal position of women within the maternity services, either as midwives or as mothers, or both. The medical model has imposed upon women a structure that makes the combination of motherhood and midwifery untenable unless she has a surfeit of family support and childcare. This reinforces the status of caring, cooperation and community within the birth arena as the lowest status of all. In other words, midwives have been disempowered by the institution and the system in much the same ways as have childbearing women. Even the ongoing professionalisation of midwifery is double-edged, because it demands of those training to enter the profession often-impossible levels of commitment, and this from cohorts of students increasingly composed of older women with families, children, and significant domestic responsibilities. Yet these very women often enter the profession through a desire to improve the experiences of childbearing women because they understand the significance of the transition to motherhood and the importance of the care women receive during this time. This kind of experiential knowledge is not recognised as a valid component of the overall evidence-based spectrum of midwifery and obstetrics.

INFORMED CHOICE?

It has long been a theme of maternity care that women should be offered informed choice, and that they should knowingly consent to all the care and interventions provided for them during their childbearing journey. However, while choice and consent are ongoing 'buzzwords' of the maternity services, midwives and obstetricians offer only an illusion of choice. Ultimately, a woman cannot exercise informed choice because the information that is given is controlled and restricted by the institution (i.e. the NHS), the medical profession, and the majority of midwives she will encounter. Furthermore, the information and descriptions that are provided to women do not allow them to exercise an informed choice, because the language can only be understood by the initiated (Foucault 1976).

Women are choosing medical interventions, and requesting caesarean sections for first pregnancies, not understanding the interventions, the procedures, or their implications for their childbearing experience and future health and fertility. True choice is not offered, and the only real options are those related to a technological labour and birth, because the concept of risk defines whether or not a woman can be 'allowed' to have a normal birth. Normal labour now consists of electronic monitoring of fetal heart rate, promotion of epidurals, and routine use of medical and surgical interventions to speed up the process. The key to all of these occurrences is the 'risk' associated with deviations from a standard or norm that is defined by the obstetric profession and implemented and enforced by the midwifery profession. Normal labour therefore involves removing the woman from her familiar surroundings and her usual support network, or informing her that if she deviates from the 'norm' she is under threat of this occurring. The woman is then placed in a clinical setting where every appliance, uniform and explanation speaks of science, medicine, doctors, and control and disempowerment. Choice, in this context, would not appear to be between natural and interventionist birth, but between normal medical labour and complicated medical labour.

What is most important is that midwives do not overlook the fact that it is women who give birth, and women are subject to the ongoing legacy of patriarchal systems, which have become entrenched within the new rhetoric of risk. The critical issue is that some women are choosing medical birth themselves, sometimes even elective caesarean births, because they too are being acculturated into a 'risk culture' that does not support any alternative choices.

RISK, RISK MANAGEMENT AND THE SURVEILLANCE AND REGULATION OF MATERNITY CARE

The notion of risk is central to the demarcation between midwifery and medical obstetrics. Women who are deemed low-risk (by parameters set by the medical profession) are the province of midwives, while any women deemed high-risk come under the management of obstetricians. There can be no doubt that women should receive the best possible care from the most appropriate personnel, and that they should be treated promptly and appropriately, and guidelines and structures that support this are the foundation of good maternity care. The difficulty for midwives with this view is that the foundations of maternity services are not solely built on impartial evidence, but on medico-patriarchal ideologies, which do not always recognise the 'people' element of the healthcare (and risk) equation. Student midwives are taught in terms of what is high risk, and what is low risk, and there seems to be no grading of risk between these two extremes other than what seem to be increasingly narrow parameters of low risk, and broadening parameters of what is considered high risk.

The centrality of risk as a concept has led to a reorientation of healthcare services around risk management. Risk management emerged from the industrial sector in response to reviews of major industrial disasters that identified what factors affected the outcomes, and what should have been done instead (Thompson and Owen 2005).

Within healthcare services, it arose first within the USA as a response to the pervasive influence of the legal profession and substantial litigation claims, and other Western nations subsequently followed suit (Thompson and Owen 2005). It began as a means of measuring 'adverse clinical events' and evaluating how well hospitals and other healthcare providers complied with risk management standards (Thompson and Owen 2005).

Cottee and Harding (2008) define risk management as 'a vital tool in preventing repetition of errors which are costly to patients, staff and institutions' (p. 155). This suggests a common goal that can be satisfied by managing risk, by controlling it. It also suggests that there is, within the obstetric and health services, the ability to control risk, even though those of us who work within these services are aware that risk reduction is the best that can be hoped for. Risk management and risk reduction (in obstetrics) is ultimately aimed at reducing the number of cases of litigation taken out against the maternity services, which continues to be a dominant proportion of those taken out against the NHS in general (Cottee and Harding 2008). All healthcare professionals are expected to understand and engage with the policies, practices and procedures of risk management in an effort to reduce these cases of compensation by ensuring that mistakes do not occur, that the best standards of care are given, and that all the guidelines have been adhered to. But the problem with this is that the guidelines are not developed within woman-centred or midwifery paradigms; they are developed within medical paradigms, using evidence-based practice protocols, which are in turn based on scientific evidence that does not encompass the human domain of childbearing. Systematic procedures have been introduced within the NHS and (with great enthusiasm) within the maternity services, which set specific questions and parameters of risk and risk management, and prescribe the procedures and actions that must be taken to address risk (Cottee and Harding 2008).

Midwives in the UK are accustomed to surveillance and regulation of their role, as the history of the profession demonstrates, but this has become embedded in practice and in the ideologies of the NHS through risk-oriented surveillance, explicitly linked to the aim of reducing the amount of clinical negligence insurance – in terms of premiums – payable by trusts. The Clinical Negligence Scheme for Trusts (CNST) is one such form of surveillance, and is viewed by many (perhaps rightly) as nothing more than ticking the right boxes to save the Trusts money (Thompson and Owen 2005). And after all, saving money would mean more resources for the patient, surely? Yet the resources that are most vital and most stretched – those at the frontline of care – may be further compromised by maternity departments' obsessive quests to achieve higher and higher standards of CNST appraisal, because it means they are then viewed as more successful by their Trusts. This may also represent a reorientation of midwifery philosophies towards viewing women in terms of risk rather than viewing them as individual women in the context of their differing lives and experiences. This may be in part due to the increasing awareness of the consequences of the near-misses and mistakes, which are highlighted through risk management, but also due to the ongoing erosion of the status of midwifery and the status of women in childbearing. This may be compounded by the socialisation of each successive generation of student midwives into these medicalised models of maternity care.

Risk is entrenched not only within the structures and discourses of the maternity services; all aspects of human endeavour now seem to reflect this obsession. Modern

technology – not only medical but also social and interactive technology, and information and communications technology – both reflects and augments the notion of risk.
The broadcast media, including web-based media, constantly focus on the dramatic
aspects of people's lives (and deaths) and in the case of birth dramas, focus on those
involving miraculous rescues, difficulties, and problems – the majority of which are
solved by obstetricians and other clinicians within acute hospital settings. During prime
viewing time on television, programmes (mostly American) are aired showing medical
birth stories, usually featuring hyped-up drama and tension masquerading as 'reality'.
Even in cases where the mother has planned for normal birth, the end result is usually
an emergency and their experience becomes that of a hospitalised, physician-controlled
birth. The women labour in bed, attached to electronic fetal monitors and oxytocin
drips. They have epidurals and when they do not have a caesarean, they deliver in the
lithotomy position. The fetus and its well-being are emphasised constantly, as is the use
of technology and medication. The UK-based programmes predominantly feature hospitals and hospital births, and highlight women who had aimed to have a natural birth
but were thwarted by nature, who then availed themselves of every obstetric service
available. These kinds of programmes reinforce the issue of risk as central to childbearing, and not only undermine women's confidence in their own ability to give birth, but
reinforce the medical control of women through their childbearing experience.

What are the effects on childbearing women of this repeated exposure to the
concepts of risk? First, they will inevitably view their pregnancies as inherently risky,
adhere to the party line, and come to believe that their pregnancies are fraught with
uncertainty, particularly for their unborn babies. Secondly, women will only view birth
from a medically-influenced perspective, in terms of risk, and so this kind of birth
becomes the norm. Such women are likely to then display a greater dependence on science and medicine to reassure and support them, and so will be complicit in the erosion
of their autonomy by the medical institution.

CONCLUSION

The modern environment of birth is the institution – the hospital, with its own set of
rules, standards of behaviour, language and technology. Risk and risk management are
rapidly becoming the dominant discourses within the obstetric domains of this institution. In order to function within such a system, the woman and her partner must
comply with and conform to the rules and standards, and their childbearing experience
is likely to become redefined for them in terms of risk, risk reduction and risk management. This somewhat negative approach, while laudable in terms of increasing patient
safety and positive clinical outcomes, does not address the psychosocial and individual
elements of birth, and leaves no room for non-scientific evidence or alternative modes
of birthing. Combating the entrenched norms of pregnancy and birth is a much greater
task than simplistic opposition to medical control, technological supremacy and practice
regulated by threats of risk-associated litigation, because becoming pregnant and giving
birth are complex social processes (Kent 2000). If clinical care is to be truly effective,
then it must be inclusive rather than exclusive, and should be the result of the contributory work of women who give birth, as well as those who seek to control it. But if
women are never exposed to true discourses of normality, and become proficient only
in the language of risk, there will be no opposition to medical control of the natural

processes of women's lives and bodies. Risk management is an important part of modern healthcare systems, particularly because of their complexity and the challenges of care delivery in such a context. But risk management is not the chief goal of midwifery. Being 'with women', supporting them, helping them to learn about and understand their bodies and their transition to motherhood, all in the context of women's social lives, these are the functions of midwifery. There is a need to develop a social model of birth that can intersect collaboratively with the obstetric model and meet the needs of all those requiring maternity care, whatever their associated 'risk'.

KEY POINTS

- Birth in the UK takes place within a Western medical scientific paradigm, increasingly influenced by concepts of risk and risk management.
- The divide between natural and medical birth reflects the gendered divide between obstetrics/midwifery and midwifery/motherhood.
- Women are increasingly exposed to medically dominated examples of childbearing, and so become acculturated into the obstetric 'risk' culture, perhaps to the detriment of normality within childbirth.
- Women do not have true choice and control with regard to their own childbearing. Only a reorientation of maternity care away from risk and towards a social model of birth and motherhood, with women as the central theme, would allow them to be true, informed partners in their care.

REFERENCES

Annandale EC, Clark J. (1996) What is gender? feminist theory and the sociology of human reproduction. *Sociol Health Illn.* 18: 17–44.

Ball L, Curtis P, Kirkham M. (2002) *Why Do Midwives Leave?* London: Royal College of Midwives.

Becker G, Nachtigall RD. (1992) Eager for medicalisation: the social production of infertility as a disease. *Sociol Health Illn.* 14: 456–71.

Björnsdottir K. (2001) Language, research and nursing practice. *J Adv Nurs.* 33: 159–66.

Boyle M. (2000) Childbirth in bed: the historical perspective. *Pract Midwife.* 3: 21–4.

Cahill HA. (2001) Male appropriation and medicalisation of childbirth: an historical analysis. *J Adv Nurs.* 33: 334–42.

Cottee C, Harding K. (2008) Risk management in obstetrics. *Obstet Gynaecol Reprod Med.* 18(6): 155–62.

Field PA. (1990) Effectiveness and efficacy of antenatal care. *Midwifery.* 6(4): 215–23.

Foucault M. (1976) *The Birth of the Clinic.* London: Routledge.

Haralambos M, Holborn M. (1995) *Sociology: themes and perspectives.* London: Collins Educational.

Illich I. (1976) *Limits to Medicine. Medical nemesis: the expropriation of health.* Harmondsworth: Penguin Books.

Kirkham M. (1989) Midwives and information giving in labour. In: Robinson S, Thomson A, editors. *Midwives, Research and Childbirth Volume 1.* London: Chapman and Hall.

Kirkham M, Stapleton H. (2000) Midwives' support needs as childbirth changes. *J Adv Nurs.* **32**: 465–72.

Kitzinger S. (1992) Birth and violence against women. In: Roberts H, editor. *Women's Health Counts.* London: Routledge; pp. 63–80.

Oakely A. (1990) Who's afraid of the randomised controlled trial. In: Roberts H, editor. *Women's Health Counts.* London: Routledge; pp. 167–94.

Scholefield H. (2005) Risk management in obstetrics. *Current Obstet Gynaecol.* **15**: 237–43.

Simkin P. (1996) Labour support: where has it been and where is it going? *Int J Childbirth Educ.* **14**: 22–3.

Thompson PJ, Owen JH. (2005) Risk management in obstetrics: just another inspection or improving patient care? *Fet Mat Med Rev.* **16**(3): 195–209.

Towler J, Bramall J. (1986) *Midwives in History and Society.* London: Croom Helm.

Viisainen K. (2001) Negotiating control and meaning: home birth as a self constructed choice in Finland. *Soc Sci Med.* **52**: 1109–21.

CHAPTER 12

Social support and childbirth

Christine McCourt

Social support has always been central to midwifery practice, but there is concern that its role has diminished in the recent past because of continuing fragmentation and medicalisation of care. The meaning of social support is broad and diffuse, making it difficult to define and study. Nonetheless, there is considerable evidence that levels of social support have a major impact on health and there are a number of theories and mechanisms that have been put forward to explain this. This chapter discusses the meaning of social support and related concepts, and reviews the theoretical underpinnings and research evidence as to its effectiveness. It also discusses the balance between professional interventions and ordinary sources of support, noting that the evidence does not always suggest that health professionals are the best providers of social support.

INTRODUCTION

... she was much better in a way because if there was any small problem bothering you, you go to the hospital or the GP, you think oh, should I tell her? This is what was bothering me, whereas a midwife comes to you, you are friendly and you talk to them, you have no fears or anything you can say to them, look there is something bothering me, how small it is. They don't make you feel as if you are wasting their time.

I suppose when you are pregnant you want to be, I don't think they pampered me as much as I would have liked. Although you could have five children, you still want to be seen to ... maybe they felt I knew everything and it was OK, just to leave me to get on with it. I sensed that anyway. I don't think it is they didn't care; there just wasn't a great urgency. Making sense?

These quotes, taken from a study of women's experiences of maternity care (McCourt and Pearce 2000: 149, McCourt, *et al.* 2000: 275) illustrate in a very direct way what is so important and so difficult to encapsulate about social support. They suggest that midwifery care is very important to women's feelings of being supported and that this, in turn, is important to their experiences of pregnancy, birth and early motherhood. They also illustrate how diffuse and difficult it is to define the concept, and how easily overlooked social support may be in modern maternity care.

The UK Government's National Service Framework for Children, Young People and Maternity Services (Department of Health 2004, Department of Health 2007) advocated extended roles for midwives in supporting the health of women and families. Midwives were seen as being in an ideal position to positively influence public health through their work with women before and around the time of birth. Pregnancy is acknowledged as a time when women are receptive and eager for health information and advice, and when they need particular support. This framework followed a shift in policy from the 1990s, towards attending to the issue of health and social well-being. In 1992 the House of Commons Select Committee on Maternal and Infant Health (House of Commons 1992) acknowledged some of the problems with changes that had taken place in maternity care during previous decades – such as the shift to hospital-based services – and advocated a broader, more 'joined-up' approach to policy and service provision. It noted that the influences on maternal and infant health are wider in scope than the traditional remit of healthcare, including social and economic conditions of family life. However, this emphasis was not picked up and put into practice initially. By the late 1990s, the importance of structural and social influences on health was more strongly acknowledged in government policy, and reflected in policy documents, such as Our Healthier Nation (Department of Health 1997b), which advocated a more structural and social-policy-oriented approach to health promotion. The importance of social support, and the cost of its neglect was really brought home to the UK government, however, by the 2004 report of the Confidential Enquiry into Maternal and Child Health, entitled Why Mothers Die (Lewis 2004). This report highlighted that the major causes of maternal death in the UK (and probably in many resource-rich countries) were now social exclusion, social disadvantage and mental health problems among women.

Much of the theoretical evidence supporting this shift in policy thinking rests on concepts such as those of social support, social inequality and more recently defined concepts such as social capital. This chapter focuses on social support and its relationship with the health of mothers and through this, their children. It explores the meanings and applications of the concept and the research evidence that underlines its importance. It then critically examines the historical and current relationship between the concept and the practice of midwifery and suggests some indications for the future of midwifery care.

WHAT IS SOCIAL SUPPORT?

Social support is a rather flexible concept – so broad that its meaning can easily be assumed, or bent to different purposes, rather than explicitly attended to. This produces problems in researching social support since the underlying assumptions or theoretical frameworks of the work are not always spelt out. Midwives often discuss social support as being essential to their role, and one of the things that distinguishes midwifery from obstetrics, beyond the traditional normal/abnormal division of labour that was instituted in the Midwives Act of 1902. The old English meaning of midwife – *mid wif*, meaning 'with woman' – is seen as a fundamental root of midwifery practice.

Consequently, much of the midwifery literature in recent decades has focused on the withdrawal of much of this supporting and 'presencing' role (Mander 2001) as services became increasingly organised around a fragmented, production-line model of hospital-centred care (Robinson 1990, Davis-Floyd 1994).

Social support has been defined as:

> . . . an exchange of resources between at least two individuals perceived by the provider or recipient to be intended to enhance the well-being of the recipient. (Schumaker and Brownell 1984: 13)

However, such a definition is so broad that it remains difficult to pinpoint what social support is, or is not. The problem with many definitions is that they may appear tautological, implying simply that social support is a relationship or action perceived as supportive. It is helpful, therefore, to break such general definitions down into different attributes. The simplest distinction commonly drawn is by describing social support as either emotional or practical. Key components of social support can be summarised as:

- **Emotional support** – the term implies a warm or caring relationship, but emotional support may be as simple as presence or companionship and willingness to listen. Some definitions include 'conveying esteem' and 'providing security' in emotional support.
- **Informational support** – providing good information and advice is widely perceived as being supportive. It underlies the ability to make positive choices, increases confidence and sense of security. It may also help to increase personal sense of control.
- **Practical or tangible support** – the type of practical or instrumental support may vary widely and its importance should not be underestimated. It may include financial support for a pregnant woman or physical comfort measures during labour and birth, for example.

Any of these attributes could reflect support provided by an individual (or individuals) or a network of relationships, which not only provides support but may also provide a feeling of membership in a group of people who share interests and social activities (Dykes, *et al.* 2003).

PERCEIVED AND RECEIVED SUPPORT

This distinction is useful since the effects of social support are likely to depend heavily on personal perception. Different people will view different things as supportive, influenced by personal circumstances and preferences as well as cultural and social factors that guide norms and expectations. For example, the needs of first and second time parents are likely to differ; some people may have adequate personal sources of support so they do not value professional support equally; some may perceive offers of support from professionals as intrusive while others may wish for much more professional support to be available. Additionally, to be experienced as positive, a means of support should not incur extra costs (such as excessive time, or demeaning the self) that would counter the intended benefits.

There is evidence from psychological research that support which is given, but not perceived as such, may be ineffective (Cohen and Wills 1985) or can even have negative effects. It is the perceived adequacy and appropriateness of support that has been found, in some studies, to relate positively to mental or physical health (Barrera 1986, Hirsch and Rapkin 1986). Indeed, a number of researchers since then have gone on to develop the theory that social support itself works particularly through people's perceptions – that feeling supported is a basic aspect of attachment that is fundamental for a person's sense of being esteemed or valued, and for their sense of agency or ability to control what happens to them.

Support is likely to be perceived negatively if it is overprotective or lacking understanding. In many instances, health professionals may offer support or care that is not helpful. Oakley, for example, in discussing the value of trials to test the effects of health and social interventions, cited several examples of interventions that were intended to help but had counter-productive effects (Oakley 1998). Such evidence is a useful reminder that social ties or relationships (personal or professional) cannot always be assumed to be beneficial. Similarly, offering interventions that raise expectations but do not meet them, may also be unhelpful. Such considerations have particular resonance for maternity care, which often fails to deliver the kinds and levels of support it seems to promise, particularly in postnatal services (Ball 1994, Garcia, *et al.* 1998, Proctor 1998, Beake, *et al.* 2006). Nonetheless, as this chapter will discuss, social support has been shown to be very important in maternity care, with both emotional and more practical forms of support being highly valued.

SOURCES OF SOCIAL SUPPORT

Sources of social support can be divided into two main categories: formal (e.g. professionals and paid helpers), and informal (e.g. family, friends, neighbours, community groups and so on).

It is important to remember that professionals are not the main source of social support, except for very isolated people. Abrams, in his seminal study of neighbourhood care (Bulmer 1986) argued that kin, friendships and neighbourhood relationships are of overwhelming importance in social support, and that public services should seek to facilitate such support networks where possible (and avoid undermining or by-passing them), and should consider focusing specific interventions on those who lack good support networks.

RELATED CONCEPTS
Care

The enduring importance of *care* in health service provision reflects the nature of health needs, including the need for social support. As Oakley has highlighted (1993), the use of the placebo (from the Latin 'to please') in medical research highlights the importance of providing care and support for people's health and illuminates the enduring importance of *care* as an aspect of all healing. The ways in which placebo effects have been understood in biomedicine reflect an artificial dichotomy between pleasing the patient and benefiting the patient. Evidence that levels of social support influence health outcomes cuts across such a dichotomy. However, *care* is often distinguished from *cure* as a way of encapsulating perceived differences between the roles of medicine and midwifery or nursing. Care is perceived as more holistic and long-term, an essential but undervalued aspect of healthcare, possibly due to its gendered nature.

Care has been described as having two key forms (Bulmer 1987, *see* also Leininger 1988):

- caring *for* – which may include physical tending or providing material and psychological resources, depending on the person's need, and
- caring *about* – which may not mean providing direct care but involves concern which is supportive, on an individual or a more general level.

From these definitions we can see that the concept of care is closely related to that of social support and such notions are often used interchangeably. However, care tends to imply something given or provided to a person – used in the sense of caring for – while social support may be more indirect.

Social capital

The term *social capital* refers to the kinds of resources that are essential underpinnings of social and community life. The use of the word *capital* draws on the notion that social relationships can be regarded as a kind of resource, without which people and communities are unable to function effectively and achieve well-being. Although the growing use of the term in much recent social policy has been critiqued (Morrow 2001) it can be argued that it represents an attempt to move away from more individualised approaches to health. For example, while UK Government policy for health promotion during the 1980s and early 1990s tended to locate health problems within the individual (Department of Health 1992) this was reformed in the late 1990s to focus more on the social conditions for health (Department of Health 1997a, b).

This more structural focus is reflected in a number of recent UK policy initiatives that are relevant to health. The New Deal for Communities, for example, funded regeneration schemes in deprived neighbourhoods that cut across institutional boundaries such as housing, leisure, employment, food, education and healthcare. Healthy Living Centres, while more specifically health focused, encompass a range of potentially health promoting facilities and activities that could be described as forms of social support. Similarly the Sure Start initiative is intended to promote the health and well-being of families with young children. The initiatives implicitly recognise the considerable evidence that the social networks and resources that people have available to them, not only personally but also within their local environment, can make a difference to health.

Social networks

The concept of social capital relies to some extent on earlier work of anthropologists and sociologists on social networks, through the theory that the extent and quality of social networks are related to the health of individuals and populations.

Network analysis has been useful for getting around the methodological problems incurred by asking people to rate their levels of social support in a way that is not simply tautological – where those with good health and well-being are more likely to rate their social support more positively. Network analysis requires researchers and respondents to be more specific about the relationships involved. Social networks can be classified or measured in various ways including:

•• extent – the number of ties or relationships and how far ranging they are
•• density or interconnectedness – the degree to which people in the network are linked to each other
•• quality – the nature and significance of relationships and whether close or distant
•• types – types of relationships involved, for example whether formal or personal
•• frequency – how often contacts are made
•• duration or durability – how stable relationships are
•• direction or symmetry – for example, whether relationships are mutual or involve dependency in one direction
•• reciprocity – the degree to which relationships are reciprocal, acknowledging that lack of balanced reciprocity can have negative effects on individuals' social status and self-esteem.

Individual and groups can be asked to map their relationships as networks using such principles to provide a detailed picture of the degree and kind of social support they may offer. Since effectiveness of different interventions may depend on the degree to which support is appropriately targeted, network analysis may be a useful tool for researchers or practitioners to explore where or what types of support are needed. Surkan, *et al.* (2006) for example used network mapping to study the relationship between social support and well-being, finding independent associations between both social support and social networks, and women's scores on postnatal depressive symptoms.

THEORIES OF SOCIAL SUPPORT

It is important to understand the nature of social support and how its effects may operate. There are several key theoretical frameworks for understanding potential mechanisms of effectiveness. Although they offer different, potentially competing theories, it is possible that, in explaining such complex phenomena, they are complementary.

The mechanisms by which social support 'works' – for example, to have a positive impact on health – are not clearly understood, but there is a great deal of evidence that they work on a number of levels. This should not be surprising since health is multi-faceted and influenced by a wide range of physiological, environmental and social factors. The approach of biomedicine has been rooted in a paradigm that tends to view such issues as separate. However, research into social support and health adds weight to the alternative view that such factors are closely inter-related: what some commentators have described as an ecological view of health (Arney 1982, Scheper-Hughes and Lock 1987).

Psychological theories

Psychological theories tend to be individually oriented – focusing on the impact of various influences on the perceptions, feelings and behaviours of individuals. Key psychological theories include the *stress buffering*, *coping* and *effect on health behaviour* hypotheses:
•• that social support acts as a buffer against stress (Cobb 1976)
•• that it assists the development of coping strategies that support health (Wheatley 1998)
•• that it influences behaviours that impact on health (Culpepper and Jack 1993).

Social support, therefore, is widely viewed as protective against the negative effects of psychosocial risk factors on health and is often mediated through responses to stress. The 'buffering' hypothesis suggests that psychosocial supports can help counter, or decrease the negative impact of risk factors (Wheatley 1998). Some recent commentators have argued that the person's sense of control is a key aspect of such buffering effects (Mander 2001).

Stress is part of everyday life, and is increased in periods of considerable change, such as pregnancy, changing home or job, or bereavement (Murray-Parkes 1971, Marris 1974) even where the change is viewed positively. Such psychological risk factors appear to play a role in reducing the person's ability to cope with stress, or encourage responses to stress that may not benefit health. For example, in a study of what influences women's health behaviour during pregnancy, Aaronson (1989) found that both perceived and received support had independent positive effects on women's ability to modify behaviours such as drinking alcohol or smoking, and in a more recent study, Cannella (2006) similarly found that social support was independently related to positive health practices in pregnant women. Another important theoretical strand comes from cognitive psychology: the view that beneficial effects of support are cognitively mediated. This theory proposes that perceptions of support may influence a person's interpretation of stressors, their knowledge of coping strategies and self-concept (Cohen and McKay 1983).

A number of recent studies have lent weight to psychological theories that social support helps to protect women from the negative effects of stress and difficult life events (Robertson, *et al.* 2004). Giurgescu, *et al.* (2006) for example, in a study of the relationships between social support, uncertainty and prenatal coping concluded that social support had a significant direct effect on preparation for motherhood. Strong associations have been found between levels of support, stress and incidence of problems such as ante- and postnatal depression, particularly in women with other risk factors and in adolescent mothers. Similarly, Howell, *et al.* (2006) in a cross-sectional study, found that women with a high level of depressive symptoms postnatally were more likely to be non-white, have lower income and educational qualifications, report less social support and have lower self-efficacy scores. Similar results were reported by Jesse, *et al.* (2005), who found higher levels of stress and lower levels of social support and self-esteem were associated with higher levels of depressive symptoms. Research focused on adolescent mothers in particular has highlighted the importance of the esteem aspects of social support to the well-being of new mothers (Gaff-Smith 2004, Harris 2006, Logsdon, *et al.* 2005, Nirattharadorn, *et al.* 2005).

Sociological theories

Sociological theories give greater focus on the influence of social and cultural environment on health and on the individual's capacity to cope with stressors and maintain healthy behaviours. Such theories are supported by a large body of evidence about the negative health effects of inequality and poor social and environmental conditions, which is discussed in more depth in Chapter 3.

In a sense, sociological theories build on rather than contradict psychological theories, and address some of the limitations of a more individually-oriented approach. It is likely that psychological theories underpin sociological ones by exploring and explaining ways in which the effects of social conditions may operate on the individual, and why some people may cope better with difficult conditions than others.

Different sociological theories suggest that social support:

- has a protective effect on health by making the experience of stress less likely in the first place
- can facilitate recovery from illness
- protects against the negative effects of psychosocial risk factors on health.

Again, these factors are likely to be linked and iterative, and therefore self-confirming. Broadhead and colleagues argued that social support is both an outcome of healthy social competence and a contributing cause of good health: those with good health or social resources are more likely to obtain social support, encouraging a cycle of positive health benefits (Broadhead, *et al.* 1983). Conversely, those who lack such social resources are less likely to be able to obtain the support they need. This is endorsed by research into maternity care that suggests socially disadvantaged women tend to receive poorer quality of support from service providers (McCourt and Pearce 2000, Lewis 2004, 2007). Similarly, Oakley's trial of social support for pregnant women suggested that women offered additional support were more likely to gain additional support from their partners (Oakley, *et al.* 1996).

Physiological theories

Research is beginning to identify complex physiological mechanisms for the relationships that have been identified between social support and health. These have immense potential value in breaking down the dichotomous approach to natural and social sciences that has tended to prevail in health research: the disjuncture between 'mind' and 'body' and between the 'social' and the 'physical' body. They address the question: given the considerable evidence that social support (or stress) affects people's health, how does this work within the body? The developing evidence supports those psychological and sociological theories that propose direct as well as indirect effects on people's health.

Much of the research is endocrinological, supporting the view that hormonal mechanisms play an important role in responses to stress or support, with direct long-term effects on health. Much of this work draws on the physiology of stress responses developed by Selye (1976). This work suggested that the physiological responses to stress, involving the hypothalamic–pituitary–adrenal axis, are normally protective: once the source of stress is removed, the body systems return to their normal level. However, with prolonged or chronic stressors, the prolonged exposure to raised levels of hormones such as cortisol can be damaging (Selye 1976). A full exploration of physiological theory is beyond the scope of this chapter; hence it focuses on some key examples of research that is informative with regard to social support and pregnancy.

Anxiety and umbilical cord blood flow

Teixeira, *et al.* (1999) investigated the physiological relationship between anxiety and low birthweight by looking at the potential impact of raised anxiety levels on umbilical cord blood flow. Drawing on evidence from endocrinology, they hypothesised that raised anxiety levels resulting in increased levels of stress hormones, such as noradrenaline, would restrict blood flow from the mother; such a mechanism could account, at least in part, for low birthweight, since blood flow has a direct effect on fetal development. Such an effect would work in a similar way to smoking, which has been shown to have a negative influence on fetal blood supply and on birthweight. They found significant associations between anxiety levels and umbilical cord blood flow, supporting the hypothesised relationship between stress, anxiety and low birthweight.

The authors noted in their discussion that it was unclear how strong the associations were with current or long-term anxiety – since most women with raised anxiety had high scores on both trait (general) and state (current feelings) levels. This would have implications for considering social support interventions: if long-term anxiety is the key factor, the effects of short-term interventions in pregnancy may be limited.

Possible hormonal factors: oxytocin

There is considerable indirect evidence to suggest a complex relationship between stress and anxiety, and the hormone oxytocin, which plays an important role in pregnancy and labour. Animal studies have suggested that oxytocin itself may have an anxiety-reducing effect, but also that stress levels may affect the synthesis of oxytocin in the body (Uvnas–Moberg 1998). Research on childbirth suggests relationships between anxiety, oxytocin synthesis and women's needs for oxytocic augmentation of labour and pharmacological pain relief (Haddad 1989). Such findings have led to increasing interest in the possible role of endogenous oxytocin on anxiety and pain threshold during pregnancy and labour, and in specific interventions to enhance oxytocin synthesis during the latter half of pregnancy. The evidence of a relationship between anxiety levels and oxytocin suggests that interventions would need to be directed towards reducing women's anxiety – through their responses to stress and the life events and difficulties that contribute to raised anxiety.

Role of massage

Physiological experiments have also shown that a variety of sensory stimuli such as touch – including massage and baby holding – have endocrinological effects that decrease blood pressure and stress responses. Historically, massage has been used by traditional birth attendants and a variety of therapists in a wide range of cultures. Jordan (1993) cites the example of the Mayan traditional midwife who massages the woman's abdomen during pregnancy and labour. Many midwives and mothers in the UK use massage to provide comfort, relaxation and pain relief during pregnancy and labour. Additionally, a number of massage specialists now teach infant massage techniques to mothers and there is a growing body of research evidence to suggest benefits for mother–infant interaction, especially for premature babies. The evidence of effects on pregnancy and childbirth is more limited, but some small trials have found beneficial effects of massage on pain in a range of groups (Field, *et al.* 1997, Kimber, *et al.* 2008). Some studies also found differences in anxiety levels between groups receiving massage and control groups. Kimber, *et al.*'s pilot randomised, controlled trial found differences in women's sense of control during childbirth. While massage may have direct effects (e.g. through synthesis of oxytocin), its influence may also be indirect and mediated through effects on stress and anxiety that result in secondary hormonal responses.

RESEARCH ON SERVICE USERS' VIEWS OF SOCIAL SUPPORT

In researching perceptions of social support Gottlieb (1978, cited in Oakley 1992) found that what ordinary people valued most were:

- emotionally sustaining behaviours – for example, listening, showing concern, conveying intimacy
- problem solving behaviours – for example, material and financial help.

Similarly, studies of women's experiences and perceptions of pregnancy and birth are highly consistent in indicating what they see as supportive maternity care, namely:
- good communication – not only being given information but also being listened to
- being treated as individuals – feeling known and understood
- being given a sense of choice and control over what happens to them
- being given a sense of trust and confidence both in themselves and those caring for them
- perceiving professionals as sensitive and caring (e.g. Oakley 1993, Green, *et al.* 1988, Brown and Lumley 1994, Proctor 1998, McCourt, *et al.* 1998, McCourt and Stevens 2006).

Studies of women in different social classes and ethnic groups (Handler, *et al.* 1996, Laslett, *et al.* 1997, Hirst, *et al.* 1998, McCourt and Pearce 2000, Harper-Bulman and McCourt 2002) suggest that such core principles are relevant to a wide range of women, rather than confined to an articulate minority. Women's specific concerns about support do vary, however, as do their specific experiences of healthcare, with many women in minority groups, for example, experiencing greater communication problems with service providers, and women in lower social class groups receiving poorer information from service providers (Reid and Garcia 1989, McLeish 2005, Walker, *et al.* 1995).

In a survey of Finnish mothers' perceptions of maternity care, Tarkka and Paunonen (1996) found that in pregnancy, women saw partners, family and friends (respectively) – rather than professionals – as their main sources of support. However, midwives were the most important source of support during birth. The support given by midwives in labour was valued most in the domain of affect (emotional support), and this was also associated with positive birth experiences. Issues particularly important to mothers' experience were:
- their reception and treatment by staff
- encouragement
- sense of security
- alleviation of pain
- individuality of treatment
- continuity.

In a USA study by Bryanton, *et al.* (1994) of mothers' views of maternity support, the women regarded all the categories of help as important, but behaviours categorised as emotional support were perceived as the most helpful. These were:
- feeling cared about as an individual and treated with respect
- praise
- staff appearing calm and confident
- assistance with breathing and relaxing.

A study of Hong Kong Chinese women's views of labour support, by Yin-King, *et al.* (1998), highlighted the degree to which the perceived supportiveness of particular behaviours may vary culturally. As in many other studies, information and emotional support rated most highly, with tangible support the least. In keeping with Chinese cultural norms about presentation of self, being praised was rated most highly, while being touched was rated as least helpful.

EFFECTS OF SOCIAL SUPPORT: THE PSYCHOLOGICAL EVIDENCE

In an overview of evidence on the health effects of social support, Cobb interpreted social support as information leading the subject to believe that he [sic] is cared for and loved, that he is esteemed and valued and that he belongs to a network of communication and mutual obligation (Cobb 1976: 300). Drawing on Nuckolls' research on pregnancy as a significant life event, Cobb suggested that the interaction of levels of social support and levels of stressful life events is crucial. In Nuckolls' study of 'army wives' it was the group with both high levels of 'life change' and low levels of social support who had an excessive level of pregnancy and birth complications. Women with high support had significantly fewer complications. For women with low levels of 'life change', levels of support appeared to matter less (Nuckolls, *et al.* 1972). A study of asthma patients using a similar methodology showed comparable effects: patients with high 'life change' and low social support scores needed significantly higher doses of steroids to control their symptoms. Patients with high 'life events' but high levels of support did not need more medication than those with lower 'life event' scores – suggesting a protective effect of support (de Araujo, *et al.* 1973).

In another study reviewed by Cobb (1976), Egbert and colleagues randomised surgical patients to two groups one of which received additional supportive care from the anaesthetist in a way that was concealed from the surgeons involved. They found this group needed lower levels of pain relief and were discharged earlier than the control group (Egbert, *et al.* 1964). This replicated similar findings obtained for children undergoing tonsillectomy (Jessner, *et al.* 1952). The findings of such early studies have been established in healthcare principles to the extent that not providing patients, including children, with appropriate information is widely regarded as poor practice.

EFFECTS OF SOCIAL SUPPORT: THE SOCIOLOGICAL EVIDENCE

A seminal sociological study pointing to the effects of social support was the Brown and Harris (1978) study of women and depression. The authors found a very high prevalence of depression among women, particularly those at home with young children and those not in paid work. On this basis, they hypothesised that much depression among women has social origins and is linked to social isolation and lack of support.

A series of qualitative studies by Oakley also highlighted the problems associated with women's gender roles and the impact of social isolation on many women as housewives and mothers (1979, 1980). These studies led Oakley to investigate further the issue of social support, with a trial of the effects of social support in pregnancy, which is discussed below.

In her account of this trial, Oakley (1992) reviewed a range of studies providing evidence that social support influences physical and psychological health. Among these, a large-scale, community-based study of patterns of mortality in the USA (Cohen and Syme 1987) showed that long-term survival was correlated with social support independently of other potentially related factors such as initial physical health, social status or habits like smoking. Generally, social involvement predicted better survival, although the types of involvement that mattered differed for men and women.

In an early qualitative study of 41 middle- and upper-class mothers, Abernethy (1973) examined the effects of a tight or loose social network in predicting a woman's attitude to her children and her response to the demands of the maternal role. She concluded that women in loose networks appeared to suffer from insufficient feedback and were therefore likely to be exposed to a confusing variance in childrearing theory. Women embedded in a tight network were more likely to have confidence in their maternal competence, while those in loose networks were more likely to be frustrated by motherhood and to feel unsure of how to relate to their children.

As will be seen in the following section, such studies highlight that social support is far broader than the remit and power of health services – the most important sources are likely to be in people's personal and community networks and these vary greatly. Hence the findings of studies of the impact of maternity care may vary according to the nature of the support offered and how it is targeted and received.

EFFECTS OF SOCIAL SUPPORT: THE MIDWIFERY EVIDENCE
Pregnancy
An early overview covering 14 trials of social support interventions in maternity care identified key features associated with increased support:
- reduced anxiety (e.g. confidence, nervousness, fear or positive feelings regarding birth)
- reduced psychological and physical morbidity
- increased satisfaction with care and communication (in most cases)
- increased sense of control (Elbourne, *et al.* 1989).

There was no significant impact on labour interventions or outcomes, but the authors concluded that, given the positive impact of social support on women's feelings about pregnancy and birth, and the lack of negative effects found in these trials, such support should be seen as integral to good maternity care, rather than some kind of optional extra. They highlighted that increasing fragmentation of care and obstetric focus in services had made this more difficult.

Following this, a series of trials were conducted to consider the potential impact of social support in pregnancy on birthweight (Oakley, *et al.* 1990, Oakley 1992, Oakley, *et al.* 1996, Villar, *et al.* 1992, Norbeck, *et al.* 1996). Birthweight has been repeatedly selected to test the effects of social support since it is seen as a relatively reliable, valid and readily measurable indicator of maternal and infant health (Barker 1998).

The intervention tested in Oakley and colleagues' trial was a series of home visits by research midwives plus telephone support offered to women with a previous low birthweight baby (<2500g). The study also used a range of secondary outcome measures that were possible indicators of maternal and infant well-being and gathered both quantitative and qualitative data.

Although the study did not find a statistically significant increase in birthweight there were fewer very low birthweight babies, fewer antenatal hospital admissions, a lower use of epidural pain relief, more spontaneous labours, and more spontaneous vaginal births. There was no significant difference in the number of babies needing special care, but those in the support group required less invasive resuscitation methods and less intensive care. Mothers reported better physical health for themselves and their babies, and less use of health services, six weeks after birth. Their views were positive about the intervention, emphasising the importance of the midwife listening to them.

In a long-term follow-up study – something that is unusual due to difficulties with finance and keeping in touch with research participants – mothers reported fewer health problems in their children, fewer concerns about their social well-being, greater personal well-being and greater ability to obtain social support from others, particularly their partners (Oakley, *et al.* 1996).

Although this study indicated certain benefits of social support it had a number of drawbacks that highlight the difficulty of conducting trials to test the effects of complex interventions, especially of concepts such as social support that may be poorly defined and extend far beyond the reaches of healthcare. Not least, it did not establish a significant difference in the primary outcome measure chosen – incidence of low birthweight.

In the Cochrane overview of trials studying the association between birthweight and social support intervention in pregnancy, Hodnett and Fredericks (2003) found no evidence of significant differences in perinatal outcomes, but did find a reduced rate of caesarean births overall, and improvements in immediate maternal psychosocial outcomes, or increases in uptake of pregnancy termination, in those trials that included such measures. Their discussion raised a number of cautionary points:

- such interventions are short-term and may not be adequate to counter the well researched effects of poverty and social disadvantage on health
- the underlying mechanisms linking social support to health outcomes are still not well understood
- researchers' ability to identify and include the women at most risk, and most likely to be helped by such support, is limited
- the trials covered a wide range of interventions all classed as social support – including education and practical help – some of which may not have been perceived as supportive by the recipients.

These cautions are illustrated well by a large multi-centre Latin American trial of effects of social support on birthweight (Villar, *et al.* 1992), which was included in the review's meta-analysis. The support was home-based, provided by social workers, included an educational focus as well as support, and targeted towards women at high 'psychological and social risk' (Langer, *et al.* 1996). This was conceived as an ecological model of social support where health education and social support would function synergistically. No difference in birthweight was found. However, women's views of the intervention were not specifically studied and it was not clear whether they perceived the intervention to be supportive. Langer and colleagues concluded from their trial that psychosocial interventions solely during pregnancy and on a scale possible within public services in poorer countries, would not counter the adverse effects of psychosocial distress. In another included trial (Spencer, *et al.* 1989) the majority of those randomised to additional social support did not accept it, suggesting that not all interventions trialled were perceived as supportive, or were truly accessible by the intended recipients.

Discussing the differences found in caesarean birth rates, Hodnett and Fredericks

(2003) noted the similarity of this finding to those on caregiver support during labour, discussed below. In relation to termination of pregnancy, they hypothesised that increased information and awareness might have accounted for women making different decisions.

In another overview – of trials of home visitation programmes offering support to socially disadvantaged mothers – Bennett, *et al.* (2007) found few differences in outcomes. The studies reviewed were disparate in aims, nature of the intervention and outcome measures and they noted that the visits may not have been sufficient, or sufficiently well targeted, to make a difference. Many socio-economically disadvantaged parents, for example, do not need help with parenting. This might especially apply in countries like the UK where there already is a universal home-visiting service, provided by health visitors and targeted to some degree at those needing more support. In countries like the USA, where there is not a universal service, they observed that the interventions were limited and visits tended to be geared towards teaching parenting skills – interventions that perhaps do not address the underlying issues affecting child outcomes, such as poverty. They quoted the authors of one trial (Hardy and Streett 1989) who concluded their intervention was too limited and short term to make a difference, and noted that the home visitors often entered general crisis situations – such as threat of eviction or loss of electricity supply – which they were not able to address. The reviewers, therefore, questioned whether the interventions studied were 'fit for purpose'.

A parallel review of home visiting support for teenage mothers (Macdonald, *et al.* 2007) found somewhat more evidence of benefits. For example, in two trials, mothers were significantly more likely to have returned to education at the end of the study period. In the one trial that measured this, their infants had improved physical growth (Field 1982) and they also scored more highly on motor and mental development. In another trial, the Elmira Study (Olds, *et al.* 1998), mothers reported significantly fewer problems of crying, conflict and scolding their infants and long-term follow-up suggested lower documented incidence of child injury, abuse and neglect, while in the Memphis study (Olds, *et al.* 1998, 2004) mothers showed less punitive attitudes towards their infants.

The finding of differences was possibly because these studies focused on a group with more specific disadvantages, and the programmes appeared to be more intensive and practical than those offered in the adult-mother studies. Additionally, all but one of the studies were based in the USA, where universal home-based support is not provided. Nonetheless, the authors drew similar conclusions about the need for such intervention studies to clarify more carefully their underlying assumptions and the nature and extent of the interventions offered. They noted, for example, that although the results of the Field (1982) study showed some evidence of benefits, in another arm of this study mothers who were given training placements as teachers' aides in the medical school nursery had even better outcomes than the home-visiting group.

Several descriptive studies have looked at the impact of peer support – with encouraging findings. The 'Mentoring Mothers Program' studied by Navaie-Waliser, *et al.* (1996) trained mature local women as volunteer mentors to young socially-disadvantaged pregnant women within a continuing caring one-to-one relationship. The programme targeted three communities known to have a high incidence of low-birthweight and recruited 42 volunteers. It was described as a community-empowering approach.

Although this was not a trial – so had no formal comparisons – the outcomes for the mothers involved were positive in the light of general outcomes for this community and they reported a decrease in sense of isolation. Additionally, they reported positive responses from the volunteer women themselves, including enhanced self-esteem and motivation. Although not designed to formally test the outcomes of an intervention, the study provides an example of the way in which professionals can facilitate the provision of ordinary sources of social support within a community, in a way that may be more enduring than any health service-based intervention.

Labour and birth

A number of trials have also tested the potential impact of labour support on birth outcomes, including continuous support during labour by lay (doula) or professional companions.

In a Cochrane review of trials of continuous support in labour, Hodnett, *et al.* (2007) looked at the impact of *continuous* one-to-one support, either by trained or untrained people. Elements of such support included emotional support, information and comfort measures. The review included 16 trials in a wide range of cultural and medical settings, some of which excluded other companions. The meta-analysis showed:

- reduced duration of labour
- lower likelihood of medication for pain relief
- lower rate of caesarean birth
- higher rate of spontaneous vaginal birth
- less dissatisfaction with birth.

In addition, some trials found evidence of:

- lower use of electronic fetal monitoring
- fewer women feeling lack of control
- less postnatal depression, anxiety and difficulty in mothering.

Subgroup analysis (to control for factors such as different environmental conditions) showed that benefits tended to be greater when the supporter was not a member of hospital staff, where companions were not routinely permitted, and in settings where epidural pain relief was not routinely available. Differences were also stronger where support had begun before the onset of active labour. The reviewers noted that it was not possible to identify particular underlying reasons for these differences, but they noted that it may be more difficult for social support to make a difference in environments where labour is routinely actively managed. Similarly, they noted that professional care providers may be influenced by factors such as divided loyalties, competing work demands, self-selection, and the constraints of institutional policies and routine practices.

The review included two early and influential trials in Guatemala in a busy public hospital where companions were not normally admitted and one-to-one professional support was not the norm (Sosa, *et al.* 1980, Klaus, *et al.* 1986).

Klaus and colleagues' (1986) trial, which replicated the earlier study on a larger scale, included healthy women admitted, without a companion, in early but established labour. Those randomised to the intervention group were supported by a doula while control group women received standard care. They found significant reductions in the duration and augmentation of labour, caesarean sections, admission to the neonatal unit and perinatal complications. Additionally, regression analysis suggested that the effects were greater in women living alone. The study indicated that very large differences could be achieved with 'poor women who routinely undergo labour alone on a crowded ward' (Klaus, *et al.* 1986: 586).

The trial was then replicated in a North American (USA) context, in a busy, obstetrically oriented unit with high prevailing intervention rates but greater access to pain relief. As in the Guatemalan context, it included a large proportion of women who were socially disadvantaged and non-English speaking. The labour supporters were bilingual local women with personal experience of a normal birth, who were given three weeks of preparation. Similar results were obtained (Kennell, *et al.* 1991).

This study included both an observed group without support (observed unobtrusively by a researcher) and a control group assessed by review of hospital notes after birth. Interestingly, similar differences, but of a smaller magnitude, were found between the control group with review of notes only and the group observed by a researcher. This unexpected finding suggested that even continuous presence, without active engagement or support, could have a protective effect although the authors noted that the reason for this difference was unclear – and could equally be explained by the researcher's presence having an effect on hospital staff behaviour.

A similar trial in Canada by Hodnett and Osborn (1989) examined the impact of continuous support by a familiar, trained caregiver, using self-employed 'coaches' who were either 'lay' or student midwives. This Canadian teaching hospital cared for mainly white, middle class women, who were routinely allowed the companionship of their husband or partner. As in the US unit there was a high level of routine intervention in labour, but good staff-to-patient ratios. The study found significant reductions in use of pain relief medication and episiotomy but not in major outcomes such as mode of birth. The authors noted the difficulty of conducting such a trial in a context where actively managed and accelerated labour was the norm: only 8 of 103 women included in the trial laboured with no intervention.

The findings of this overview highlight the need to take context as well as type of intervention into account when studying the effects of social support. In the later trials in more 'developed' medical settings, the women selected were not those likely to be in the highest need of social support from professionals, and companions were normally allowed, but the settings also placed limitations on the capacity of supportive care to influence interventions in birth.

MODELS OF MIDWIFERY AND MATERNITY CARE

The report Changing Childbirth (Department of Health 1993) advocated a shift in the organisation of maternity care to enable a more woman-centred approach. Recognising the impact of fragmentation of care on women's experiences, a number of schemes were piloted to improve continuity of care and carer. Studies of such schemes suggest that continuity of care and carer are important to women's feelings that care is supportive.

An overview of trials of continuity of carer indicated beneficial effects on use of pain relief and episiotomies and women were more satisfied with their care (Hodnett 2000). Continuity of midwifery carer is often provided in models of care that also introduce midwife-led care for those women on the midwife's caseload who are of low medical risk. Consequently, a subsequent Cochrane review focused on midwife-led care, including continuity of midwife carer, which identified similar and additional benefits such as reduced rates of antenatal admission and early fetal loss, and women feeling greater sense of control (Hatem, *et al.* 2008). Other studies indicate that greater continuity in the relationships between mothers and midwives facilitates mothers' confidence in the midwife and in themselves (McCourt, *et al.* 2006). In interviews, mothers described the importance of a known midwife being with them throughout labour and birth in terms of feeling understood and respected, being relaxed and confident, and feeling comforted (McCourt and Stevens 2006). Women who lacked such continuity of support were more likely to describe feelings of anxiety, fear and confusion in their accounts of pregnancy and birth, and this was particularly the case for those who were socially disadvantaged or in minority groups, who tended to receive less information and less supportive care in the health services.

It could be argued that these mothers' accounts are primarily about feeling supported by their midwife carers, support that should be achievable by ensuring a consistent approach rather than needing known carers – or simply by 'good midwives'. However, the relative lack of such accounts by women receiving shared or conventional consultant-led maternity care, suggest that the supportive or caring qualities of midwives cannot be readily separated from the organisation and environment of their work. The manner in which services are organised and provided may have an important impact on the levels or forms of support that midwives are able to offer women.

Postnatal support

A number of studies have indicated the importance to women of postnatal social support, but also the lack of supportive care found in current health systems. The major study by Ball (1994) highlighted how hospital practices often worked *against* the provision of social support. These included:

- unnecessary separation of mother and baby soon after birth
- (once maternal–infant bonding was recognised as an issue) 'rooming in' coupled with loss of practical support
- fragmentation of care
- task- rather than person-based work and routines
- didactic style when giving help or advice
- care focused mainly on physical examination of the mother and feeding of the baby
- inadequate support for breastfeeding.

Compounding this, she found a mismatch between midwives' summing up of women's emotional states and their more specific comments, for example, on the numbers of women who had been crying or showing sleep or appetite disturbances – suggesting that they either see this as 'normal' or give low priority to emotional states.

Her study showed that emotional well-being and satisfaction with motherhood were associated with:

- antecedent factors (in the woman's own background for example)
- other stress factors
- self-confidence on return home.

The experience of 'other stress factors' was strongly influenced by postnatal care prac-tices, the key factors being feelings at the time of birth, self-image in feeding the baby in hospital and conflicting advice or lack of rest in hospital.

What is particularly disappointing is that studies conducted since then (Garcia, *et al.* 1998, Beake, *et al.* 2006, Redshaw, *et al.* 2006), suggest little change in postnatal care despite Changing Childbirth policy (Department of Health 1993).

A number of maternity interventions have been piloted to offer additional postnatal support to women, such as the home-visit schemes reviewed by Bennett, *et al.* (2007) and discussed above. This evidence is limited in its applicability, however, as most were in the USA where there is no routine postnatal midwifery home care and they tended to be geared towards prevention of child abuse, and child health or service utilisation problems, and only rarely focused on general psychosocial or physical health effects for mothers. Nonetheless, some schemes using the skills of experienced mothers living in local communities may provide less expensive and more culturally sensitive support than professional, hospital-based programmes.

A recent trial in the UK of additional postnatal visits by a support worker (Morrell, *et al.* 2000) did not result in any significant differences in women's psychological or general health, or in breastfeeding rates. As with studies of antenatal care and low-birthweight, this study provides a caution against assuming that additional sup-portive maternity care will necessarily make a significant impact on women's health. However, like some of those trials, the intervention was not targeted towards women who lacked ordinary sources of support. It might be argued that additional support offered to those who do not need it may decrease or at least delay their ability to take up the informal sources of help available to them. Similar warnings may be found in the research on breastfeeding, which has suggested that professional support is not necessarily or always helpful or effective (Renfrew, *et al.* 2000). In contrast, a trial of a more focused and flexible approach to postnatal midwifery care (MacArthur, *et al.* 2002) identified significant differences in outcomes for mothers, including reduced postnatal depression symptoms, when midwives used several tools to assess the type and level of women's needs, and were then given the scope to design flexible care packages accord-ing to need, for up to three months. The more positive findings of this study suggest that postnatal social support may be most effectively provided through a service that is both universal – routinely available to all – and flexible, so that it can be centred on each individual's needs.

CONCLUSIONS

This brief overview has indicated that social support is an important concept, with clear implications for health and general well-being and highly relevant to maternity care. Midwives' have traditionally combined a number of roles focused on supportive care around the transitional period of childbirth, However, socio–medico–political changes throughout the twentieth century have undermined the degree to which 'support' has been integral to the midwife's role (Tew 1998, Mander 2001).

This chapter has discussed how the concept of social support is very difficult to define or measure – despite the considerable evidence of its fundamental importance in health and healthcare. But it is the very flexibility and breadth of the concept that may be an undeniable aspect of its power. On the one hand, such concepts need to be 'unpicked' so that they can be viewed critically and researched effectively, but on the other hand such unpicking may undermine their integration of a range of functions and thereby hinder effective analysis. Additionally, it must be recognised that the highly subjective meaning of support, for the recipient, is a crucial aspect of its effectiveness. What is supportive for one person may not be so for another, even though clear patterns can be discerned and have been demonstrated in the research on women's experiences of maternity and healthcare.

Related concepts, such as reciprocity, are highly relevant here since they show that being the receiver of a gift or service can mean loss of power or status, unless the form of reciprocity is appropriately balanced (Benson and Carter 2008). This provides a warning to health professionals that 'giving' – providing services – is not as straightforward a 'good' as it might appear. It may also explain the degree to which the evidence reviewed in this chapter suggests that 'lay' or 'peer' models of support may be as effective, if not more so, than professional models. This suggests that professional thinking about ways of providing support needs to change, and should be increasingly geared towards underpinning, facilitating and promoting non-professional sources and towards more individualised approaches that can be easily tailored to individuals' needs. Additionally, the needs should be identified in partnership with the person, since the evidence shows that social support is strongly linked to subjective perceptions. The concept of social capital – the networks and social cohesion of local communities or other social groups – is also relevant here, but critical work on social capital highlights the difficulties of aiming for community empowerment amongst people who are substantially deprived. High levels of deprivation undermine people's capacity to form, sustain and participate in networks of support. Nonetheless, networks of support have been shown to be important to well-being.

The research on mechanisms of social support is building up a picture of ways in which it may work to enhance health, or at least reduce the negative health effects of a range of stressors or threats. Such work also demonstrates clearly a traditional rationale of midwifery – that mind and body are not separate and that effective care must address physiological, psychological and environmental factors in an integrated fashion – what is often called 'holistic care'.

The varied and sometimes disappointing findings of research on the effectiveness of health professional interventions to offer social support, highlight the need for caution in planning services. It is tempting, for professionals and policy makers, to see social support interventions as solutions to what are often structural and deep-rooted problems, such as social inequality. Such interventions might instead be seen as complementary to social policies to support good housing, education, employment, nutrition and a range of community resources and facilities. It is also tempting for professionals and policy-makers to design and deliver what they see as needed support, rather than taking the more complex approach of involving individuals and communities in designing and delivering support interventions.

While planners are presented with challenges of targeting and designing support interventions appropriately, and researchers with continuing to tease out and identify what seems to work best, and for whom, it seems wise to echo Elbourne's (1992) sentiments – that support should be seen, quite simply, as part of providing good midwifery care. That this is not always the case, and for all women, is the challenge to midwives in the twenty-first century.

KEY POINTS

☞ The concept of social support is broad and difficult to define, and careful attention to definitions and meanings is needed when researching the effects of interventions.

☞ There is evidence for a positive impact of some maternal health interventions, especially those targeted towards mothers with low social support and perceived as supportive by mothers themselves.

☞ Appropriate social support has a positive impact on general health and well-being.

☞ Professionals should remember that most of the social support is provided by friends, family and community, not by professionals or formal interventions.

☞ Organising and providing midwifery care in different ways can have an important impact on the levels of supportive care provided.

REFERENCES

Abernethy VD. (1973) Social network and response to the maternal role. *Int J Sociology Family.* **3**: 86–92.

Arney W. (1982) *Power and the Profession of Obstetrics.* Chicago: University of Chicago Press.

Ball J. (1994) *Reactions to Motherhood: the role of postnatal care.* Cambridge: Cambridge University Press.

Barker DJP. (1998) *Mothers, Babies and Health in Later Life.* Edinburgh: Churchill Livingstone.

Barrera M. (1986) Distinctions between social support concepts, measures, and models. *Am J Community Psychol.* **14**(4): 413–45.

Beake S, McCourt C, Bick D. (2006) Women's views of hospital and community-based postnatal care: the good, the bad and the indifferent. *Evidence Based Midwifery.* **3**(2): 80–6.

Bennett C, Macdonald GM, Dennis J, *et al.* (2007) Home-based support for disadvantaged adult mothers. *Cochrane Database Syst Rev.* **3**: CD003759.

Benson M, Carter D. (2008) Nothing in return? Distinctions between gift and commodity in contemporary society. *Anthropol Action.* **15**(3): 1–7.

Broadhead WT, Kaplan BH, James SA, *et al.* (1983) The epidemiological evidence for a relationship between social support and health. *Am J Epidemiol.* **117**(5): 521–37.

Brown GW, Harris T. (1978) *Social Origins of Depression: a study of psychiatric disorder in women.* London: Tavistock.

Brown S, Lumley J. (1994) Satisfaction with care in labor and birth: a survey of 790 Australian women. *Birth.* **21**(1): 4–13.

Bryanton J, Fraser-Davey H, Sullivan P. (1994) Women's perceptions of nursing support during labor. *J Obstet Gynecol Neonatal Nurs.* **23**(8): 638–44.

Bulmer M. (1986) *Neighbours: the work of Philip Abrams.* Cambridge: Cambridge University Press.

Bulmer M. (1987) *The Social Basis of Community Care.* London: Allen and Unwin.

Cannella B. (2006) Mediators of the relationship between social support and positive health practices in pregnant women. *Nurs Res.* **55**(6): 437–45.

Cobb S. (1976) Social support as a moderator of life stress. *Psychosom Med.* **38**(5): 300–14.

Cohen S, McKay G. (1983) Social support, stress and the buffering hypothesis: a theoretical analysis.

In: Baum A, Singer JE, Taylor S, editors. *Handbook of Psychology and Health, Volume 4*. Hillsdale, NJ: Erlbaum.

Cohen S, Syme L. (1987) *Social Support and Health*. New York: Academic Press.

Cohen S, Wills TA. (1985) Stress, social support, and the buffering hypothesis. *Psychol Bull*. **98**: 310–57.

Culpepper L, Jack B. (1993) Psychosocial issues in pregnancy. *Primary Care*. **20**(3): 599–619.

Davis-Floyd R. (1994) The ritual of hospital birth in America. In: Spradley JP, McCurdy DW. *Conformity and Conflict: readings in cultural anthropology*. New York: Harper-Collins.

De Araujo G, van Arsdel PP, Holmes TH, *et al.* (1973) Life change, coping ability and chronic intrinsic asthma. *J Psychosom Res*. **17**(5): 359–63.

Department of Health. (1992) *The Health of the Nation*. London: HMSO.

Department of Health. (1993) *Changing Childbirth (Cumberledge Report): the report of the expert advisory committee*. London: HMSO.

Department of Health. (1997a) *The New NHS: modern, dependable*. Cmd 3807. London: Department of Health.

Department of Health. (1997b) *Our Healthier Nation: a contract for health*. Cmd 3852. London: The Stationery Office.

Department of Health. (2004) *National Services Framework for Children, Young People and Maternity Services*. London: The Stationery Office.

Department of Health. (2007) *Maternity Matters: choice, access and continuity of care in a safe service*. London: The Stationery Office.

Dykes F, Moran VH, Burt S, *et al.* (2003) Adolescent mothers and breastfeeding: experiences and support needs: an exploratory study. *J Hum Lactation*. **19**(4): 391–401.

Egbert LD, Battit GE, Welch CE, *et al.* (1964) Reduction of post-operative pain by encouragement and instruction of patients. *N Engl J Med*. **270**: 825–7.

Elbourne D, Oakley A, Chalmers I. (1989) Social and psychological support during pregnancy. In: Chalmers I, Enkin MW, Keirse MJNC, editors. *Effective Care in Pregnancy and Childbirth*. Oxford: Oxford University Press; pp. 221–35.

Field T, Hernandez-Reif M, Taylor S, *et al.* (1997) Labour pain is reduced by massage therapy. *J Psychosom Obstet Gynaecol*. **18**(4): 286–91.

Field T, Widmayer S, Greenberg R, *et al.* (1982) Effects of parent training on teenage mothers and their infants. *Pediatrics*. **69**(6): 703–7.

Gaff-Smith M. (2004) Attachment, self-esteem and social support in rural adolescents during pregnancy and early motherhood. *Birth Issues*. **13**(4): 139–45.

Garcia J, Redshaw M, Fitzsimons B, *et al.* (1998) *First Class Delivery: a national survey of women's views of maternity care*. Abingdon: Audit Commission/National Perinatal Epidemiology Unit.

Giurgescu C, Penckofer S, Maurer MC, *et al.* (2006) Impact of uncertainty, social support and prenatal coping on the psychological well-being of high-risk pregnant women. *Nurs Res*. **55**(5): 356–65.

Green JM, Coupland VA, Kitzinger JV. (1988) *Great Expectations: a prospective study of women's expectations and experiences of childbirth*. Cambridge: Childcare and Development Group, Cambridge University.

Haddad F. (1989) Effect of anxiety in pregnancy. *Contemp Rev Obstet Gynaecol*. **1**: 123–32.

Handler A, Raube K, Kelley MA, *et al.* (1996) Women's satisfaction with prenatal care settings: a focus group study. *Birth*. **23**(1): 31–7.

Hardy JB, Streett R. (1989) Family support and parenting education in the home: an effective extension of clinic-based preventive healthcare services for poor children. *J Pediatr*. **115**(6): 927–31.

Harper-Bulman K, McCourt C. (2002) Somali refugee women's views and experiences of maternity care in West London: a case study. *CPH*. **12**(4): 365–80.

Harris JG. (2006) *Self-esteem, Family Support, Peer Support and Depressive Symptomatology: a descriptive correlational study of pregnant adolescents*. Pittsburgh, PA:Georgia State University. Health Sciences Library System; Publication #3208769.

Hatem M, Sandall J, Devane D, *et al.* (2008) Midwife-led versus other models of care for childbearing women. *Cochrane Database Syst Rev.* **4**: CD004667.

Hirsch BJ, Rapkin BD. (1986) Social networks and adult identities: profiles and correlates of support and rejection. *Am J Community Psychol.* **14**(4): 395–412.

Hirst J, Hewison J, Dowswell T, *et al.* (1998) Antenatal care: what do women want? In: Clement S, editor. (1998) *Psychological Perspectives on Pregnancy and Childbirth.* Edinburgh: Churchill Livingstone.

Hodnett ED. (2000) Continuity of caregivers for care during pregnancy and childbirth. *Cochrane Database Syst Rev.* **4**: CD000062.

Hodnett ED, Fredericks S. (2003) Support during pregnancy for women at increased risk of low birthweight babies. *Cochrane Database Syst Rev.* **3**: CD000198.

Hodnett ED, Gates S, Hofmeyr GJ, *et al.* (2007) Continuous support for women during childbirth. *Cochrane Database Syst Rev.* **3**: CD003766.

House of Commons. (1992) *Maternity Services: government response to the second report from the health committee, Session 1991–2.* London: HMSO.

Howell EA, Mora P, Leventhal H. (2006) Correlates of early postpartum depressive symptoms. *Matern Child Health J.* **10**(2): 149–57.

Jesse DE, Walcott-McQuigg J, Mariella A, *et al.* (2005) Risk and protective factors associated with symptoms of depression in low-income African American and Caucasian women during pregnancy. *J Midwifery Wom Heal.* **50**(5): 405–10.

Jessner L, Blom GE, Waldfogel S. (1952) Emotional implications of tonsillectomy and adenoidectomy on children. *Psychoanalytic Study Child.* **7**: 126–69.

Jordan B. (1993) *Birth in Four Cultures: a cross-cultural investigation of childbirth in Yucatan, Holland, Sweden and the United States.* Long Grove, IL: Waveland Press.

Kennell J, Klaus M, McGrath S, *et al.* (1991) Continuous emotional support during labour in a US hospital: a randomised controlled trial. *JAMA.* **265**(17): 2197–201.

Kimber L, McNabb M, McCourt C, *et al.* (2008) Massage or music for pain relief in labour: a pilot randomised placebo controlled trial. *Eur J Pain.* **12**(8): 961–9.

Klaus MH, Kennell JH, Robertson SS, *et al.* (1986) Effects of social support during parturition on maternal and infant morbidity. *BMJ.* **293**: 585–7.

Langer A, Farnot U, Garcia C, *et al.* (1996) The Latin-American trial of psychosocial support during pregnancy: effects on mothers' well-being and satisfaction. *Soc Sci Med.* **42**(11): 1589–97.

Laslett A, Brown S, Lumley J. (1997) Women's views of different models of antenatal care in Victoria, Australia. *Birth.* **24**(2): 81–9.

Leininger MM. (1988) *Caring: an essential human need.* Detroit, MI: Wayne State University Press.

Lewis G, editor. (2007) *Saving Mothers' Lives: reviewing maternal deaths to make motherhood safer – 2004–2005.* The Seventh Report of the Confidential Enquiries into Maternal Deaths in the United Kingdom. Confidential Enquiry into Maternal and Child Health (CEMACH). London: CEMACH. Available at: www.cemach.org (accessed 12 Mar 2009).

Lewis G, Drife J, editors. (2004) *Why Mothers Die: 2000–2002.* The Sixth Report on Confidential Enquiries into Maternal Deaths in the United Kingdom. CEMACH. London: RCOG Press.

Logsdon MC, Birkimer JC, Simpson T, *et al.* (2005) Postpartum depression and social support in adolescents. *J Obstet Gynecol Neonatal Nurs.* **34**(1): 46–54.

MacArthur C, Winter HR, Bick DE, *et al.* (2002) Effects of redesigned community postnatal care on womens' health 4 months after birth: a cluster randomised controlled trial. *Lancet.* **359**(9304): 378–85.

Macdonald G, Bennett C, Dennis J, *et al.* (2007) Home-based support for disadvantaged teenage mothers. *Cochrane Database Syst Rev.* **1**: CD006723.

Mander R. (2001) *Supportive Care and Midwifery.* Oxford: Blackwell.

Marris P. (1974) *Loss and Change.* London: Routledge and Kegan Paul.

McCourt C, Hirst J, Page L. (2000) Dimensions and attributes of caring: women's perceptions.

In: Page L, editor. *The New Midwifery: science and sensitivity in practice*. Edinburgh: Churchill Livingstone.

McCourt C, Page L, Hewison J, *et al.* (1998) Evaluation of one-to-one midwifery: women's responses to care. *Birth*. 25(2): 73–80.

McCourt C, Pearce A. (2000) Does continuity of carer matter to women from minority ethnic groups? *Midwifery*. 16: 145–54.

McCourt C, Stevens T. (2006) Continuity of carer: what does it mean and does it matter to midwives and birthing women? *Canadian Journal of Midwifery Research and Practice*. 4(3): 10–20.

McCourt C, Stevens T, Sandall J, *et al.* (2006) Working with women: continuity of carer in practice. In: Page L, McCandlish R, editors. *The New Midwifery: science and sensitivity in practice*. 2nd ed. Oxford: Churchill Livingstone.

McLeish J. (2005) Maternity experiences of asylum seekers in England. *Br J Midwif*. 13(12): 782–5.

Morrell CJ, Spiby H, Stewart P, *et al.* (2000) Costs and benefits of community postnatal support workers: a randomised controlled trial. *Health Tech Assess*. 4(6): 1–100.

Morrow G, editor. (2001) *An Appropriate Capital-isation? Questioning social capital*. London: London School of Economics.

Murray-Parkes C. (1971) Psychosocial transitions: a field for study. *Soc Sci Med*. 5: 101–15.

Navaie-Waliser M, Gordon SK, Hibberd ME. (1996) The mentoring mothers program: a community-empowering approach to reducing infant mortality. *J Perinat Educ*. 5(4): 47–58.

Nirattharadorn M, Phancharoenworakul K, Gennaro S, *et al.* (2005) Self-esteem, social support and depression in Thai adolescent mothers. *Thai Journal of Nursing Research*. 9(1): 63–75.

Norbeck JS, DeJoseph JF, Smith RT. (1996) A randomised trial of an empirically-derived social support intervention to prevent low birthweight among African American women. *Soc Sci Med*. 43(6): 947–54.

Nuckolls KB, Kaplan BH, Cassel J. (1972) Psychosocial assets, life crisis and the prognosis of pregnancy. *Am J Epidemiol*. 95: 431–41.

Oakley A, Hickey D, Rajan L, *et al.* (1996) Social support in pregnancy, does it have long-term effects? *J Reprod Infant Psychol*. 14: 7–22.

Oakley A, Rajan L, Grant A. (1990) Social support and pregnancy outcome: report of a randomised controlled trial. *Br J Obstet Gynaecol*. 97: 155–62.

Oakley A. (1979) *Becoming a Mother*. Oxford: Martin Robertson.

Oakley A. (1980) *Women Confined: towards a sociology of childbirth*. Oxford: Martin Robertson.

Oakley A. (1992) *Social Support and Motherhood: the natural history of a research project*. Oxford: Blackwell.

Oakley A. (1993) *Essays on Women, Medicine and Health*. Edinburgh: Edinburgh University Press.

Oakley A. (1998) Experimentation in social science: the case of health promotion. *Soc Sci Health*. 4(2): 73–88.

Olds D, Henderson C Jr, Kitzman H, *et al.* (1998) The promise of home visitation: Results of two randomized trials. *J Community Psychol*. 26(1): 5–21.

Olds DL, Kitzman H, Cole R, *et al.* (2004) Effects of home-visiting on maternal life course and child development: age 6 follow-up results of a randomized trial. *Pediatrics*. 114: 1550–9.

Proctor S. (1998) What determines quality in maternity care? Comparing the perceptions of childbearing women and midwives. *Birth*. 25(2): 85–93.

Redshaw M, Rowe R, Hockley C, *et al.* (2006) *Recorded Delivery: a national survey of women's experience of maternity care*. Oxford: National Perinatal Epidemiology Unit.

Reid M, Garcia J. (1989) Women's views of care during pregnancy and childbirth. In: Chalmers I, Enkin M, Keirse M, editors. *Effective Care in Pregnancy and Childbirth*. Oxford: Open University Press.

Renfrew M, Woolridge MW, Ross McGill H. (2000) *Enabling Women to Breastfeed: a structured review with evidence-based guidance for practice*. London: The Stationery Office.

Robertson E, Grace S, Wallington T. (2004) Antenatal risk factors for postpartum depression: a synthesis of recent literature. *Gen Hosp Psychiatry*. 26: 289–95.

Robinson S. (1990) Maintaining the role of the midwife. In: Garcia J, Kilpatrick R, Richards M, editors. *The Politics of Maternity Care*. Oxford: Clarendon.

Scheper-Hughes N, Lock MM. (1987) The mindful body: a prolegomenon to future work in medical anthropology. *Med Anthropol Q.* **1**: 6–41.

Schumaker S, Brownell A. (1984) Towards a theory of social support: closing conceptual gaps. *J Soc Issues*. **40**(4): 11–36.

Selye H. (1976) *Stress in Health and Disease*. London: Butterworth.

Sosa R, Kennell J, Klaus M, *et al.* (1980) The effect of a supportive companion on perinatal problems, length of labour, and mother–infant interaction. *N Eng J Med*. **303**: 597–600.

Spencer B, Thomas H, Morris J. (1989) A randomised controlled trial of the provision of a social support service during pregnancy: the South Manchester family worker project. *Br J Obstet Gynaecol*. **96**(3): 281–8.

Surkan PJ, Peterson KE, Hughes MD, *et al.* (2006) The role of social networks and support in postpartum women's depression: a multiethnic sample. *Matern Child Health J*. **10**(4): 375–83.

Tarkka MT, Paunonen M. (1996) Social support and its impact on mothers' experiences of childbirth. *J Adv Nurs*. **23**(1): 70–5.

Teixeira J, Fisk N, Glover V. (1999) Association between maternal anxiety in pregnancy and increased uterine artery resistance index: cohort-based study. *BMJ*. **318**: 153–7.

Tew M. (1998) *Safer Childbirth? A critical history of maternity care*. 3rd ed. London: Chapman and Hall.

Uvnas-Moberg K. (1998) Anti-stress pattern induced by oxytocin. *News in Physiological Science*. **13**: 22–5.

Villar J, Farnot U, Barros F, *et al.* (1992) A randomised trial of psychosocial support during high-risk pregnancies. *N Engl J Med*. **327**: 1266–71.

Walker J, Hall S, Thomas M. (1995) The experience of labour: a perspective from those receiving care in a midwife-led unit. *Midwifery*. **11**(3): 120–9.

Wheatley S. (1998) Psychosocial support in pregnancy. In: Clement S, editor. *Psychological Perspectives on Pregnancy and Childbirth*. Edinburgh: Churchill Livingstone.

Yin-King L, Holroyd E, Pui-yuk LW, *et al.* (1998) Hong Kong Chinese women in labour: implications for midwives. *Pract Midwife*. **1**(11): 26–8.

CHAPTER 13

Fathers and childbirth

Tim Blackshaw

Historically, fathers have played a variable role in the birth and aftercare of their children, but currently, fathers attend the birth of their children in unprecedented numbers. This chapter describes how industrialisation and the hospitalisation of birth contributed to both the absence and the subsequent attendance of fathers at births. Socio-cultural and historic contexts and discourses that have contributed to the present levels of attendance, are explored. In critically examining the how and why of fathers' birth attendance, emphasis is placed on the possible consequences that may accrue from attendance. These include the impact that attendance may have on the parents' sexuality and well-being, the possibility of a relationship between fathers' attendance and the increased incidence of instrumental deliveries, and what parents and healthcare professionals think about fathers attending the birth. Finally, a brief discussion will examine how fathers feel midwives can best help them in supporting their partner.

INTRODUCTION

Not so long ago, most fathers-to-be would have spent the hours preceding their child's birth in a state of banishment. They might have been found pacing the well-worn carpet of some maternity unit waiting-room, striding up and down a hospital corridor chain-smoking, or down at the 'local', waiting for a telephone call, protected from the perceived gruesome reality of childbirth. Indeed, where 'Dad' was and what he was doing when you were born passed into family folklore, as may be the case for some readers of this chapter.

However, for those younger readers with children, it is far more likely that the father was present at the birth. Furthermore, the younger the reader, the greater the likelihood that the father was both present and actively involved throughout the pregnancy (Smith 1999b). This could be dismissed as a vaguely interesting anecdote were it not for the fact that the increase in the number of fathers attending and participating at the birth of their children has been meteoric over the last 40 years. Furthermore, it is globally and historically unprecedented (Burgess 1997a). In the past, fathers who wanted to attend the birth were regarded as potentially deviant, and only 5% of fathers attended hospital births in the 1950s (Smith 1999a). Today, attendance is seen as *de rigueur* (Newburn 2000), with 97% of fathers attending hospital births in the 1990s (Smith 1999b). Watts goes so far as to describe this as a 'badge of manhood' (1995: 59).

This transformation has been supported by a number of interested parties, including the Maternity Alliance, the Fatherhood Institute and the National Childbirth Trust, and it has the New Labour Government seal of approval. In demonstrating its backing for a more 'hands-on' approach to fatherhood, the Government has funded the largest ever survey of first-time fathers in the UK – *Becoming a Father* (National Childbirth Trust 2000). The survey portrays some fathers as feeling poorly informed, unsupported and ignored by health professionals, despite their desire to be involved from the beginning of the pregnancy. The Government has responded by announcing that its proposed £100 million improvement and refurbishment of maternity units will include facilities for fathers and families (Carlowe 2001).

The absentee father is now a rarity – a 'statistical deviant'. In the present consumer-orientated health service, healthcare professionals would want to be certain that they could justify the exclusion of a father from the birth of his child. Although the changing professional and societal attitudes are clear, the transformation has not gone unopposed. Childbirth has been regarded by some as one of life's great mysterious experiences from which fathers since the beginning of time should be excluded. For others, concern is expressed in terms of stereotypes that rest upon the propensity for fathers to faint, panic, behave inappropriately – e.g. wielding a camera/camcorder – (Thomas 2000) or require support from the midwife that should be going to the woman in labour.

The leading polemicist of the 'anti-fathers-at-the-birth movement' is a French obstetrician, Dr Michel Odent. He believes that men are emotionally unintuitive and too rational during the labour, thereby impeding women from getting on with the primal business of giving birth. Fathers, he posits, distract their partners, which leads to a delay in the birth, resulting in women requiring more analgesia, more interventions such as epidurals, and more caesarean sections (Boseley 2000).

In order to gain a balanced perspective it is necessary to examine the interplay between cultural and social change in the attitudes of men and women with regard to men's involvement at the birth. The beliefs, values and attitudes of fathers, their partners, midwives and other health professionals are critically examined. In contextualising the father's birth experience, a range of social science perspectives is used with a view to addressing what is said to be the important question. Is the presence of fathers at the birth a good thing, and if so, for whom? However, what will best enable readers to draw their own conclusions are the *how* and the *why* of fathers' birth attendance.

The chapter begins with a social historical account and a comparative cultural overview of fatherhood, fathers and birth attendance prior to the twentieth century. It then examines how the rise of the biomedical model in obstetric practices and new social movements and discourses transformed the birth process and fathers' birth attendance throughout the twentieth century to the present time. Finally, the consequences of the new orthodoxy of fathers' attendance are examined.

FATHERHOOD AND THE SOCIAL CONTEXTS OF BIRTH

For thousands of years and in the majority of cultures, women have facilitated the birth process (Turner 1995). Fathers have been absent for two key reasons, namely, the manner in which gender and parental roles have been socially constructed, and specific cultural taboos relating to women, pregnancy and birth within particular social contexts. However, fathers' absence from the *birth* does not mean that they were not in the vicinity of the birth or actively involved both physically and emotionally.

Anthropologists have documented the diversity of received beliefs that exist among differing cultures about conception, pregnancy and birth. Hahn and Muecke (1987) call such belief systems the *birth culture*. This birth culture informs a society's members about the nature of conception, the proper conditions of procreation and childbearing, the nature of pregnancy and labour, and the rules and rituals of pre- and postnatal behaviour.

Globally, the presence or absence of fathers at the birth can be partly explained by reference to the birth culture of the particular social group. Anthropological work has largely focused on the differences between fathers in industrialised and low- or non-industrialised societies. In so doing, anthropologists and historians have demonstrated that birth cultures in non- or low-industrialised contexts are predominantly derived from lay and/or theological bodies of knowledge (Helman 1993). Kitzinger (2000) notes that the core cultural values of societies are revealed in the beliefs and rituals surrounding birth and death. The more technologically orientated a society is, the more technological the birth culture will be.

For fathers in Western society (with the exception, to this day, of the Netherlands), it was the onset of modernity in the late eighteenth century, with the advent of industrialisation, that heralded the demise of the home and its environs as the place of work and living. Fathers' (and later mothers') workplaces were increasingly geographically distinct from the home. Furthermore, salaried work was more and more a contributory factor in the gendering of social roles, relationships and identities (Burgess 1997a). This, together with an increase in cultural secularity, facilitated the rise of a medicalised scientific discourse concerning conception, pregnancy and specifically the place and process of birth (Mishler 1981).

As such, it marks the beginning of the absent father. As late as the 1960s, fathers were commonly refused admission to hospital births, and in 1975 one in three obstetricians still excluded fathers (Burgess 1997a). However, this does not mean that British fathers had not wished to or had not attended births prior to this time. Nor indeed was it necessarily the case that they had limited parental input, contrary to the popular image of the father in times past.

FATHERS, FATHERHOOD AND BIRTH ATTENDANCE: PRE-MODERNITY

In order to explain why birth was primarily a 'women–only' business until the mid-eighteenth century, it is necessary to understand the ways in which the roles of men and fathers have been socially constructed, and to identify the ideologies and belief systems that underpin these constructions.

The ways in which masculinity and fatherhood have been constructed by differing discourses and ideologies have shaped men's perceptions and behaviour during pregnancy, birth and subsequent paternal activity in terms of childcare and domestic labour.

Burgess (1997a) describes images of the father and fatherhood that were prevalent during the last few centuries, from the distant, godly patriarch of pre-enlightenment times to the distant, rational patriarch of the enlightenment. There is also the gradual emergence (post industrialisation) of the 'new dad', from the playful post-war father to the so-called co-parent of the 1990s.

Although there is a lack of hard data on what fathers in past times did with regard to birth, labour and child rearing, the diaries, journals and writings of just a few hundred fathers offer us what Burgess (1997a) describes as a tantalising glimpse into their lives. She suggests that general trends emerge, and specifically the patterns of paternal involvement. At present there are no official central UK Government records documenting fathers' birth attendance (Draper 1997).

For example, Ralph Josselin, a seventeenth-century English country vicar, noted in his diary all manner of details about the progress of his babies. He specified the dates, time and circumstances of their births, even noting when he and his wife had decided to wean their babies, and his feelings about the death of his young son (MacFarlane 1970).

In his novel *Amelia* (published in 1751), the English novelist/dramatist Henry Fielding describes conflicting ideas as to what men should be doing during the labour:

> I thought the best husbands looked on their wives lying-in as a time of festival and jollity. 'What! Did you not even get drunk in the time of your wife's delivery? Tell me honestly, how did you employ yourself at this time?' 'Why then honestly', replied he, 'and in defiance of your laughter, I lay behind her bolster and supported her in my arms.' (Kitzinger 1987: 150)

The writings of Josselin and Fielding would appear to challenge some of the stereotypical images of the father of past times. From these and other historical texts, several observations can be made as to how social and working life prior to industrialisation impacted broadly on fathers as parents, and more specifically their availability and location during labour and birth.

The most striking observation is the day-to-day availability of the father. This, at different periods in time, occurred for several reasons. From the time of the Tudors most families' incomes were partly derived from piecework, with only a minority of parents working away from the home. This symbiotic relationship between domestic and economic organisation required the presence of the parent(s) to create and maintain the family and home as an economic unit.

The late seventeenth century saw the rise of retailing occupations as a source of income. Once again the family was the agency of training, with the home and business being either geographically close to each other or one and the same. It is reasonable to assume that younger children, given the lack of formal schooling, would play or work around their fathers for most of the day: 'Playing in the village street and fields . . . hanging around the farmyards . . . thronging the churches . . . crowding around the cottage fires'. Laslett (1983) notes that 'the perpetual distraction of childish noise and talk must have affected everyone almost all of the time'.

Even a well-to-do household with servants did not prohibit paternal involvement. In 1668, the Earl of Lauderdale offered a graphic description of the night his daughter gave birth, his wife being ill in bed. He notes that he was in:

... troublesome governance going to and from one sick to another [At this point his newly born grandson] took convulsions and the smallpox ... Sure I slept little [because] my babe Charles slept ill all night, was most impatient for the breast, and was in cruel heat [and] all this while the mother and grandmother knew nothing, for the physician positively forbade it ... I sent my excuse to the King, compelled by my wife's sickness and my daughter's lying-in to stay here. (Pollock 1983)

Lewis-Stempel (2001) has documented the existence of childcare manuals that were written in the sixteenth and seventeenth century specifically for fathers. This is not surprising given that between 1599 and 1811, a quarter of children under 16 years of age lived in lone-father households, and one-third of the fathers managed without any live-in female help (Burgess 1997b).

Furthermore, architectural evidence does not support the myth that prior to the late nineteenth century all children of the rich were raised in a nursery wing, separate from their parents (Hardyment 1982). The worlds of work and social interactions were family focused, with the nature of the built environment creating close proximity between fathers and children. In most homes there was no separation between adult and child space, or for that matter between working, eating and sleeping space. This is significant, given that until the earlier part of the twentieth century the home was the place of birth.

Although it should be emphasised that these examples in no way represent what all men were doing, they do indicate that social life prior to industrialisation was such that men were likely to be involved in family life, domestic labour and, to varying degrees, the birth of their children. By the 1920s, through the medicalisation of birth, male obstetricians were increasingly controlling of the mother, excluding the father, and prescriptive with regard to the place of birth and the dynamics of the parents' relationship and roles, specifically during labour.

RITES AND RITUALS: BIRTH CULTURE AND THE TRANSITION TO FATHERHOOD

Although in most Western birth cultures the contemporary trend is increasingly one of fathers regarding it as their 'right' to attend the birth, in other cultures this is not the case, and childbirth and pregnancy remain both physically and socially female events. However, as in the case of pre-industrial Britain, the exclusion of the father does not mean the absence of physical or emotional involvement for him.

In many birth cultures the father's involvement takes the form of enacting specific ritual tasks during the pregnancy, birth and postpartum period. Such tasks are performed in order to protect the mother and child and facilitate an easier delivery. Heggenhougan (1980) calls these tasks *ritual couvade* (*couvade* is derived from the Basque-Spanish word *couver*, meaning 'to brood or hatch') (Helman 1993). The father is required to observe certain taboos. In some societies the parents follow similar taboos, with the father often supporting the mother during labour. In other societies he may take to his bed during labour, but subsequently take care of and 'mother' the baby.

In societies where the father is present at the birth, his role is invariably functional, with the ritual tasks being viewed as integral to the birth process. For example, tasks may take the form of rituals designed to distract or lure away evil spirits until the baby is safely delivered. Linguistically, in societies where childbearing is regarded as involving both parents, the phrase 'to bear a child' is applied to men as well as women (Helman 1993).

Some examples of 'ritual couvade' incorporate the belief that by enacting specific rituals the father is creating his child's spirit/soul. Rivière (1974) cites an extreme example in which the mother is perceived as a mere vessel or conduit for the baby, whereas the father is considered to be the sole creator of the baby. In addition, rituals have protective functions and also facilitate the expression of empathy for the mother and baby.

Rituals exist in all societies, and are a means by which humans structure, maintain and reproduce social life. Furthermore, they facilitate the management of potentially dangerous and polluting phenomena, and in essence allow for the creation of order in the presence of 'chaotic nature' (Douglas 1966). Okely (1983) states that for British traveller-gypsy men and fathers, birth is viewed as a major source of potential 'pollution'. Therefore it is common practice that if the birth takes place in obstetric units (which are regarded as already polluted), the father does not attend or participate, even to the extent of not subsequently discussing the birth with the mother.

Some rituals are specific to social transitions, such as becoming a father. Van Gennep (1960) called these rituals 'rites of passage'. Such rituals connect the changes in the human life cycle to the attendant change in the social hierarchy, thus uniting the physical and social aspects of the individual's biography. Rites of passage have three stages, namely rituals of separation, transition and incorporation. In essence, 'ritual couvade' can be regarded as 'rites of passage', facilitating/celebrating the transitional journey into fatherhood (Lester and Moorsom 1997). This transition begins in pregnancy, moving through birth and into new fatherhood (Goldberg 1988). Utilising Van Gennep's concepts, these rituals are illustrated in relation to contemporary fatherhood in Figure 13.1.

Seel (1987) has suggested that fathers' attendance in Western birth cultures is a modern *couvade* ritual. As social and family structures have changed during the last 50 years, there has been a decline in 'traditional' ritual practices, a proliferation of divorce, and the reconstitution of families. The father's presence at the birth is now seen as an official way of announcing paternity (Hearn 1984).

In 1968, the anthropologist Mary Douglas forecast that these changes in family structure would lead to fathers increasingly being present at the birth of their children. Although this theory had a pertinence at the time, she could not have foreseen the impact that DNA analysis would have in effectively establishing paternity, nor could she have predicted the widespread acceptance of cohabitation. However, neither of the above has deterred fathers from attending births. An interesting exception to this trend is to be found in Japan, where most women leave their partner and return to their mother's home before the birth (Boseley 2000).

Fathers in the UK and other Western societies are increasingly participating in antenatal classes as well as breastfeeding and natural childbirth workshops. While some regard these activities as appropriate manifestations of Western 'ritual couvade' behaviour (National Childbirth Trust 2000), for others they are merely 'fashion' statements (Heiney 1986, Eagle 1988). During the last 20 years, research into an age-old phenomenon called *couvade syndrome* has suggested that such rituals, whether old or

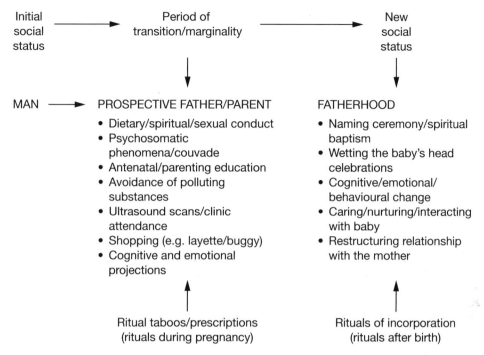

Initial social status → Period of transition/marginality → New social status

MAN → PROSPECTIVE FATHER/PARENT — FATHERHOOD

PROSPECTIVE FATHER/PARENT
- Dietary/spiritual/sexual conduct
- Psychosomatic phenomena/couvade
- Antenatal/parenting education
- Avoidance of polluting substances
- Ultrasound scans/clinic attendance
- Shopping (e.g. layette/buggy)
- Cognitive and emotional projections

FATHERHOOD
- Naming ceremony/spiritual baptism
- Wetting the baby's head celebrations
- Cognitive/emotional/behavioural change
- Caring/nurturing/interacting with baby
- Restructuring relationship with the mother

Ritual taboos/prescriptions (rituals during pregnancy)

Rituals of incorporation (rituals after birth)

FIGURE 13.1 Contemporary rites of passage: the social transition to fatherhood

new, have significance for the well-being of the father-to-be. Couvade syndrome is more commonly known as *sympathetic pregnancy*. In the UK it has been construed as a humorous eccentricity, as exemplified by Charles Hawtrey in the 1968 cinematic gem *Carry On Doctor*. Researchers have described cultures in which 'ritual couvade' is not practised or conducted 'appropriately', with some prospective fathers reporting physical and psychological symptoms during the mother's pregnancy, birth and postpartum period (Helman 1993).

In Lipkin and Lamb's study of couvade syndrome, 22.5% of the 267 partners of expectant mothers suffered from the syndrome (Lipkin and Lamb 1982). Many of their symptoms had characteristic vagueness and non-specificity (e.g. feeling 'low', 'run down', 'weakness'), but there were also more 'pregnant' symptoms (e.g. backache, fluid retention, genital/retrosternal burning, abdominal cramps and dizziness). Klein (1991) describes expectant fathers who presented with a range of bodily symptoms, such as indigestion, altered appetite, weight gain, altered bowel function, headache and toothache. Masoni, *et al.* (1994) also noted nausea and insomnia. Such symptoms typically appear during the third month of the pregnancy, with increasing symptomatology in the last two months of the pregnancy. The symptoms typically resolve at the time of the birth. Khanobdee, *et al.* (1993) also reported identical findings in Thai fathers.

Significantly, researchers noted that the symptoms had no obvious physiological basis. However, a range of psychological explanations have been offered, including the somatisation of anxiety arising from concern about the mother, the baby and role transition, ambivalence about fatherhood, and a statement of paternity. Less flatteringly, pseudo-sibling rivalry and parturition envy have also been suggested (Klein 1991). Masoni and colleagues concluded that although there is a lack of data to support a physiological explanation for couvade syndrome, 'we think that some male experiences, which constitute a peculiar imaginary and behavioural reality of the father-to-be, do exist' (Masoni, *et al.* 1994: 130).

An interesting caveat to the purported lack of a physiological explanation for couvade syndrome is to be found in an intriguing study conducted in 2001. It suggests that fathers experience dramatic hormone changes after the birth. The author, Dr Wynne-Edwards from Kingston, Ontario, Canada, claims to have not only demonstrated a reduction in testosterone and cortisol levels but also, crucially, increased levels of oestradiol, as measured in the saliva samples of a group of men attending pre- and postnatal classes, and a control group. Although multiple studies have demonstrated that women's hormones are altered during and after pregnancy, only two studies have explored the biochemical effects of parenthood on the father. Wynne-Edwards' study confirms and expands the results of the only previous study (Lewis-Stempel 2001). She states that the finding of raised levels of oestradiol, which were detected in a larger proportion of the samples from fathers than in those from a control group, is 'ground breaking' (cited in McVeigh 2001).

Although she was unable to offer an explanatory mechanism for the changes, Wynne-Edwards suggests that it could occur as a result of fathers experiencing increased exposure to the hormone from the mother. Both the tabloids and the broadsheets have been quick to suggest that such hormonal changes 'transform the toughest unreconstituted fathers into big softies' (McVeigh 2001), thereby explaining the behaviour of so-called 'celebrity dads' such as DJ 'Fat Boy Slim', the Gallagher brothers (Oasis), the former British Prime Minister Tony Blair, the film director Guy Ritchie, the footballer David Beckham, and the rap-star and film actor Will Smith (Stevenson 2001).

On a more academic note, Dr Malcolm Carruthers, who treats men who experience the menopause, suggests that oestradiol, which makes women 'broody', could exert a similar effect on men. Further research is needed, and although oestradiol has long been known to be significant in mammalian maternal behaviour, no animal research has found changes in male mammals. It could be that the human father is unique (McVeigh 2001).

FATHERS' BIRTH ATTENDANCE IN THE TWENTIETH CENTURY

By the 1930s, birth in the USA had become streamlined and mechanistic, incorporating a range of surgical and pharmacological interventions (Mishler 1981). Britain was not slow in replicating this approach to birth management. Such interventions required hospitalisation, and this process occurred rapidly in this country. Between 1927 and 1946 the rate of hospital births increased from 15% to 54%. After the war, a succession of Government publications, namely the *Guilleband Report* (published in 1955), the *Cranbrook Report* (Ministry of Health 1959) and the *Peel Report* (published in 1970) promoted hospital births (Tew 1998). Since then hospitalisation has continued unabated – the rate increasing from 64.4% in 1957 to 99% in 1984 (Open University 1992), with little decline thereafter.

Throughout this period the dominant obstetric discourse maintained that the presence of the father at the birth:

- was an increased infection risk
- was perverse and sadistic
- would inhibit future sexual relations between the couple
- created a nuisance due to the father interfering or fainting (Bedford and Johnson 1988).

These ideologies embodied a pseudoscientific rationale for denying admission to fathers, and offered a practical mechanism for avoiding the complex psychodynamics involved in having to relate to both parents (Henslin and Biggs 1971). Complexities arising from the increasingly invasive 'clinical intimacy' during the birth process, and subsequent concerns about complaint or litigation, arguably also had an influence.

It therefore came to be regarded as normal and 'appropriate' professional practice to exclude fathers, and subsequently this was integrated into both lay and professional health beliefs and behaviours, albeit with regional variations. The 1959 British Medical Association (BMA) publication *You and Your Baby* is a good example of public exposure to medical beliefs about fathers and the birth:

> The last requirement of all for a successful delivery at home is the husband – the poor father. If he is of the right mentality, and very few are, he may sustain his wife's morale during the first part of her labour. Otherwise he is best employed making tea, keeping the kettles boiling, and answering the front doorbell. (Kitzinger 1987: 150)

The fact that a father might wish to be present on his own account alone was not considered reason enough; even the most progressive obstetricians contended that the father had to be of use. In the late 1940s and early 1950s, the American obstetrician Robert Bradley agreed that husbands should be involved in the birth experience. He therefore developed the *Bradley Method* or *Husband-Coached Childbirth*. This focused on educating the couple so that the husband could serve as a 'coach' during labour. In 1947, American fathers were first allowed to attend the birth, on the condition that they acted as labour coaches (Burgess 1997a).

Despite the efforts of some obstetricians and midwives to create a more 'natural' approach to childbirth, which was inclusive of the father, the vast majority of practitioners adopted and reinforced the ideology of excluding fathers, and not just for the reasons cited above. Increasingly, the dire structural and material constraints under which the maternity services were operating created additional reasons for excluding fathers.

Before World War Two (1939–45), women in the higher socio-economic groups in Britain had given birth at home or in a nursing home. After the war, young middle-class couples found themselves with less space and domestic help. Home birth became inconvenient and was regarded less favourably as hospitals offered women analgesia in labour, as well as a period of recuperation after the birth (Squire 2000). As the numbers of women experiencing hospital births increased, so did the diversity of the parents, reflecting the changing socio-economic, cultural and ethnic context and their different expectations. This stimulated the re-attendance of fathers at the birth of their children.

A new 'breed' of mother, unused to the routine condescension, minor humiliations and poor physical surroundings endured by the public patients, now sought hospital care. Cohen observed that 'This type of woman, informed, articulate, and perhaps of a higher social grade than the midwives, did not take kindly to regimentation; she was a 'difficult patient', and she wrote to the papers or joined a mysterious league to reform the whole maternity service' (Cohen 1964: 93). In the maternity services, these influential women and their husbands/partners experienced the common touch and did not like it. What they disliked was the inability of the service to cope with two problems, namely, waiting in antenatal clinics and 'frightened loneliness in labour' (Cohen 1964: 95). The former problem objectified women in the time–squandering humiliations of the clinic with its 'batch management' ethos (Goffman 1961). The latter problem was a direct consequence of the prohibitive visitation and attendance policies operated by labour wards, particularly those relating to fathers.

The idea of expectant fathers partnering the midwifery team evoked strong emotions. Many midwives 'felt there was no place for husbands during the second stage of labour'. Some hospitals conceded that 'if there was a specific request, each case would be considered on its merits' (Cohen 1964: 97). This begs the question of what constituted 'merit'. Unsurprisingly, there were few 'specific requests'. Some London hospitals (Queen Charlottes' Hospital, Charing Cross Hospital and University College Hospital) began to encourage husbands to support their wives during birth. At the latter two hospitals about 50% of all fathers attended (Cohen 1964).

In 1961, Mrs Groves wrote:

> I have recently returned home from having my second child within two years at Queen Charlotte's . . . When my elder daughter was born, my husband visited me in the labour ward during official visiting hours, 7–8 p.m. I was in labour 55 hours and recall it as a time of great loneliness and tedium. This time, however, my husband was admitted without preamble to the labour ward and remained with me until I requested him to leave. (Beech and Thomas 2000: 7)

Not all obstetricians were convinced of the benefits of fathers attending. When asked what he thought, a distinguished obstetrician at Queen Charlotte's Hospital responded 'What do I feel about this?', paused for a moment, and then with the grim hesitation adopted by someone describing an atrocity, he asked 'Have *you* ever seen a woman give birth?' (Cohen 1964: 97).

The trend of allowing fathers to attend births snowballed during the 1960s, mirroring the social changes that were occurring in work patterns and traditional social roles and identities. Such changes, underpinned and augmented by the 'political' gains of second–wave feminist groups, challenged the assumptions that men held about women, and men's own social roles.

By the late 1970s a clear culture of fathers' birth attendance had emerged, as had the term 'birthing rooms'. Increasingly, hospitals had made pragmatic changes. Recognising that labouring mothers required psychological support, while tacitly acknowledging that midwives and nurses had little time to give it, they allowed and encouraged men to assume active roles in the care of their partners (Enkin, *et al.* 1995). Thus they acknowledged the importance of parent and baby bonding and the father's support of the mother during the birth. The old 'rationales' that had justified excluding fathers from the birth were being challenged both academically and politically (Summersgill

1993), and a new 'rationale/discourse' emerged that championed the fathers' presence. The obstetrician Peter Huntingford typifies this new thinking:

> Why should he not share responsibility with his partner, and her medical attendants, for her care? Why should he be sent out of the room when treatment is given and examinations made during labour? These symbols of the barrier that is erected to male participation in childbearing mean that there is less chance for fathers to share the sensations and emotions of birth. (Huntingford 1978)

Women were enthusiastic about the 'natural birthing' campaigns that were promoted in the 1970s and 1980s by obstetricians such as Frederic Leboyer and Michel Odent. Maternity departments responded further by providing a less institutional experience for the mother, that was inclusive of the father. However, although they were beginning to give parents what they wanted, the hospitals did not relinquish power over the major procedures used in birth (Porter 1999). By the 1980s, the majority of fathers were attending births. It had been the response of the public and of parents to these ideologies, set against changing social contexts and material constraints, that transformed fathers' birth attendance.

THE NEW ORTHODOXY OF ATTENDANCE: IS THE PARTICIPATION OF THE FATHER AT THE BIRTH DANGEROUS?

From the few atypical parents of the 1950s, fathers' birth attendance has now become normative, and a new 'negotiated order' (Strauss, *et al.* 1963) between practitioners, fathers and parents has emerged. However, as fathers' attendance has become widely accepted, questions have arisen.

Michel Odent speculates that fathers' birth attendance may be 'dangerous' (Odent 1999: 23). He believes that the dawn of the twenty-first century signifies a new phase in the history of childbirth, the current turning point being the fast development of evidence-based obstetrics and midwifery. This new phase represents a unique opportunity to reconsider many theories and preconceived ideas, and to make an inventory of the questions that we must raise.

> Where the participation of the father at birth is concerned, we must raise at least three questions. Can the participation of the father at the birth influence the sex life of the couple afterwards? Can all men cope with the strong emotional reactions that they may have while participating in the birth? Does the participation of the father aid or hinder the birth? (Odent 1999: 24)

In addition, one could ask what benefits might occur as a result of the father's presence, or why most fathers want to attend. These questions, arising from the lived experience of practitioners and fathers attending births, will now be addressed.

SEXUALITY AND BIRTH ATTENDANCE

From the earliest times sexuality and gender constructs have influenced the exclusion of fathers from the birth. In many cultures the locating of birth in a specific place, administered by women, could be interpreted as overtly desexualising the birth process. However, it is possible that there is a covert assumption that men's sexuality and 'gaze' inherently threaten the birth process, based on the notion that men regard birth as a potentially erotic situation, and only conceptualise women's secondary sexual characteristics as sites of (male) pleasure, as opposed to 'functional organs'. This underpins a popular but unsubstantiated belief that couples who experience problems with their subsequent sexual relationship, do so primarily as a result of the father being present at the birth; such a belief ignores possible previous sexual difficulties.

Although changing notions about sexuality, gender roles and relationships contributed to fathers' presence in the delivery room in the 1960s and 1970s, it would be incorrect to assume that sexuality is no longer a pertinent issue. As one tabloid subtly observed, 'Is it good for the rest of us (fathers) to see much industry taking place in an area once laced with Janet Reger?' (Young 1994: 43).

Indeed, this is one of the central tenets of those who would like to reverse the trend of attending fathers. According to Michel Odent:

> There are issues about the future sex life of the couple . . . Older women who gave birth when men were expected to stay in the pub are often appalled at the idea of their partner witnessing the physical spectacle of delivery . . . Sexual attraction is mysterious . . . Perhaps it needs a bit of mystery . . . I have seen so many couples who had wonderful births according to present criteria, yet several years later they divorced. They have remained good friends, but not sexual partners any more. (Boseley 2000)

Seel (1994) notes that sex therapists working with 'sexually dysfunctional' couples have observed that the man's experience of what was for him a traumatic labour/birth can subsequently stifle any sexual feelings for his partner. As one man described it:

> Suddenly this part of Angela that had been terribly private was being stared at by five other men. She didn't mind . . . in fact, she said that while it was going on the whole world could have watched and she wouldn't have given a damn . . . but I did. I felt it was a grotesque intrusion into our lives. And there was so much blood it shocked me, it was like seeing the person you love most on a battlefield. I had nightmares about it for weeks afterwards, and that affected the way I saw her as a sexual being. (Craig 1993: 131)

Jackson (1997) calls this 'post-traumatic parturition syndrome', and reasons that it can occur in men as the onlookers as well as in women as the receivers. She likens this to the well-documented feelings of violation that are experienced after rape (Raphael-Leff 1991, Walton 1994).

On the surface this appears to be a hard case to answer. However, closer analysis suggests that although there is little doubt that witnessing a birth can be traumatic for some men, it is not the case for the majority of them. People experience problems with their sexual relationships for a multiplicity of reasons, which can be grouped as being linked to biological factors (Hulme 1993) and physical and psychological factors (Walton 1994).

Given the significant social role transformations that occur on becoming a parent and which require immediate adaptation, it is not surprising that problems occur within a relationship. As Walton has observed:

> Sexuality is a fundamental aspect of life and so must be involved in the momentous adjustments that are made by men and women on becoming parents, and that change which started with the pregnancy continues in the postnatal period onwards. (Walton 1994: 97)

Problems can therefore occur as a consequence of roles adopted by the parents and the socio-cultural context of the relationship. For example, the division of domestic and salaried labour, and the relationship between the father, the mother and the baby are other significant factors.

Riley (1989) claims that, following the birth of their first child, two-thirds of couples have not resumed sexual intercourse within six weeks. The evidence suggests that for many men and women their experience of sexuality is not related solely to sexual activity, and therefore a narrow focus on sexuality as sexual activity is misleading, as it ignores the totality of human sexuality, as well as the impact of roles and societal values on the couple's sexuality. Given the diverse and complex reasons that people give to explain difficulties in their sexual relationships after birth, it is untenable to suggest, given the lack of supporting data, that the father's presence at the birth is the main source of such problems. Sexuality during early parenthood is only *one* factor in the ongoing process of negotiating relationships and roles after the birth (Curtis and Dunn 1994).

Michel Odent further speculates on the existence of male postnatal depression:

> Are we sure all men can cope with the strong emotional reaction they can have when their wife is in labour? . . . Most cultures have rituals for keeping a man busy while his partner is in labour . . . modern birthing practice makes little allowance for this. (Boseley 2000: 5)

A National Opinion Poll stated that 4% of men in the UK and 10% of men in London believe that they suffer from 'postnatal depression'. Although some of the physical symptoms could be attributed to altered hormone levels, as discussed earlier, Steve Jamieson of Men's Health Forum believes that this recently recognised phenomenon has a variety of contributory 'causes', including the sudden extra responsibility and financial burden, a lack of preparation for the role change, and acute/chronic tiredness. Many fathers who believed that they were depressed had witnessed the birth and found it 'off-putting' (BBC 1999).

Although the presence of the father at the birth would appear to impact on sexual relationships and contribute to depressive feelings in some fathers, this is not the case for the majority of them. However, this suggests that some fathers may want or seek support from midwives.

ATTENDING FATHERS: HELP OR HINDRANCE?

Perhaps the most serious concern that has been raised with regard to fathers' attend-ance at births is that in some way their presence has contributed to the sharp increase in the number of caesarean sections and medically assisted births. Odent believes that this has occurred in part because fathers become anxious and distressed at seeing their partners in pain, and they therefore try to talk to them, asking rational questions about what is happening. This requires the mother to respond using the intellectual as opposed to emotional side of the brain. This, he argues, inhibits the woman's ability to manage labour emotionally, and leads her to opt for analgesia and more interventionist approaches in the management of her labour (Boseley 2000).

In aiming to protect his partner, a father might request that she have an epidural or even a caesarean birth in order to avoid experiencing too much pain. Odent attributes this to men's respect for technology and gadgets to solve the 'problems' of natural child-birth: 'men feel happier knowing that their wives are getting as much medical attention as possible' (Walters 2000). Indeed, he speculates that this may be responsible for the upsurge in caesarean sections, and that fathers are sometimes inclined to celebrate the birth too soon, distracting the woman before the vital delivery of the placenta.

The six-fold increase in the number of caesarean sections in parts of England, Wales and Northern Ireland during the last 30 years means that one in five of all births (21.5%) is via caesarean section. In London and Wales the figure is as high as one in four (24.2%) (Department of Health 2001). These data require some unravelling. Is it possible that the father's presence at the birth could have contributed to the increase in medical interventions?

The two periods of greatest increase were the 1970s and the 1990s. Although the 1970s represent the period during which fathers started to attend births in significant numbers, Odent's hypothesis does not stand up to scrutiny. In the National Sentinel Caesarean Section Audit 2001, the main reasons offered by clinicians for performing caesarean sections were fetal distress, failure to progress in labour, breech presentation, previous caesarean section and the mother's specific request. However, these reasons need to be viewed in the light of the audit's key findings, which are summarised below (Boseley 2001).

- Women are still restricted in their movements during labour because they are attached to oversensitive and inaccurate fetal heart monitors.
- Drugs are too frequently used to induce labour when the pregnancy has run to term.
- Labouring women do not receive continuous attention, with one-third of all units unable to offer one-to-one care, and midwives in 5% of units could be caring for two to three women at any one time.
- There is an increase in the age of women who are having babies.
- There is a high rate of hospital births.
- There is lack of agreement between the World Health Organization and the Royal College of Obstetricians and Gynaecologists as to what constitutes 'a high rate of caesarean sections'.
- There is an increased number of 'defensive' caesarean sections arising from fear of litigation.
- There is an increased number of elective procedures (most notably in private practice) at the mother's request, in the absence of clinical indications.

The presence of fathers is noticeably absent as a contributory factor (although it may not have been considered). Odent is aware that he is challenging what has become an orthodoxy, and he does publicly acknowledge that 'there is little scientific evidence for his view that men can be a hindrance rather than a help' (Boseley 2000).

HERE TO STAY: WHY DO FATHERS WANT TO ATTEND?

Although the majority of fathers willingly attend the birth, some do so reluctantly for a variety of reasons, including squeamishness, uncertainty about their role, previous life experiences and personal beliefs (Robertson 1993). Is it possible that a minority of men are being 'forced' into the labour room? Seel (1994) believes that this new orthodoxy puts enormous pressure – from women, partners, staff or other men – on fathers who are reluctant. One prospective father commented on how he was finding it particularly difficult to receive support from his colleagues: 'My mates keep skitting me about it . . . it does make me feel a bit guilty' (Lavender 1997: 94). For some men this creates a 'Catch-22' situation: 'There are so many people expecting you to be at the birth, yet nobody really asks you if you want to be' (Lavender 1997: 94).

In essence, the father's attendance has come to be construed as part of the expression of the ideal closeness and mutual dependence of contemporary relationships, and his intention to be a 'father' to the child. Therefore it is not uncommon for the father who does not witness the birth to be viewed as an incompetent father and an inadequate man, who has shirked his duty to the child and denied the mutuality that is so necessary for relationships. Worse still, his partner is to be pitied.

The literature suggests that only a few men encounter this dilemma, and given that high levels of attendance have persisted for over 20 years, this not a passing fad, but one which is likely to be continued by the future generation of fathers (O'Brien and Jones 1995). It would appear that fathers are in the birthing room to stay. Therefore it is pertinent at this stage to examine why men want to attend the birth, the expectations and experiences of the couple, and what fathers have felt enabled them to be supportive of their partners during the birth.

Although fathers have different reasons for wanting to attend the birth, Richman (1982) describes them collectively as having a 'kaleidoscopic pattern of motives'. Birth attendance is the culmination of months of preparation for fatherhood. A study of new fathers showed that 93% of them wanted and had planned to be present at the birth (Royal College of Midwives 1995). Fathers want to be close to and supportive of their labouring partner, and to witness the birth of a new life (Draper 1997). They equate attendance with developing a close relationship with the baby, which enables them to express loving feelings towards him or her. Attendance at the birth also facilitates their involvement in the daily care of the baby, and makes it clear that they are parents with the associated responsibilities (Palkovitz 1987). Some fathers were aware that their presence served to remind healthcare workers that childbirth could not be viewed entirely as a medical event (Beail and McGuire 1982).

EXPECTATIONS AND EXPERIENCES OF ATTENDANCE

Despite having differing expectations of childbirth, fathers generally reported that labour and birth were stressful events for them, with anxiety arising from their concern about the physical and emotional well-being of their labouring partner (May and Perrin 1985). Doubts about their ability to be supportive of their partner while trying to hide their own feelings (Berry 1988), and uncertainty about their roles during the labour and birth (Bothamley 1990) were additional stressors. Chandler and Field (1997) have illustrated how these stressors and the consequent anxiety had different foci, duration and intensity, which were determined by where the couple was on the 'labour path'.

Consistent with the unique motives and expectations that fathers have for attending the birth, they also adopt different roles during labour and the birth. From the behaviours that fathers display, Chapman (1991) identified three commonly adopted roles, namely coach, team mate and witness.

'Coaches' actively assisted their partner, and had a strong need to feel in control of themselves and the labour experience. Their partners wanted them to be physically involved in the labour, regarding this as crucial to their own ability to maintain control.

'Team mates' assisted their partner in response to requests for physical or emotional support, occasionally leading. These fathers saw themselves as a member of the birth team, and were less concerned with issues of control. They focused on the needs of their partner, who wanted them there both for their presence and for their willingness to follow directions.

'Witnesses' described their primary role as being a companion who provided emotional and moral support. These fathers witnessed the birth of the baby, but believed that there was little they could do to help their partner. Therefore they looked to others to take charge of the situation, and were often seen reading or watching television. This role was viewed as creating 'togetherness without the pressures of having to be in control' (Chapman 1992).

Irrespective of the roles adopted during the labour and birth, the most important role for the partner of a labouring mother is just 'being there' (Flint 1986). Many mothers benefit from the supportive presence of the father – the very fact of him being there meant that the mother had access to physical and emotional support as required. Although some fathers may have been of little practical help, their mere presence was supportive (Stolte 1987), even if fathers did not get it right all of the time. As one mother commented, 'I wasn't particularly amused at being offered fish and chips . . . That's just trying to help' (Somers-Smith 1999: 106).

However, many mothers stated that the presence of their partner could alleviate the loneliness, pain and uncertainty during the delivery, and gave them strength to endure their suffering as well as share their joy. The presence of the father meant 'communion' to the mother, and this communion emanates from the partners caring for each other and their baby. For the mothers, their partner was not only a support person, but also above all the father-to-be – a double and sometimes paradoxical role (Bondas-Salonen 1998).

Some studies have described an enhanced positive emotional experience of the birth for the mother (Entwhistle and Doering 1988). May (1982) noted that the shared experience of the birth had a positive impact on the couple's relationship, and more recently it was reported that 80% of couples did not anticipate any adverse effects on their future personal relationship (Szevérenyi, et al. 1998). Mothers experienced less pain and required less analgesia (Henneborn and Cogan 1975, Niven 1985), while Chopstick, et al. (1986) identified a reduction in the frequency of epidurals for mothers who had the father's support.

In being present at the birth, fathers felt that they were valuing, caring for and appreciating their partners, and were pleased with the support that they had given (Somers–Smith 1999). Fathers experienced immense joy, relief and overwhelming emotions both during and after the birth of the child, and what Hall (1995) describes as 'love at first sight'. Many fathers complete the experience with an enhanced respect for their partner, and feel that they have introduced themselves personally to the child (Chandler and Field 1997). Furthermore, fathers who have involved themselves in the pregnancy, birth and subsequent care of the child often describe feelings of elation and enhanced self-esteem (Lewis 1986, Bedford and Johnson 1988).

ENABLING FATHERS TO BE SUPPORTIVE AT BIRTH

Midwives have been known to complain that fathers are 'useless' in the labour ward (Robertson 1999: 21). While stereotypes may contain a grain of truth, the majority of fathers want to help their partners during the birth, and to bond with the child. If the father is to provide practical help and emotional support, and to make the most of the opportunity, he will need insight, information and support from the midwife.

In antenatal classes, fathers valued an emphasis being placed on the 'whole birth thing'. The 'whole birth thing' was an awareness that just learning the medical facts and having a technical knowledge of labour was not enough, and implied that those lead-ing the classes saw birth as a series of biological processes and medical procedures – a literal lack of wholeness. What was of most help to fathers was a clear acknowledgement of the father's supportive role, clear guidance on what he could do, practical tips and balanced insights into life with a baby. The 'whole birth thing' emphasises that labour and birth are part of the transition to parenthood, but does not assume that all fathers will be present at the labour, or that they will adopt similar roles.

This suggests a need to allow fathers to explore what being present at the birth means, in 'men only' forums (Smith 1999b). Midwives need to be aware of the need to avoid stigmatising non-attendees, as this can lead to inappropriate care (May 1982), and to avoid focusing solely on the father's perceived role as a 'labour coach', which could mean neglecting his psychological or other needs – antenatally or during the birth (Draper 1997). Lester and Moorsom (1997) consider this to be a 'golden opportunity' for midwives to provide information and emotional support for fathers throughout the pregnancy, birth and postnatal period. Midwives should permit emotional catharsis, acknowledge 'couvade syndrome', and be as flexible as possible with regard to their working hours to allow for fathers' work commitments. In terms of obtaining informa-tion, the consensus of opinion among fathers was that midwives are the people to ask (Lavender 1997). This is not surprising. Bothamley (1990) observed that some fathers felt inhibited in the hospital environment, even with regard to performing simple tasks such as moving a chair. She maintains that fathers need to be informed about what is happening, and about the hospital setting itself. It is through the 'presencing' and 'being there' that the father is enabled to feel that he is welcome, valued and integral to the birth team.

This can be exemplified as follows:

> We decided to have Ricky at home, and initially I didn't like the idea . . . had all logical reasons why I didn't want to do it, about being safe in hospital . . . But once we embarked upon it, it was a brilliant experience. We had this wonderful midwife.

I think she really liked me. She did something she said she had never done, and she has delivered over 1000 children, but she got me to get hold of his head and pull him out. And then she let me cut the cord! (Ralph, 37-year-old father of three) (Burgess 1997a: 123–4)

CONCLUSION

Enabling fathers to be supportive of their partners through the births of their children is important and rewarding for both the couple and the midwife. Contrary to popular perceptions, fathers have historically been active in birth and childcare, prior to industrialisation and the hospitalisation of childbirth. Therefore the present trend of fathers attending births is not a totally new phenomenon, but rather the re-emergence of an old one – 'reconstructed'. The forces that have shaped and moulded this transition, and the subsequent outcomes, have been described and critically examined. Given that the high levels of attendance are set to continue, it is hoped that these insights into to the how and why of fathers attending the birth will enable midwives and other healthcare workers in their practice with the mother, the baby and the father.

KEY POINTS

- ↪ The present high numbers of fathers attending the birth of their child represent a relatively recent phenomenon. However, historically, fathers have been involved in the birth of their children and their subsequent care.
- ↪ Although for Western fathers the norm is one of attendance at the birth, globally this is not the case. In other societies, birth is administered by women, while the transition to fatherhood is enacted through couvade rituals.
- ↪ The hospitalisation of birth in the latter half of the twentieth century first prevented and then encouraged the attendance of fathers at the birth. However, concerns have been expressed about the merits and demerits of this phenomenon.
- ↪ The majority of fathers wish to attend the birth. Collectively, they have diverse motives for attending, and different experiences and expectations of themselves, their partner and the birth.
- ↪ Midwives can enable fathers to be supportive of their labouring partner by acknowledging the significance of the father's role at the birth for the couple, and through antenatal education that is practically orientated and allows the father to be emotionally expressive.

DEDICATION

For Sharon, Jake and Poppy, without whom I would not have had the privilege of being a father.

REFERENCES

BBC. (1999) *Men suffer from baby blues*. London: BBC News (online); 4th May. Available at: http://news.bbc.co.uk/2/hi/health/334735.stm (accessed 1 Jan 2009).

Beail N, McGuire J. (1982) *Fathers: psychological perspectives*. London: Junction Books.

Bedford V, Johnson N. (1988) The role of the father. *Midwifery*. **4**: 190–5.

Beech B, Thomas P. (2000) Forty years ago: men in the labour wards. *Adv Midwif Sci* J. **12**: 7–8.

Berry L. (1988) Realistic expectations of the labour coach. *J Obstet Gynecol Neonatal Nurs*. **17**: 354–5.

Bondas-Salonen T. (1998) How women experience the presence of their partners at the births of their babies. *Qual Health Res*. **8**: 784–801.

Boseley S. (2000) *Anxious fathers may be bad for the birth: 'Keep them away from the delivery room', advises childbirth guru*. Manchester: Guardian; 17 January 2000: p. 5.

Boseley S. (2001) *Caesarean births soar to one in five: survey puts UK way above WHO limits*. Manchester: Guardian; 26 October 2001: p. 13.

Bothamley J. (1990) Are fathers getting a fair deal? *Nurs Times*. **86**: 68–9.

Burgess A. (1997a) *Fatherhood Reclaimed: the making of the modern father*. London: Vermilion.

Burgess A. (1997b) *Carlton Parenting Campaign: fathers' booklet*. London: Carlton Television.

Carlowe J. (2001) *Birth control*. London: Observer magazine; 2 December 2001: p. 49.

Chandler S, Field P. (1997) Becoming a father: first-time fathers' experience of labour and delivery. *J Nurse Midwifery*. **42**: 17–24.

Chapman L. (1991) Searching: expectant fathers' experiences during labor and delivery. *J Perinat Neonat Nurs*. **44**: 21–9.

Chapman L. (1992) Expectant fathers' role during labor and birth. *J Obstet Gynecol Neonatal Nurs*. **21**: 114–20.

Chopstick S, Taylor K, Hayes R, *et al.* (1986) Partner support and the use of coping techniques in labour. *J Psychosom Res*. **30**: 497–503.

Cohen GL. (1964) *What's Wrong with Hospitals?* Harmondsworth: Penguin.

Craig A. (1993) *Sex after stitches: will your love life ever be the same?* She magazine; September: pp. 130–2.

Curtis P, Dunn K. (1994) *How's the Love Life? sexuality and early motherhood*. Paper presented to the Annual Conference of the British Sociological Association, Sexualities in Social Context, March 1994, Preston, UK.

Department of Health. (2001) *National Sentinel Caesarean Section Audit*. London: The Stationery Office.

Douglas M. (1966) *Purity and Danger*. Harmondsworth: Penguin.

Draper J. (1997) Whose welfare in the labour room? a discussion of the increasing trend of fathers' birth attendance. *Midwifery*. **13**: 132–8.

Eagle R. (1988) *Bedside man*. Vogue magazine; March: pp. 330–1.

Enkin M, Keirse MJNC, Neilson J, *et al.* (1995) *A Guide to Effective Care in Pregnancy and Childbirth*. Oxford: Oxford University Press.

Entwhistle D, Doering S. (1988) The emergent father role. *Sex Roles*. **18**: 119–41.

Flint C. (1986) *Sensitive Midwifery*. London: Heinemann.

Goffman E. (1961) *Asylums: essays on the social situation of mental patients and other inmates*. Harmondsworth: Pelican Books.

Goldberg WA. (1988) Introduction: perspectives on the transition to parenthood. In: Michaels GY, Goldberg WA, editors. *The Transition to Parenthood*. Cambridge: Cambridge University Press.

Hahn RA, Muecke MA. (1987) The anthropology of birth in five US ethnic populations: implications for obstetrical practice. *Curr Prob Obstet Gynecol Fertil.* **10**: 131–71.

Hall EO. (1995) From fun and excitement to joy and trouble: an explorative study of three Danish fathers' experiences around birth. *Scand J Caring Sci.* **9**: 171–9.

Hardyment C. (1982) *Dream Babies: childcare from Locke to Spock.* London: Jonathan Cape.

Hearn J. (1984) Childbirth, men and the problem of fatherhood. *Rad Commun Med.* **17**: 9–19.

Heggenhougan HK. (1980) Fathers and childbirth: an anthropological perspective. *J Nurse Midwifery.* **25**: 21–6.

Heiney P. (1986) *Fathers voting against forced labour.* London: The Times; 21 July: p. 11.

Helman CG. (1993) *Culture, Health and Illness.* Oxford: Butterworth-Heinemann.

Henneborn WJ, Cogan R. (1975) The effect of husband participation on reported and probability of medication during labour and birth. *J Psychosom Res.* **19**: 215–22.

Henslin JM, Biggs MA. (1971) The sociology of the vaginal examination. In: Henslin M, editor. *Down to Earth Sociology: introductory readings.* New York: Free Press.

Hulme H. (1993) Grin and bear it. *Nurs Times.* **89**: 66.

Huntingford P. (1978) *The Baby Book for Fathers.* London: Fenwick and Fenwick.

Jackson KB. (1977) Paternal presence at delivery. *Br J Midwif.* **25**: 682–4.

Khanobdee C, Sukratanachaiyakul V, Gay JT. (1993) Couvade syndrome in expectant Thai fathers. *Int J Nurs Stud.* **30**: 125–31.

Kitzinger S. (1987) *The Experience of Childbirth.* Harmondsworth: Penguin.

Kitzinger S. (2000) Some cultural perspectives on birth. *Br J Midwif.* **8**: 746–50.

Klein H. (1991) Couvade syndrome: male counterpart to pregnancy. *Int J Psychiatr Med.* **21**: 57–69.

Laslett P. (1983) *The World We Have Lost: further explored.* London: Routledge.

Lavender T. (1997) Can midwives respond to the needs of fathers? *Br J Midwif.* **5**: 92–6.

Lester A, Moorsom S. (1997) Do men need midwives? Facilitating a greater involvement in parenting. *Br J Midwif.* **5**: 678–81.

Lewis C. (1986) *Becoming a Father.* Oxford: Oxford University Press.

Lewis-Stempel J. (2001) *Fatherhood: an anthology.* London: Simon & Schuster.

Lipkin M and Lamb GS. (1982) The couvade syndrome: an epidemiological study. *Ann Int Med.* **96**: 509–11.

MacFarlane A. (1970) *The Family Life of Ralph Josselin.* Cambridge: Cambridge University Press.

McVeigh T. (2001) *Tough guys get the baby blues, too.* London: Observer; 24 June: p. 7.

Masoni S, Maio A, Trimarchi G, *et al.* (1994) The couvade syndrome. *J Psychosom Obstet Gynaecol.* **15**: 125–31.

May K. (1982) Three phases of father involvement in pregnancy. *Nurs Res.* **51**: 337–42.

May K, Perrin S. (1985) Prelude: pregnancy and birth. In: Hanson S, Bozzet F, editors. *Dimensions of Fatherhood.* Beverly Hills, CA: Sage.

Ministry of Health. (1959) *Report of Maternity Services Committee: Cranbrook Report.* London: HMSO.

Mishler EG. (1981) *Social Contexts of Health, Illness and Patient Care.* Cambridge: Cambridge University Press.

National Childbirth Trust. (2000) *Government-funded Study of 'Blair Fathers' Demands Better Support for New Dads.* Available at: www.midirs.org (accessed 22 May 2001).

Newburn M. (2000) *Head to head: fathers and childbirth.* London: BBC News Online. Available at: http://news.bbc.co.uk/2/hi/health/607005.stm (accessed 1 Jan 2009).

Niven C. (1985) How helpful is the presence of the husband at childbirth? *J Reprod Infant Psychol.* **3**: 45–53.

O'Brien M, Jones D. (1995) Young people's attitudes to fatherhood. In: Moss P, editor. *Father Figures: fathers in the 1990s.* London: HMSO.

Odent M. (1999) Is the participation of the father at birth dangerous? *Midwifery Today.* 51: 23–5.

Okely J. (1983) *The Traveller-Gypsies.* Cambridge: Cambridge University Press.

Open University. (1992) *Health and Well-Being.* Milton Keynes: Open University.

Palkovitz R. (1987) Fathers' motives for birth attendance. *Matern Child Nurs. J.* **16**: 123–9.

Pollock LA. (1983) *Forgotten Children: parent–child relations from 1500–1900*. Cambridge: Cambridge University Press.

Porter R. (1999) *The Greatest Benefit to Mankind: a medical history of humanity from antiquity to the present*. London: Fontana Press.

Raphael-Leff J. (1991) *Psychological Processes of Childbearing*. London: Chapman and Hall.

Richman J. (1982) Men's experience of pregnancy and childbirth. In: McKee L, O'Brien M, editors. *The Father Figure*. New York: Tavistock Publications.

Riley AJ. (1989) Sex after childbirth. *Br J Sexual Med*. **16**: 185–7.

Rivière PG. (1974) The couvade: a problem reborn. *Man*. **9**: 423–35.

Robertson A. (1999) Get the fathers involved! The needs of men in pregnancy classes. *Pract Midwife*. **2**: 21–2.

Robertson I. (1993) Birth pains. *BMJ*. **307**: 687.

Royal College of Midwives. (1995) RCM survey (summary): men at birth. *Midwives*. **108**: 18.

Seel R. (1987) *The Uncertain Father*. Bath: Gateway Books.

Seel R. (1994) Men at the birth. *New Generation*. **13**: 16–17.

Smith J. (1999a) Antenatal classes and the transition to fatherhood: a study of some fathers' views. *MIDIRS Midwif Digest*. **9**: 327–30.

Smith N. (1999b) Men in antenatal classes: teaching 'the whole birth thing'. *Pract Midwife*. **2**: 23–6.

Somers-Smith MJ. (1999) A place for the partner? Expectations and experiences of support during childbirth. *Midwifery*. **15**: 101–8.

Squire C. (2000) Pain relief: past and present. In: Yerby M, editor. *Pain in Child-Bearing: key issues in management*. London: Baillière Tindall.

Stevenson S. (2001) *Why new fathers are such softies*. Metro; 25 June: p. 14.

Stolte K. (1987) A comparison of women's expectations of labour with the actual event. *Birth*. **14**: 99–103.

Strauss AL, Schatzman L, Ehrlich D, *et al.* (1963) The hospital and its negotiated order. In: Friedson E, editor. *The Hospital and Modern Society*. London: Free Press.

Summersgill P. (1993) Couvade: the retaliation of the marginalised fathers. In: Alexander J, Levy V, Roch S, editors. *Midwifery Practice: a research-based approach*. Basingstoke: Macmillan.

Szeverényi P, Póka R, Hetey M, *et al.* (1998) Contents of childbirth-related fear among couples wishing the partner's presence at delivery. *J Psychosom Obstet Gynecol*. **19**: 38–43.

Tew M. (1998) *Safer Childbirth?* London: Chapman and Hall.

Thomas C. (2000) *Childbirth scares men too*. BBC News Online. Available at: http://news.bbc.co.uk/2/hi/health/673294.stm (accessed 1 Jan 2009).

Turner BS. (1995) *Medical Power and Social Knowledge*. London: Sage.

Van Gennep A. (1960) *The Rites of Passage*. London: Routledge and Kegan Paul.

Walters C. (2000) *Millennium Babies: current research on the health of the unborn generation*. Families Magazine (online). Available at: www.familiesonline.co.uk/article/articleview/19/1/9/ (accessed 1 Jan 2009).

Walton I. (1994) *Sexuality and Motherhood*. Hale: Books for Midwives Press.

Watts J. (1995) *Gendering One, Gendering Two*. Unpublished paper.

Young J. (1994) *Birth day blues of a dad*. London: Daily Mail; 28 April: p. 43.

CHAPTER 14

Unhappiness after childbirth

Christine Grabowska

This chapter critically appraises the circumstances of women's transition into motherhood, based on social norms and cultural expectations. It is proposed that some women find the transition difficult because of the value and status attached to earning an income. The imagery to which women are exposed prior to having their first child is romanticised and often unrealistic.

The social need for competition and why that skill is inappropriate for all intimate relationships and is thus the cause of unhappiness is discussed. The effects of overworking when a woman is trying to take on the roles of mother, lover, housewife and career woman can leave her feeling out of control, particularly if she does not feel satisfied with her involvement in any of these areas. It is arguable that these feelings of loss and being out of control may be considered as normal and actually aiding the transitions a woman makes when becoming a mother.

Post-traumatic stress syndrome following childbirth has now been recognised. The incidence of the condition appears to be increasing in mothers, manifested as a form of extreme anxiety. Women with the syndrome will find every area of their lives affected. They often cannot function effectively, and this results in the disruption of their lives and those of their family. Consideration of women during the maternity experience needs to be prioritised by service provision and Government policy. The chapter concludes by asking for political solutions in the short-term, but ultimately a radical change in behaviour and social expectations is needed in order to support the mothering role.

INTRODUCTION

Women have often been blamed for causing their own suffering and unhappiness. They are told by knowledgeable others that their feelings are caused by their hormones, unrealistic expectations of childbirth, having an idealised image of motherhood, listening to too many stories and so on. This blaming culture increases the woman's internalisation of her own unhappiness and she is left with no other recourse but the knowledge that if she created it she must deal with it. Society is thus absolved of any responsibility for the creation of each woman's unhappiness so no social or political resolution needs to be instituted. Society therefore does not support motherhood – mothers are left to do this themselves.

Women are surviving traumas of their everyday life and coping. Motherhood changes their whole being and the way they see themselves as well as how they are viewed by others (Buultjens and Liamputling 2007, Patel, *et al.* 2005). It is a birth into a new social role, a transition from a woman's former self into what could be seen as a personally fulfilling experience in the development of a person. Many women go through this transition and emerge excited and fulfilled at being mothers. However, for some it is one trauma they will not survive or be able to cope with. It may be viewed with feelings such as contempt, bewilderment, sadness, anger and resentment. It may be a transition that was neither anticipated nor wanted (Brotherson 2007, Lupton 2003). These feelings are not dependent on the decision to have a baby (Nicolson 1998), but rather they result from the outcome of childbearing (Frost, *et al.* 2006, Oakley 2005)). The explanation of why some women have reached such a place in their lives will often depend on their history and their present cultural surroundings. All women need to find some form of contentment or even happiness in becoming mothers, which will aid their confidence and abilities.

The aim of this chapter is to propose that mothers are integral to the continuing functioning of society, and that therefore society has a responsibility to support the mothering role. It is suggested that unhappiness, for some mothers, is socially created (Gilbert 1992, Pilgrim and Bentall 1999, Johnston and Swanson 2003, Kitzinger 2005). Ussher (2004) on the other hand looks at the experience of unhappiness as a normal response to becoming a mother and therefore should be expected.

HISTORY

Women who have felt loved throughout their lives have the greatest chance of happiness when they become mothers. However, Gilbert (1992) points out that historically, societies have been more concerned about success in promoting the social ideal rather than about individual happiness. Odent (1999) agrees that in the past, love was put on the back burner and mothers were positively discouraged from openly displaying love for their children in order to produce aggression and competitiveness, particularly among male children. This creates the initial conflict of interests for women entering motherhood. Social success is defined through the capitalist economy for all Western societies, and people are defined by the amount of money they are able to generate. Motherhood does not create wealth and may therefore be regarded in a lowly way by such societies (Korten 2007).

Many authors (Sheppard 1997, Hope, *et al.* 1999, Reading and Reynolds 2001, Nicolson and Ussher 1992, Harris 2001, Bernazzani and Bifulco 2003) refer to the classic study by Brown and Harris (1978) of depression in order to highlight the circumstances of women's lives that may have contributed to their unhappiness. Brown and Harris (1978) identified four vulnerability factors that predispose women to the onset of unhappiness:

●● lack of a confiding relationship with their partner
●● presence at home of three or more children under the age of 14 years

➻ loss of their own mother before the age of 11 years
➻ absence of outside employment.

Lack of a confiding relationship with their partner

The sharing of daily experiences, regardless of their worth and value, is a way of debriefing and thus coping with the next onslaught of experiences with greater calm and ease. It enables an individual to move through life with courage. Courage is enhanced by encouragement (Smail 2001) which people have a greater chance of receiving when relating to others, and in turn others' lives gain fulfilment by this contribution to mothers. For many people it is difficult to be this relaxed about themselves, and thus it is difficult for them to be open and vulnerable, because generally speaking people have been taught as children, to present 'a good image' or 'not to wash their dirty linen in public'. Equally, as individuals interact with each other, they may have seen others take advantage of this vulnerability, including their partners, therefore to allow vulnerability involves being confident in oneself. Confidence develops when someone else is confident in you (Smail 2001). It is believing in the new mother, her love of the baby and her capabilities that potentially creates the difference in the way that she is feeling and thus trusting of herself.

The confiding relationships that a woman has, involve trust and love. It is where others see the woman's worth and value that will determine the woman's confidence in herself as a mother. Being able to confide in someone on a regular basis is nurturing to the mother, who will in turn be able to nurture her young. However, some women have no such confiding relationships.

People often embark on relationships that are based on lust, and sometimes friendship has no place in those relationships; they can become competitive with each partner feeling that they constantly have to prove their own worth and value in order to be liked. This leaves no room for vulnerability, openness and honesty, and may be the source of a breakdown of relationships due to lack of communication. Romito, *et al.* (1999) believe that unless the relationship is considered to be good or even better, it is preferable to be a single parent.

Why do people behave competitively in relationships? Is it because this is the nature of the world in which they live? In order for business to function, profit has to be made, and thus competition is created to vie for profit. People are exposed to this on a daily basis and it is considered to be normal behaviour. Often people find that they cannot change their behaviour easily, especially if competition is the socially preferred way of behaving (Navarro and Schwartzberg 2007, Smail 2001).

People may have been children in families where competitive behaviour was seen and encouraged, and therefore being open and vulnerable will cause fear and avoidance. Inter-collegial socialising and networking are often interpreted as developing friendships. However, these tend to be competitive gatherings where much mutual evaluation, resourcing and 'taking what you can get from it' is going on (Navaro and Schwartzberg 2007). People often form relationships from such gatherings, but behavioural changes away from these interactions then become difficult, as they are frightened of loving, mutual dependency, sharing, caring and availability when competition, independence and teamwork are valued. Teamwork here means that everyone is assigned a specific area of responsibility that will link with the whole, not spending the working day making time available to listen to colleagues. Often people will be 'advised' to take time off 'sick' with stress, when all they want to do is to debrief.

This study by Patel, *et al.* (2002) showed that even in countries such as India where marital relationships may be created for economic reasons, unhappiness stemmed not just from a poor relationship with the woman's husband. It often resulted in pathological mental health when combined with poor financial resources, violence from the woman's husband and hunger. However, this was causally offset with the number of years' education the woman had received and if her husband was gainfully employed. Expectations of relationships vary between individuals and their experiences of these interactions. Thus unhappiness may be integral to some relationships, born of the initial relationships from which the mother originated and compounded by the birth of her own child.

The way in which individuals behave in relationships is influenced by the way in which they were socialised through life experiences. In motherhood, the woman has a baby who is open and vulnerable. The mother will experience basic human emotions for which she may have had no training or preparation. She may turn to the relationship with her partner for support. However, her partner may well have had no training in supporting others up to this point. He may deal with this situation by withdrawing from the relationship, trying to give practical help or trying to find practical solutions, such as the employment of domestic help. On the other hand, he may start to listen to his partner and deepen their relationship, leading to total acceptance of the other (Navaro and Schwartzberg 2007).

The presence, at home, of three or more children under the age of 14 years

The demands of children are relentless. For many parents this may feel like a one way system in which they give to the children but receive very little. The younger the children are, the more demanding they tend to be, and needless to say the more of them there are, the more likely it is that their demands may become insurmountable.

What help does a family have to enable it to cope with these demands? Sometimes there are relatives living nearby who are willing to help out, but generally the culture in the UK promotes the nuclear family. Geographical mobility underpins the capitalist market economy. People make themselves available to this market in order to earn an income, and because this is seen as a priority, being available to the family takes a back seat. This leaves the children with limited support from adult carers – and some of those carers will be paid to care. Thus, according to Korten (2007), priority is given to the exchange of money instead of a genuine regard for other human beings and caring for each other. However, many families require two incomes in order to have an adequate standard of living, and some women choose to work in order to maintain their mental health.

This attitude of viewing caring as a job and not as a social expectation is manifested in the rise of 'caring' social organisations. There are organisations specifically created to take caring out of the home and virtually all of them charge a fee for their services. Consider old peoples' homes, nurseries, respite care, childminding and so on. There are very few voluntary or Government funded organisations. The cultural norm has become an expectation of the exchange of money for services rendered. Perhaps the meaning of the word 'caring' needs to be reconsidered. It involves more than physical minding, and it is usually women who put the love into caring of others. Consequently, a woman might very well be unhappy that her services to her child go unrecognised – not just in monetary terms but also in emotional terms – by the other people in her life as well as by the children (Flacking, *et al.* 2006).

There is a social expectation that mothers will behave favourably and respond to their children's needs with total disregard for their own needs (Flacking, *et al.* 2006). This expectation is inconsistent with all of a woman's learning about social behaviour and the satisfaction of personal needs as a priority (Brock 1998). The larger the family, the less likely it is that the mother will have time for other interests, and therefore her life choices will be reduced, including the option of employment outside the home, as the costs of childcare can be prohibitive (Rachman 1998). The materialist culture promotes choice. Through advertisements, the public are urged on a daily basis to choose between products in order to boost consumerism. The mother has to live with another conflict in that she is admonished for reducing her consumer capacity (largely due to financial circumstances) while at the same time finding little support to make choices for her own life (Graham 2007, Johnston and Swanson 2003).

Unhappiness was further compounded for mothers who had problems breastfeeding (Patel, *et al.* 2002), or whose babies were admitted to neonatal units (Flacking, *et al.* 2006); and for those who produced baby girls there was a considerable increase in a low emotional mood. Significantly, despite marital violence, women reported lower rates of unhappiness where the baby was a boy. In this scenario, cultural factors are crucial in provoking negative feelings; the meaning given to birthing female children is not universal.

The loss of their own mother before the age of 11 years

A woman often gains a greater understanding of her own mother when she takes on this role herself, and often their relationship changes at this point. Early loss of her own mother and the grief that probably resulted, may re-surface at the time when she becomes a mother herself. The social attitude of 'life goes on' following a death may mean that grieving was inhibited or disturbed. Role modelling by a mother will have been limited, but more importantly, a loving, nurturing relationship may also have been missing (Deaves 2001). Showing and feeling love towards a child enables the growth of that person. It allows them to develop the confidence to fulfil a wide range of social roles. When children feel supported, they can 'test out' the environment from a safe place knowing the security of their relationship with their mother and that she will protect them. Children know they can find approval and acknowledgement in this relationship, and their exploration of and learning about the world is done from a safe base (Smith and Cowie 1998). However, if this is missing from a child's life, they may be afraid to take risks in life and possibly lack confidence. The mother may also re-experience the pain of grieving for her own mother, as well as being aware of the lack of support for her own mothering role. Motherhood – one of the greatest rides in life – may not be safe for this child, who is now herself the mother, and she may hit the crash barrier. She may have been unprepared for taking this risk, but now there are no buffers in sight.

The absence of outside employment

Outside employment is familiar to those who have worked outside the home prior to motherhood. It is a place where people generally feel valued, if only in the sense that they receive monetary reward (Simmel and Frisby 2004). Many people value monetary reward highly because of the goods and services that they can buy with it. People may feel powerful when they can control what they want in life through money (Johnston and Swanson 2003). This view is supported by the capitalist economy in which mothers are living their lives (Smail 2001). The interpretation that is often made of wanting the best for their baby is in materialist terms – the 'best' pram, the 'best' cot, the 'best' clothes, the 'best' milk – commodities that are usually costly and exacerbate the culture of separatism between the mother and her child. For example, a pram or cot will take the baby out of his or her mother's arms, and by giving the baby formula milk the mother is allowing others to feed the child, thus depriving him or her of the 'best' food. Employment often separates the mother from her baby for many hours, yet the social expectation is that mothers will return to paid employment – so this is the choice that women often make. It may be inconsistent, but it is here that she regains her esteem based on the high value that is attached to earning an income – motherhood has no such rewards.

The study by McKim, *et al.* (1999) showed that mothers who were working and wanted to do so were happier than mothers who chose to stay at home to care for their own babies. One of the advantages of employment is that it can prevent loneliness, in that people socialise and debrief at work. Outside employment can also raise self-esteem because personal identity is closely linked with employment. For example, 'Sally the midwife' has a different meaning to 'Sally the mother'. In other words, greater social value is attached to career status than to family position (Hope, *et al.* 1999). Interestingly, the value changes, depending on the total amount of personal income, with higher values being accorded to those who receive higher salaries (Virtanen, *et al.* 2008). Children are socialised into understanding the value of different careers, and they are often encouraged to choose a career on the basis of the status and power attached to it, rather than because of a personal preference for a particular job.

MOTHERHOOD AS A LOSS

Most women have no awareness of the factors in society that mitigate against their role as mothers. What they do know, however, is that they can feel a deep sense of loss. Patel, *et al.* (2005), Ussher (2004) and Brock (1998) consider that unhappiness at the start of motherhood is a normal state and will aid the transition to this new role because it is a major life event requiring substantial psychological adjustment. The beginning of motherhood can be a form of bereavement (Nicolson 1998) in that the woman is grieving the loss of her former self and the lifestyle to which she had become accustomed. Hochschild (1983) refers to motherhood as 'hurting an illusion' (the public image of motherhood that does not match the reality). As the mother yearns for the 'illusion' and her previous lifestyle, she begins to feel unhappy with the reality. The constant tiredness during the first three months after the birth may make the losses seem insurmountable.

Dalton (1980) describes the mother as having lost not only happiness and sleep, but also her interests, enthusiasm, energy, security, pleasure, adequacy, insight, clear thinking, libido, memory, concentration, bowel movement, weight and appetite. Analysing one of these areas, loss of libido, reveals many new areas of difficulty and conflict that the mother now has to deal with. Larme (1998) has postulated that extramarital affairs increase during the postnatal period. It is easy to blame the woman's loss of libido, which could be the direct result of exhaustion, but there is also the question of the basis of the relationship. This is a time when the woman needs love, support and nurturing (Lee, *et al.* 2004), but what she in fact faces is rejection. If sexual activity had been regarded as the main measure of closeness and caring love in the relationship, when one partner is unable (for whatever reason) to take part in this physical act, the other may take it to mean that love and caring have gone from the relationship.

These meanings are not purely individual; they come from the prevailing cultural and social values. For example, advertising aims to persuade individuals to spend their money, and sex, in the form of barely clad people, is often used to promote products – the message is about satisfying personal needs by buying the product (Jenkins, *et al.* 1990, Johnston and Swanson 2003). Films often depict sex as being the only expression of love, and magazines and books are full of stories about the priority that sex has in loving. It is questionable whether many couples spend most of their time together making love, yet the media imagery is very powerful.

If people depend on society to guide them in creating a loving relationship, one of the predominant influences will be media images whose priority is profit, not the promotion of loving relationships. Even the definition of what is a sexual 'turn on' is socially mediated (Oakley 2005). In Western culture the breast is often depicted as a sexual organ, whereas in other cultures, where women's bodies are rarely seen, an ankle could fulfil the same role. The capitalist culture makes use of this socially constructed knowledge.

Many people lose 'friends' at the point of having a first baby because their interests change dramatically. People (including the mother's partner) get bored with listening to what colour the nappies are, although this may very well be the mother's current concern. Some interpret such conversation as being somewhat shallow when they would prefer to discuss the economy, for instance. Going to visit friends may involve arranging babysitting and having a disposable income in order to be able to enjoy a 'night out'. Having subsequent babies, when one is already part of a network of friends with children, may involve having children's parties in the middle of the day. So the mother's whole way of socialising has now changed. If the couple previously used to enjoy an evening out together followed by lovemaking, and the baby breaks this routine, then the nature of the relationship will change and some partners may find this adaptation difficult, or refuse to accept that a baby can alter one's life so dramatically. For the mother, however, caring for her children takes priority over most other matters (Navaro and Schwartzberg 2007), as it is here that she may feel that she can make a difference.

Having a baby is exhausting, and being exhausted can impair mind and body functions (Huang and Mathers 2001). The mother will sense changes (Ussher 1992) such as a loss of concentration, loss of memory, loss of a quick response time, loss of regular bowel motions, loss of appetite and loss of motivation, amongst other things (Tisdall 1997). How does this state of existence fit in with having sex? It seems obvious that one way for the mother to reduce her exhaustion is to have help. The help that is chosen is often dependent on family and friends, but their availability may be limited by, for example, geographical distance or daily employment. If one is wealthy, a nanny or childminder can be employed. The idea is to maintain some degree of 'normality' – that is, to try to achieve the lifestyle one had prior to motherhood.

SUPERWOMEN

Women are expected to manage not only their families, but also their careers and domestic chores. Many women, due to the limited number of hours that are available in a day, may feel anxious and guilty because they are not managing any of these areas to the best of their ability (Oakley 2005, Nicolson 1998). This situation is often exacerbated by such factors as poor housing, poor financial resources, poor relationships, poor social support and low income. Women even take on self-blame for living in poor social circumstances (Smail 2001, Flacking, *et al.* 2006). The risk of becoming unhappy is now increasing (Sheppard 1997, Romito, *et al.* 1999, Saurel-Cubizolles, *et al.* 2000, Beran 2000, Reading and Reynolds 2001). This is further exacerbated if the mother has a negative self-image and impression of others (Williamson, *et al.* 2002).

The woman risks becoming over-worked when there is an unequal distribution of domestic tasks (Graham 2007) and childcare (Um and Dancy 1999). Yet, in a patriarchal society, there is a social expectation that women will take on the bulk of the domestic chores and childcare (Johnston and Swanson 2003, Brown and Siegal 1988). Men are often described as 'helping' women and do not see the inequality in their relationship. The role is often modelled from the family of origin or is taken for granted as the role ascribed within a heterosexual partnership in a patriarchal society (Nicolson and Ussher 1992, Navaro and Schwartzberg 2007).

Men receive much in return for entering into personal relationships with women. They often have their housework, ironing, washing, childcare, cooking and dishwashing done for them. They will expect and often receive help with their work and entertaining of colleagues, and their biological urge to reproduce is satisfied by their partner. This is one area of the social order in which money is not exchanged for services. Many women feel that they need to have sex because it is part of 'earning their keep', while on the other hand feel that they would like to or need to care for their partner because, after all, that is their role! The paternalistic structure of society means that women often subordinate their own needs to those of their male partners (Gilbert 1992, Brock 1998, Graham 2007).

Nicolson states that motherhood is 'the key means of women's oppression in patriarchal societies' (Nicolson 1998: 7). Many mothers will feel dissatisfied, but often they do not realise why this is so. The family needs add an extra burden to the mother's ability to provide services, and the lack of material and verbal recognition for the provision of such services, most of which are repetitive and boring, can generate great frustration and unhappiness in a woman's life.

WHAT IS A GOOD MOTHER?

Mothers thus have to cope with feelings of anxiety and guilt (Oakley 2005, Flacking, *et al.* 2006). Most mothers have conflicting feelings about returning to work because they fear for their child. When they are away from their child, at work, they can only hope that he or she is being cared for adequately, and they may become anxious and feel guilty (Nahas and Amasheh 1999). Many of the sentences that they will use in their everyday language, in relation to their child, will be punctuated with 'if only', and thus the feeling of guilt arises (Smail 2001, Beran 2000). Feelings of anxiety and guilt are caused by the social image of a good mother (Gilbert 1992, Flacking, *et al.* 2006).

A good mother is portrayed as being self-sacrificing, with no needs or wants of her own (Graham 2007). She is totally available to her children, and this availability is often extended to her partner as well. The image of martyrdom is not generally associated with people who are not mothers. The way in which people are socialised into being selfish, competitive and resourceful within the capitalist economy makes no allowance for working alongside anyone, let alone giving up the self completely, with no material reward, to work for the family. Perhaps, as Price (1988) suggests, mothers should aim no higher than being 'good enough', and that still requires a considerable degree of self-sacrifice.

Unconditional love is something that many people resist. The expectation is to receive as well as to give. Many people talk about a relationship as being 50:50. Does this mean that they are willing to give only 50% of themselves, their time and their energy, or that they are only in the relationship for 50% of the time? Yet motherhood requires 100% of the mother to be available to the child. If adults cannot give to each other (as well as receive), where will they learn to do this for their children?

There are so many conflicts that women face during their development as mothers. For some women the conflicts are unbearable, their resources are limited and they cannot adapt to motherhood with ease – only with dis-ease. Ussher believes that 'it is the society which is sick, not the woman'. (Ussher 1991: 20). This is reiterated by Miller (2002) and Lee, *et al.* (2004) who point out that there are differences in the rates of unhappiness from one culture to another. The unifying difference in these rates is directly dependent on the amount of support that a mother receives (Danaci, *et al.* 2002, Huang and Mathers 2001). Lee, *et al.* (2004) go further to suggest that traditional cultural rituals to mark the transition into motherhood mobilised the needed postpartum support. Needless to say, birthing and postnatal rituals have mainly disintegrated in most cultures and with that, support networks have diminished leaving mothers alone and unhappy.

POST-TRAUMATIC STRESS DISORDER (PTSD)

The possibility of PTSD should now be considered following a traumatic birth (Welford 1998). PTSD is included in this chapter because it is thought that those who care for women throughout their pregnancy and birth experience, may have a part in its creation (Creedy, *et al.* 2000, Kitzinger 2005) and it is possible that action taken by the professionals could prevent its occurrence. Women's narratives are widely available to read in journals such as 'Association for Improvements in the Maternity Services (AIMS)' or 'New Generation' and these narratives indicate those areas about which women feel aggrieved. The action that is required is often to consider and be respectful of the woman and her individuality, rather than following routines and procedures (Hall 2005, Lupton 2003).

Woods states that PTSD 'may be a normal adaptive reaction to abnormal, extreme stress' (Woods 2000: 311). However, the trauma will be personally interpreted, as it will affect the way in which the mother feels about and within herself. Previously, PTSD was defined as being applicable to veterans and survivors of torture, assault and rape (Michaels, *et al.* 1999, Beck 2006). However, it is now recognised that as some women narrate their labour story they will use the same or similar words as those of rape survivors (DiBlasio and Ionio 2002).

PTSD has been recognised for about 20 years (Rogers and Liness 2000) as a classification of anxiety that causes major 'changes in behaviour, cognitions (thoughts, and the way that we think) and physiology (physical feelings of anxiety). It can also affect a person's daily life, including work, relationships, hobbies and interests'(Rogers and Liness 2000: 48). This is a step beyond mere unhappiness. Rachman tells us that anxiety is 'a feeling of uneasy suspense . . . tense anticipation of a threatening but "vague event"' (Rachman 1998: 25), and while depression may be the result of unresolved anxiety it should not be labelled as depression. It has to be recognised that treating a woman for clinical depression, when the latter is not present, will not resolve the initial trigger for her anxiety.

Rogers and Liness (2000) explain that during the first four weeks following the trauma the condition will be classified as acute stress disorder, and if there is no resolution, then the classification of PTSD is applied. It is easy to see how the postpartum woman is likely to be labelled as 'depressed' at this time, because giving the label of PTSD would shift the onus of responsibility away from the woman and pass it on to the professionals. If it is not the woman's hormones that are causing the way she feels, could it be the way in which she was treated during labour?

Factors that contribute to PTSD include a violent birth, fear for the baby, stillbirth, pre-eclampsia, very low birthweight (Beck 2006), postpartum pain, low energy levels, disturbed sleep, worry, being sexually abused while pregnant, excessive vomiting during pregnancy, ectopic pregnancy, hospital treatment for miscarriage, macrosomia, preterm labour (Miller 2002), and recurring episodes of preterm labour although the mother gives birth at term (Seng, *et al.* 2001). Olde, *et al.* (2006) propose that PTSD as a result of birth trauma has long-term, serious and negative mental health effects.

Laing (2001) considers that PTSD can result from loss of control and a sense of powerlessness during labour, but adds that women view that as not being treated with respect or given adequate information. Laing (2001) suggests that there are other factors that will pre-dispose a woman to PTSD such as:
- a pre-existing personality disorder or emotional disorder
- a family history of psychiatric disorders
- a poor adaptive coping style
- the severity of the actual event
- the nature of the outside support.

It is difficult to evaluate these factors because some individuals will cope better, despite having a cruel history, compared with others who appear to have had fewer life stresses. Therefore, whilst recognising risk factors for PTSD in the antenatal period, it is important to make an individual assessment of the woman as a totality.

Ayers and Pickering (2001) think that PTSD may develop in 3% of women as a result of childbirth. Beck (2006) says that the rate of PTSD as a result of birth trauma is in the range of 1.5–5.6%. However, we do not know whether the 10–15% who are diagnosed as having postnatal depression in fact have PTSD (Robinson 1999). Creedy, *et al.* (2000) mention that the classification of PTSD comes from the *Diagnostic and Statistical Manual of Mental Disorders* (American Psychiatric Association 2000), and they describe the condition as follows.

1 The stress involves an event, (i.e. labour) which could entail actual or threatened death or serious injury, or damage to the self or others. It is well known that pregnant women often think about dying during childbirth and in labour, and each

intervention is capable of resurrecting those thoughts. Narratives of women's experiences in books and journals recall the horror of their labour, together with the emotional context, and these women often wonder how they survived.

2   The woman's response involves intense fear, helplessness or horror. LeMarquand (2000) provides a narrative to demonstrate this. Loss of control is a recurring feature (Laing 2001). Axe (2000) acknowledges that women experience physical damage, stigmatisation, betrayal and powerlessness during labour.

3   There is persistent re-experiencing of the labour, with intrusive thoughts, persistent memories, nightmares and flashbacks (Bracken 2001). Michaels, *et al.* (1998) state that there can be recurring memories, which will be felt physically and visually, and even acted out. There will be no information processing in the memory storage, so no processing will have taken place.

4   There is persistent avoidance of any stimuli associated with the labour. The woman may avoid other pregnant or postnatal women, hospitals or health professionals. Fear of childbirth has the knock–on effect of sexual avoidance (Beck 2006). The woman succeeds in achieving an emotional numbing.

5   The woman will experience symptoms of increased physiological arousal that involve the fight/flight hormones, and therefore she will be in a state of heightened awareness, with extreme vigilance, insomnia and resultant irritability (American Psychiatric Association 2000). The sympathetic nervous system is called into action in the extreme, leaving little room for parasympathetic function. The physiological results of this could be manifested as irritable bowel syndrome, heartburn, digestive difficulties, bladder problems and sexual dysfunction, among other things. Beck (2006) and Madigan, *et al.* (2006) suggest that in the long term, PTSD can lead to poor maternal–infant attachment and thus defective parenting.

Creedy, *et al.* (2000) have pointed out that as the level of intervention increases, satisfaction with care decreases, and that is when the care is perceived to be inadequate. The risk of PTSD will increase at this point.

Women will often receive psychiatric referrals in order to reduce the effects of PTSD once it is suspected. However, the 2005 trial by Gamble, *et al.* of a midwifery serial counselling intervention for women who had traumatic births, was shown to significantly reduce the incidence of PTSD at three months postpartum. Perhaps consideration should be given to better preparation for the *reality* of parenthood and medicalised birth (Lupton 2003) as opposed to the glamourised versions depicted in the media that form a major source of information for potential parents (Glazener 2005, Johnston and Swanson 2003).

CONCLUSION

This chapter has discussed the realities of life underlying the unhappiness felt by some women on becoming mothers. Social factors cannot be ignored, as they are integral to the aetiology of unhappiness, and once they are recognised, solutions become obvious.

Motherhood needs to be socially and politically supported. The evolving culture needs to recognise the value of motherhood and reward mothers' contribution to society. Radical policy changes from the Government need to be instituted so that women feel valued within the cultural norm; for example, acceptance of fathers performing the traditional mothering role, and remunerating women (or men), while also allowing respite breaks from childcare. Maternity services are partly responsible for the occurrence of PTSD and need to select staff carefully and support them so that they are able to give the best care possible.

However, babies grow up and life moves on. The unhappiness may pass with time even if nothing is done; however, the long-term effects have been shown to have a negative impact on children both behaviourally and intellectually, and there is an increased incidence of non-accidental injury (Bernazzani and Bifulco 2003). The period that is spent being unhappy, and its effects on the baby and others with whom the mother is in contact, are worthy of greater consideration. There is an urgent need to radically modify attitudes towards mothers, and increase the support that is given to them, in order to produce a happier society in the future.

KEY POINTS

- Unhappiness can be a rational adaptive process to motherhood
- Mothering can reduce life choices
- Normality can exist in the procurement of a lifestyle that was maintained prior to motherhood
- Mothers may grieve for their former lifestyle
- Motherhood is regarded as a low status activity within a capitalist economy

---

USEFUL ADDRESSES

Cry-sis
BM Cry-sis
London WC1N 3XX
Helpline: 0845 1228 669
Website: www.cry-sis.org.uk

The Association of Post Natal Illness
145 Dawes Road
London SW6 7EB
Helpline: 0207 386 0868
Fax: 0207 386 8885
Email: Info@APNI.org
Website: www.APNI.org

National Childbirth Trust – Post Natal Depression Co-ordination
Alexandra House
Oldham Terrace
Acton
London W3 6NH
Tel: 0870 444 8707

REFERENCES

American Psychiatric Association. (2000) *Diagnostic and Statistical Manual of Mental Disorder.* 4th ed. Washington, DC: APA.

Axe S. (2000) Women's issues: labour debriefing is crucial for good psychological care. *Br J Midwif.* 8(10): 626–31.

Ayers S, Pickering AD. (2001) Do women get post-traumatic stress disorder as a result of childbirth? A prospective study of incidence. *Birth.* 28(2): 111–18.

Beck CT. (2006) The anniversary of birth trauma: failure to rescue. *Nurs Res.* 55(6): 381–90.

Beran CL. (2000) The pursuit of happiness: a study of Alice Munro's fiction. *Soc Sci J.* 37(3): 329–45.

Bernazzani O, Bifulco A. (2003) Motherhood as a vulnerability factor in major depression: the role of negative pregnancy experiences. *Soc Sci Med.* 56(6): 1249–60.

Bracken PJ. (2001) Post-modernity and post-traumatic stress disorder. *Soc Sci Med.* 53(6): 733–43.

Brock G, editor. (1998) *Necessary Goods: our responsibilities to meet others needs.* Lanham, MD: Rowman & Littlefield.

Brotherson SE. (2007) From partners to parents: couples and the transition to parenthood. *J Childbirth Educ.* 22(2): 7–12.

Brown GW, Harris T. (1978) *The Social Origins of Depression.* London: Tavistock Publications.

Brown JD, Siegal JM. (1988) Attribution for negative life events and depression: the role of perceived control. *J Personality Soc Psychol.* 54: 316–22.

Buultjens M, Liamputtong P. (2007) When giving life starts to take the life out of you: women's experiences of depression after childbirth. *Midwifery.* 23(1): 77–91.

Creedy DK, Shochet IM, Horsfall J. (2000) Childbirth and the development of acute trauma symptoms. *Birth.* 27(2): 104–11.

Dalton K. (1980) *Depression after Childbirth.* Oxford: Oxford University Press.

Danaci AE, Dinç G, Deveci A, *et al.* (2002) Postnatal depression in Turkey: epidemiological and cultural aspects. *Soc Psychiatry Psychiatr Epidemiol.* 37: 125–9.

Deaves D. (2001) Prevention and management of postnatal depression. *Community Pract.* 74(7): 263–7.

DiBlasio P, Ionio C. (2002) Childbirth and narratives: how do mothers deal with their child's birth? *J Prenat Perinat Psychol Health.* 17: 143–151.

Flacking R, Ewald U, Nyqvist KH, *et al.* (2006) Trustful bonds: a key to 'becoming a mother' and to reciprocal breastfeeding. *Soc Sci Med.* 62(1): 70–80.

Frost J, Pope C, Liebling R, *et al.* (2006) Utopian theory and the discourse of natural birth. *Theory and Health.* 4(4): 299–318. Available at: http://eprints.soton.ac.uk/42996/ (accessed 2 Jan 2009).

Gamble J, Creedy D, Moyle W, *et al.* (2005) Effectiveness of a counselling intervention after a traumatic childbirth: a randomised controlled trial. *Birth.* 32: 11–19.

Gilbert P. (1992) *Depression: the evolution of powerlessness.* Hove: Lawrence Erlbaum Associates Publications.

Glazener CMA. (2005) Parental perceptions and adaptation to parenthood. *Br J Midwif.* 13(9): 578–85.

Graham H. (2007) *Unequal Lives: health and socio-economic inequalities.* Buckingham: Open University Press.

Hall J. (2005) Midwifery basics: postnatal care: postnatal emotional well-being. *Pract Midwife.* 8(4): 35–9.

Harris T. (2001) Recent developments in understanding the psychosocial aspects of depression. *Br Med Bull.* 57(1): 17–32.

Hochschild AR. (1983) *The Managed Heart: commercialisation of human feeling.* Berkeley, CA: University of California Press.

Hope S, Power C, Rodgers B. (1999) Does financial hardship account for elevated psychological distress in lone mothers? *Soc Sci Med.* 49: 1637–49.

Huang Y, Mathers N. (2001) Postnatal depression – biological or cultural? A comparative study of postnatal women in the UK and Taiwan. *J Adv Nurs.* **33**(3): 279–87.

Jenkins A, Sweeney N, Potrykus C. (1990) The shock of motherhood. *Health Visit.* **63**(5): 154–5.

Johnston DD, Swanson DH. (2003) Invisible mothers: a content analysis of motherhood ideologies and myths in magazines. *Sex Roles.* **49**: 21–33.

Kitzinger S. (2005) *The Politics of Birth.* Edinburgh: Elsevier.

Korten D. (2007) Living wealth: better than money. *Yes Magazine.* Fall. Available at www.yesmagazine. org/article.asp?ID=1834 (accessed 9 Mar 2009).

Laing KG. (2001) Post-traumatic stress disorder: myth or reality? *Br J Midwif.* **9**(7): 447–51.

Larme AC. (1998) Environment, vulnerability and gender in Andean ethnomedicine. *Soc Sci Med.* **47**(8): 1005–15.

Lee DTS, Yip ASK, Leung TYS, *et al.* (2004) Ethnoepidemiology of postnatal depression: prospective multivariate study of sociocultural risk factors in a Chinese population in Hong Kong. *Br J Psychiatry.* **184**: 34–40.

LeMarquand J. (2000) 'Normal' birth in Jersey: *Association for Improvements in the Maternity Services (AIMS).* **12**(1): 13–15.

Lupton D. (2003) *Medicine as Culture.* 2nd ed. London: Sage.

Madigan S, Moran G, Pederson DR. (2006) Unresolved states of mind, disorganised attachment relationships and disrupted interactions of adolescent mothers and their infants. *Dev Psychol.* **42**(2): 293–304.

McKim MK, Cramer KM, Stuart B, *et al.* (1999) Infant care decisions and attachment security: the Canadian transition to childcare study. *Can J Behav Sci.* **31**(2): 92–106.

Michaels AJ, Michaels CE, Moon CH, *et al.* (1999) Post-traumatic stress disorders after injury. *J Trauma-Injury Infect Crit Care.* **47**(3): 460–7.

Michaels AJ, Michaels CE, Moon CH, *et al.* (1998) Psychosocial factors limit outcomes after trauma. *J Trauma-Injury Infect Crit Care.* **44**(4): 644–8.

Miller LJ. (2002) Postpartum depression. *JAMA.* **287**(6): 762–5.

Nahas V, Amasheh N. (1999) Culture care meanings and experiences of postpartum depression among Jordanian Australian women. *J Transcult Nurs.* **10**(1): 37–45.

Navaro L, Schwartzberg SL. (2007) *Envy, Competition and Gender.* London: Routledge.

Nicolson P, Ussher J. (1992) *The Psychology of Women's Health and Healthcare.* Basingstoke: MacMillan Press Ltd.

Nicolson P. (1998) *Postnatal Depression.* London: Routledge.

Oakley A. (2005) *The Ann Oakley Reader: gender, women and social science.* Bristol: The Policy Press.

Odent M. (1999) *The Scientification of Love.* London: Free Association Books.

Olde E, Van der Hart O, Kleber R, *et al.* (2006) Post-traumatic stress following childbirth: a review. *Clin Psychol Rev.* **26**(1): 1–16.

Patel RR, Peters TJ, Murphy DJ. (2005) ALSPAC Study Team: operative delivery and postnatal depression cohort study. *BMJ.* **330**: 879.

Patel V, Rodrigues M, DeSouza N. (2002) Gender, poverty and postnatal depression: a study of mothers in Goa, India. *Am J Psychiatry.* **159**(1): 43–7.

Pilgrim D, Bentall R. (1999) The medicalisation of misery. *J Ment Health.* **8**(3): 261–74.

Price J. (1988) *Motherhood: what it does to your mind.* London: Pandora.

Rachman S. (1998) *Anxiety.* Hove: Psychology Press.

Reading R, Reynolds S. (2001) Debt, social disadvantage and maternal depression. *Soc Sci Med.* **53**(4): 441–53.

Robinson J. (1999) When delivery is torture: postnatal PTSD. *Br J Midwif.* **7**(11): 684.

Rogers P, Liness S. (2000) Post-traumatic stress disorder. *Nurs Stand.* **14**(22): 47–54.

Romito P, Cubizolles-Saurel MJ, Lelong N. (1999) What makes new mothers unhappy: psychological distress one year after birth in Italy and France. *Soc Sci Med.* **49**(12): 1651–61.

Saurel-Cubizolles MJ, Romito P, Ancel PY, *et al.* (2000) Unemployment and psychological distress one year after childbirth in France. *J Epidemiol Community Health.* **54**(3): 185–91.

Seng JS, Oakley DJ, Sampselle CM, *et al.* (2001) Post-traumatic stress disorder and pregnancy complications. *Obstet Gynaecol.* **97**(1): 17–22.

Sheppard M. (1997) Depression in female health visitor consulters. *J Adv Nurs.* **26**: 921–9.

Simmel G, Frisby D. (2004) *The Philosophy of Money.* London: Routledge.

Smail D. (2001) *The Nature of Unhappiness.* London: Constable Publishers.

Smith PK, Cowie H. (1998) *Understanding Children's Development.* 3rd ed. Oxford: Blackwell Science.

Tisdall N. (1997) *Psychology of Childbearing.* Hale: Books for Midwives Press.

Um CC, Dancy BL. (1999) Relationship between coping strategies and depression among employed Korean immigrant wives. *Issues Ment Health Nurs.* **20**(5): 485–94.

Ussher J. (1991) *Women's Madness.* Hemel Hempstead: Harvester Wheatsheaf.

Ussher J. (1992) Reproductive rhetoric and the blaming of the body. In: Nicolson P, Ussher J, editors. *The Psychology of Women's Health and Healthcare.* Basingstoke: MacMillan Press Ltd. pp. 31–61.

Ussher J. (2004) Depression in the postnatal period: a normal response to motherhood. In: Stewart M, editor. *Pregnancy, Birth and Maternity Care.* Edinburgh: Elsevier Books for Midwives.

Virtanen M, Koskinen S, Kivimäki M, *et al.* (2008) Contribution of non-work and work-related risk factors to the association between income and mental disorders in a working population: the Health 2000 study. *Occup Environment Med.* **65**(3): 171–8.

Welford H. (1998) *Book of Postnatal Depression.* London: Thorsons.

Williamson GM, Walters AS, Shaffer DR. (2002) Caregiver models of self and others, coping and depression: predictors of depression in children with chronic pain. *Health Psychol.* **21**(4): 405–10.

Woods SJ. (2000) Prevalence and patterns of post-traumatic stress disorder in abused and post-abused women. *Issues Ment Health Nurs.* **21**(3): 309–24.

CHAPTER 15

Childbirth and sexual abuse during childhood

Caroline Squire

Childhood sexual abuse is an important area that midwives and healthcare workers need to confront and understand. Many women survivors will make use of the maternity services, and midwives and healthcare workers need to be fully prepared and aware of the difficulties these women may face. This chapter provides background information about the definition and prevalence of childhood sexual abuse, but the main focus is on the long-term effects and the specific issues related to pregnancy and childbirth. The relationship between childhood sexual abuse and adolescent pregnancy, preterm labour, labour and birth, language, breastfeeding, and unhappiness after birth is considered. Finally, there is a brief consideration of clinicians who have been sexually abused as children, with particular reference to the effects on their clinical judgement.

INTRODUCTION

> I was sexually abused by my grandfather and other family members from the age of two until I was approximately 12 years old . . . In the delivery room, whenever a contraction would come, I simply 'stepped out', looking right through whoever was there until the contraction subsided. My daughter was posterior and the doctor turned her . . .
>
> Finally, my baby was pulled from my body. I laid back on the bed and felt totally, utterly violated. (Christensen 1992: 34)

Childbirth can be a traumatic experience for any woman, but for women who have been sexually abused as children, the likelihood of experiencing birth as violence is increased. It is a significant trauma that is likely to have a lifelong impact on survivors. Despite the high prevalence of child sexual abuse, lack of knowledge and understanding still exists among many healthcare professionals, including midwives. This lack of understanding of the complex difficulties that survivors face during childbirth may lead to insensitive care and subsequent further emotional and psychological trauma. Many midwives will have assisted women during their births unaware that these women were sexually abused as children. On other occasions, women will disclose their tragic histories, and it is important that midwives can feel confident that they have background knowledge and understanding to support these survivors. Furthermore, there are midwives and other healthcare professionals, who themselves have experienced sexual abuse during their own childhoods and it is important that they too are supported if they decide to disclose their personal experiences. This chapter will consider definitions and the prevalence of childhood sexual abuse and, in particular, issues related to childbirth, including adolescent pregnancy, preterm labour, language and power, unhappiness after birth, and breastfeeding. It is hoped that such knowledge will help midwives to empower women who are survivors of childhood sexual abuse and so prevent further emotional trauma.

DEFINITION

Defining childhood sexual abuse is problematic for healthcare professionals and researchers. The definitions in the literature vary according to the types of activities that are considered to be 'sexual' and the age at which a child is considered competent to give 'informed consent'. Clearly, childhood sexual abuse is part of the wider issue of child abuse in general, and the official definitions that are used when children's names are placed on local child protection registers have widened. These registers, which are maintained by local authority social services departments, are lists of all children in the area for whom there are unresolved child protection issues and who are currently the subject of an interagency protection plan (Home Office, Department of Health, Department of Education and Science and Welsh Office 1991). There are currently four categories in use in England and Wales, defined as follows (Home Office, Department of Health, Department of Education and Science and Welsh Office 1991).

- **Physical injury**: actual or likely physical injury to a child, or failure to prevent physical injury (or suffering) to a child, including deliberate poisoning, suffocating and Munchausen's syndrome by proxy.
- **Neglect**: the persistent or severe neglect of a child, or the failure to protect a child from exposure to any kind of danger, including cold or starvation, or extreme failure to carry out important aspects of care, resulting in the significant impairment of the child's health or development, including non-organic failure to thrive.
- **Sexual abuse**: actual or likely sexual exploitation of a child or adolescent. The child may be dependent and/or developmentally immature.
- **Emotional abuse**: actual or likely severe adverse effect on the emotional and behavioural development of a child caused by persistent or severe emotional ill-treatment or rejection. All abuse involves some emotional ill-treatment. This category should be used where it is the main or sole form of abuse.

The problems inherent in the above general definitions are that they omit some forms of harm to children, such as child labour and the consequences of war and civil unrest, and they also require a degree of subjective judgement about the presence or absence of abuse. For example, perspectives on child abuse are culture specific, and child labour may be regarded as child abuse in one country but not in another (Hallett 1995).

In their feasibility study for a national prevalence study, Ghate and Spencer (1995) found that definitions of sexual abuse vary in terms of the following factors.

- **Type of activity**: usually distinguishing between contact and non-contact.
- **Age of victim/survivor**: in most studies the upper limit is set at 16 years.
- **Age differential between abuser and abused**: usually 5 years, with some studies specifying 5 years for children under 12 years, 8–10 years for children over 12 years, or 5-year differential for total sample, but perpetrator over 16 years of age. Definitions that set an age differential are attempting to distinguish between abusive sexual experiences and cases of sexual exploration among peers.
- **Nature of the relationship between the abuser and the abused**: in previous studies, distinctions have been made between relatives (intra-familial) and people who are not related (extra-familial). Ghate and Spencer (1995) suggest that finer distinctions are required with regard to extra-familial perpetrators, which differentiate between people in a position of trust (e.g. peers, family friends, acquaintances, babysitters) and strangers.
- **Issue of consent/responsibility/legality**: some studies probe consent, while others argue that children do not have the maturity to withhold consent.

It is clear that the different definitions employed in different studies will alter the prevalence rates and interpretations of the data.

In the UK, Creighton and Russell (1995) have used the following definition:

> . . . the involvement of dependent children under the age of 16 in a sexual activity which they do not fully understand and to which they are not in a position to give informed consent – the activity being intended to gratify or satisfy the needs of the other person. (Cited in Cawson, *et al.* 2000: 75)

This definition does not include peer sexual experimentation, but it does include the issue of informed consent.

In the US, childhood sexual abuse has been defined as any activity that engages a child in sexual activities that are developmentally inappropriate, with or without threatened or actual violence or injury. Sexual abuse does not always involve sexual intercourse or physical force. Rather, it is usually characterised by deception and coercion. Activities may include genital or anal contact, oral–genital contact and insertion of objects, and can encompass incest or sexual assault by a relative or stranger. Childhood sexual abuse is often a chronic violation rather than a single incident (Petersen 1993). This lengthy definition is useful in that it makes explicit the fact that perpetrators may be family members or strangers, contact and non-contact activities are included, and it addresses the exploitation of adult authority (and maturity) over the child. Further detail is described by Johnson (2001) in the US in terms of exposure of sexual anatomy, forced viewing of sexual anatomy, showing pornography to a child or using a child in the production of pornography.

Finkelhor (1997) suggests the following definition as being consistent with most legal and research definitions of child sexual abuse. It was formulated by the National Center on Child Abuse and Neglect (1978: 2), and it has many of the advantages of the previous definition. This definition also makes it clear that the perpetrator may be under 18 years of age.

> Contacts or interactions between a child and an adult when the child is being used for the sexual stimulation of the perpetrator or another person. Sexual abuse may also be committed by a person under the age of 18, when that person is significantly older than the victim or when the perpetrator is in a position of power or control over another child.

Cawson, *et al.* (2000) and Cawson (2002) made a distinction between abuse involving physical contact (e.g. intercourse, oral sex, touching and fondling, sexual hugging or kissing) and 'non-contact' abuse (e.g. using the child to make pornographic photographs or videos, showing the child pornography, forcing or encouraging the child to watch live sexual acts, exposing sex organs to excite themselves or shock the child). Again it is easy to see how other studies may not make the same distinction, and may therefore produce different prevalence rates and interpretations.

Scott (1996) argues that where definitions become more restrictive, prevalence rates fall, and this would partially explain the wide variations in the data on the prevalence of sexual abuse. It may be that too narrow a definition of abuse works against children's rights, while the capacity to construe almost any situation as abusive could result in the statistics being ignored and/or the issue not being taken seriously (Fitzsimons 1999).

PREVALENCE

Childhood sexual abuse occurs much more frequently than was originally believed, but as mentioned above, the prevalence rates are affected by the way in which sexual abuse is defined (Burke Draucker 2000). The reported prevalence of childhood sexual abuse is highest in studies that include subjects seeking psychiatric treatment for depression, substance abuse, suicide, post-traumatic stress disorder (PTSD), eating disorders and multiple personality disorder (Herman, *et al.* 1986, Courtois 1993). The National Society for the Prevention of Cruelty to Children (NSPCC) recently reported the findings of a survey of the childhood experiences of 2869 young people aged 18–24 years (Cawson, *et al.* 2000). The main findings are listed below. The rates of physical and emotional abuse are included here because children who are sexually abused suffer physical and emotional abuse as well.

- ➾ 7% suffered serious physical abuse as children at the hands of parents or carers, including being hit with a fist or implement, beaten up, burned or scalded.
- ➾ 6% suffered serious physical neglect at home, including being left regularly without food as a young child, not being looked after or taken to the doctor when they were ill, or being left to fend for themselves because the parents were absent or had drug- or alcohol-related problems. In total, 5% had been placed at risk by being left alone at home overnight or out overnight (their whereabouts unknown) at young ages.
- ➾ 6% suffered multiple attacks on their emotional well-being and self-confidence, including living with frequent violence between their parents, being 'really afraid'

of their parents, being regularly humiliated, being threatened with being sent away or thrown out, or being told that their parents wished they were dead or had never been born.

- 1% had been sexually abused by a parent, and 3% had been sexually abused by another relative (ranging from penetrative or oral sex to taking pornographic photographs of them).
- 1% (mainly girls, under the age of 16 years) had been forced or threatened by people known to them into taking part in sexual acts against their will.
- 25% said that there were things that had happened to them during their childhood that they found difficult to talk about. For example, only just over 25% of respondents who had been sexually abused or coerced into sexual activity had told anyone at the time that it happened.
- Childhood sexual abuse is most prevalent in the 5–14 years age group
- Overall, 11% of boys aged under 16 and 21% of girls aged under 16 experienced sexual abuse during childhood.
- The majority of children who experienced sexual abuse had more than one sexually abusive experience; only indecent exposure was likely to be a single incident.
- 16% of girls aged 12 or under experienced sexual abuse involving physical contact.

Furthermore, more than one-third (36%) of all rapes recorded by the police are committed against children under 16 years of age (Walker, *et al.* 2006). The Inter-departmental Ministerial Group on Sexual Offending (2007) also opines that child sexual abuse is more likely to be experienced by children with a disability, missing or looked after children, and children from families experiencing domestic violence. Such vulnerable children are then more likely to suffer from sexual abuse in adulthood. To date, the study by Cawson, *et al.* (2000) remains the most recent national prevalence study of childhood sexual abuse, though further prevalence rates will be published by the NSPCC in the near future (personal communication NSPCC June 2008).

Epidemiological reports from the US estimate that as many as one in four American women have been victims of sexual abuse during childhood. The number of sexually abused children during 1994 was estimated to be over 300 000, and girls were found to have been sexually abused three times more frequently than boys (Sedlack and Broadhurst 1996).

Finkelhor (1994) reviewed 21 international population studies of child sexual abuse, primarily from English-speaking and northern European countries. The prevalence rates ranged from 7% to 36% for women and from 3% to 29% for men. Despite the variation in rates, it appears that the number of people with a history of abuse is significant, with a higher prevalence for women.

Similarly, in Australia a retrospective study of 710 women randomly selected from Australian federal electoral rolls (Fleming 1997) revealed that 20% had experienced childhood sexual abuse, and that among this 20%:

- 10% had experienced either vaginal or anal intercourse
- the mean age at the first episode was 10 years (71% were under 12 years)
- 98% of the perpetrators were male; they were usually known to the child
- 41% were relatives

➡ the mean age of abusers was 34 years, with a median age difference of 24 years older than that of the abused child

➡ only 10% reported their experiences to the police, a doctor or a helping agency.

From the above listing of some of the available prevalence rates for childhood sexual abuse, it would appear that more women than men are sexually abused as children, and that only a fraction disclose their experiences to anyone. This is of great significance for midwives and healthcare professionals who work with women during pregnancy and childbirth, since most survivors will be unknown to them, rendering the notion of being 'with woman' and 'woman-centred' even more difficult.

BACKGROUND CHARACTERISTICS ASSOCIATED WITH SEXUAL ABUSE OF CHILDREN

Jehu (1988) has described the following as characteristics of the family with incestuous sexual relationships:

➡ high levels of marital conflict, often with physical abuse of the mother

➡ the father may select children as sexual objects when his sexual and emotional needs are not met within the marriage

➡ high levels of mobility, with passing of the child to one relative or another, leading to a lack of consistent stable care from the parents

➡ family often lacks social skills and is isolated from others

➡ confusion with regard to family roles and responsibilities for tasks at home.

There is now evidence of a link between childhood abuse, domestic violence and the abuse of animals (Hackett and Uprichard (2007).

Araji and Finkelor (1986) proposed four conditions that they considered to be necessary before sexual abuse could occur.

➡ The perpetrator needs to desire the child, and this may occur as a result of disinhibition due to alcohol or drugs. Yet arousal may also be partly due to a need to dominate or because of low self-esteem or immaturity.

➡ Perpetrators can often make children feel guilty and responsible for the abuse. They are sometimes able to persuade themselves that children desire sex within situations of step-parenting, because there are no biological ties and therefore the taboo is less strong.

➡ The perpetrator needs to consider external constraints. The abuser has more opportunity when the mother is out and when the child is unsupervised. Most abuse occurs when children are alone.

➡ The perpetrator needs to deal with the child's resistance, usually by threatening violence. Other adults and peers are kept away from the child in order to reduce the likelihood of discovery, and this adds to the child's isolation.

Cawson, *et al.* (2000) found that socio-economic background made no difference to the prevalence of childhood sexual abuse. This contrasted with physical abuse, which was more likely in low-income groups. In truth, there are no clear reasons why adults sexually abuse children, and offenders may commit these acts for a variety of reasons.

It is likely that both pathopsychological forces and the social structures of society form a complex mesh that may have a part in determining why some individuals engage in sexual activities with young children (Wallace 1999).

To date, it would seem that the male has been regarded as the sole possible abuser, but it is recognised that women do sexually abuse children. There is evidence of a wide variety of sexual offences known to have been committed by females either by themselves or with a male accomplice. These offences vary from voyeurism and inappropriate touching, to rape, penetration with objects and ritualistic, sadistic sexual abuse (Bunting 2005, Bunting 2007). It could be said that socialisation of males in society tends to reinforce sexually aggressive behaviour, but that socialisation of women inhibits it, so that for women to offend against children sexually, they have to deviate greatly from the accepted schema of the qualities that are considered to be female. Therefore it is extremely unlikely that as many women as men will be found to be perpetrators of child sexual abuse (Saradjian 1996).

However, the under-reporting of sexual abuse by females, especially in intra-familial situations, might be due to society's tendency to view males as aggressors and females as victims, or possibly to differences in the types of offence that are committed by female offenders. Mothers in particular are construed as a special and 'purer' form of womanhood, being virtually 'asexual' (Saradjian 1996). Offences by women may be less overt and embedded in typical parenting behaviours, such as caressing the child while bathing him or her, or becoming sexual with a child while 'cuddling' in bed (Burke Draucker 2000). Therefore it needs to be recognised that women have been the offenders in a sizeable minority of cases of children who have been sexually abused, and that the notion that the perpetrators are always men and the victims are always female is incorrect.

LONG-TERM EFFECTS

Relatively recent research has revealed that experiences of child sexual abuse are associated with numerous and varied long-term psychological, behavioural, interpersonal and physical effects (Bohn and Holz 1996, Burke Draucker 2000). Specific long-term effects with regard to pregnancy and childbirth will be discussed in more detail later in the chapter. A recurrent theme reported by survivors of childhood sexual abuse is shame and this is explored by Rahm, et al. (2006) who distinguish shame from guilt – the former being described as what one has done and the latter as who one is.

Psychological effects have been identified in several comprehensive reviews of the literature on long-term consequences of child sexual abuse (Finkelhor 1990, Polusny and Follette 1995, Young 1992). They include increased levels of depression, multiple personality disorder, suicidal ideation and suicide, as well as anxiety disorders such as phobias, panic attacks and obsessive behaviours (Bifulco, et al. 1991, Yellowlees and Kaushik 1994, Gladstone, et al. 2004, Warne and McAndrew 2005, Miller 2006, Warm, et al. 2003, Unikel, et al. 2006). There has also been found to be a correlation with the onset of PTSD in survivors assaulted below the age of 18 years (Masho and Ahmed 2007, Feerick and Snow 2005, Villano, et al. 2007). Seng, et al. (2004) found that nurses and midwives may not recognise women with abuse-related post-traumatic stress during pregnancy and childbirth and may not know how to respond to them.

A key psychological effect is dissociation, which is postulated to be a coping mechanism used by many incest survivors that allows the child to endure the pain, humiliation and rage engendered by the abuse. The child mentally leaves his or her body during the abuse and escapes to a safe place, often watching the abuse as if it were happening to someone else (Bala 1994), or else they may be able to numb body parts at will (Kendall-Tackett 1998). As adults they may later use the technique to cope with any stressful, intimate or dangerous situation. Medically intrusive procedures such as vaginal examinations or events related to previously traumatised body parts, such as childbirth or breastfeeding, may cause abuse survivors to dissociate. They may appear 'far away', may not respond to questions appropriately or may not remember parts of a discussion.

Sexual and relationship difficulties have also been reported (Mullen, *et al.* 1993, Ahmad 2006), including promiscuity, prostitution, sexual deviance, sexual dysfunction, and engaging in sexual behaviour not of their choosing for the purposes of obtaining drugs or a place to stay (Bachman, *et al.* 1988, Courtois 1993, Hendricks-Matthews 1993). Behavioural and sexual problems that are experienced by abuse survivors may change over time and vary with the age of the survivor. For example, the abused child may display self-destructive behaviour by frequently darting into streets, climbing and playing in unsafe areas, and taking physical risks, whereas the abused adolescent may run away or give sex in exchange for money or drugs.

Cohen (1995) published a preliminary report of an investigation of the maternal functioning of woman survivors of child sexual abuse. A study group of 26 mothers who were adult survivors was compared with a control group of 28 mothers with no such history of abuse. Cohen studied seven areas of parenting skills, namely role image, objectivity, expectations, rapport, communication, limit-setting and role support. She found significant differences on all seven scales, characterised by a tendency of the study group to be less skilful with regard to maternal functioning than the control group. Particularly large differences were found on the scales of role support, communication and role image. Cohen (1995) suggests that secrecy, shame and self-blame may provide a partial explanation for the study group's generally underdeveloped social skills, as well as other factors, such as age of onset, severity and age at termination of the abuse.

Female abuse survivors most frequently present for healthcare with physical complaints. They may make repeated visits with the same or varied and often vague symptoms. These complaints are often stress- or anxiety-related, or symptoms of post-traumatic stress syndrome. They include sleep disorders (with repetitive dreams and nightmares), gastrointestinal problems (e.g. nausea, vomiting, diarrhoea, constipation, irritable bowel syndrome), muscle tension, headaches, palpitations or choking sensations, and chronic pelvic pain (Hendricks-Matthews 1993, Walling, *et al.* 1994, Salmon, *et al.* 2003). Koci and Strickland (2006) also describe the relationship of childhood sexual abuse to premenstrual tension in adult life; Wallace (2007) presents a case study of a woman with incontinence and a history of childhood sexual abuse, and Lee and Tolman (2006) discuss the adverse effects childhood sexual abuse has on adult employment experiences.

The adult survivor may chain-smoke (Al Mamun, *et al.* 2007), overeat (causing bulimia and/or obesity) (Sanci, *et al.* 2008, Rayworth, *et al.* 2004, Treuer, *et al.* 2005), drink excessively or ignore basic health needs and problems (Bushnell, *et al.* 1992, Koss and Heslet 1992, Courtois 1993, Bohn and Holz 1996). Other self-destructive behaviours may include self-mutilation, suicide attempts, substance abuse and unprotected sex with multiple partners (Johnson, *et al.* 2006, Ompad, *et al.* 2005, Bohn and Holz

1996). Childhood abuse survivors are also 33–66% more likely to be assaulted and raped as adults both by strangers and by people known to them (Bohn and Holz 1996) and seem to be more likely to return to abusive relationships (Griffing, *et al.* 2005). Low self-esteem, self-hatred, guilt, a sense of unworthiness and an inability to trust their own senses and set safe boundaries may cause adult survivors to be perceived by abusers as vulnerable or easy targets.

ISSUES SPECIFIC TO PREGNANCY AND CHILDBIRTH

Research into pregnancy-related consequences of childhood sexual abuse is still in the early stages of development, and is for the most part anecdotal (Bohn and Holz 1996). However, there are a number of problems that are more likely to occur in survivors of childhood sexual abuse. They include unplanned, frequent and teenage pregnancy, spontaneous miscarriage, termination of pregnancy, hyperemesis, infertility, preterm labour, increased need for medical intervention and/or operative delivery, postpartum depression and breastfeeding difficulties (Courtois 1993, Holz 1994). Buist and Barnett (1995) and Buist (1998) found that the mother–infant relationship was impaired in women who had been sexually, physically and/or emotionally abused as children, and they were more likely to suffer from postnatal depression. Infertile women with histories of abuse may consider that they are being punished for early sexual experiences. During pregnancy, abuse survivors may report a fear of becoming fat, especially if an eating disorder is also present. Many women fear labour or are afraid that they will be unable to protect their child from abuse once it has been born, so they may require induction of labour and have to undergo the interventions which that entails (Bohn and Holz 1996). Some of these key issues are addressed below.

Preterm labour

Horan, *et al.* (2000) have postulated that early events of abuse may increase vulnerability to later experiences of unusual stress (e.g. pregnancy/childbirth), perhaps via stimulation of gene expression of corticotropin-releasing hormone (CRH) in the brain. These experiences increase the production of CRH in the brain, and elevated CRH levels have been associated with preterm labour. Stevens-Simon, *et al.* (1993) have postulated a connection between preterm labour and stress, and they have also described associations with depression, social isolation and substance abuse. Stevens-Simon and McAnarney (1994) published a study of the pregnancies of 127 poor black 12- to 18-year-old women, 33% of whom reported that they had been physically or sexually abused prior to conception. They found that these abused adolescents scored significantly worse on stress and depression scales, and they also rated their families as less supportive than did non-abused adolescents. They were more likely to report substance use during pregnancy, and they gave birth to significantly smaller and more-preterm infants. However, the possible biological connection between stress and preterm labour requires further elucidation. Hillis, *et al.* (2004) published a retrospective cohort study of 9139 women aged over 18 years, interviewed in San Diego, California in 1993–97. They found a strong link between adolescent pregnancy and adverse childhood experiences, but found that the adverse pregnancy outcomes, including fetal death, were related to adverse childhood experiences rather than adolescent pregnancy *per se*.

Adolescent pregnancy

It is postulated that childhood sexual abuse may disrupt psychosexual development in some adolescent women, and that some of them may react by voluntarily initiating sexual intercourse at a young age and becoming sexually promiscuous (Stevens-Simon and Reichert 1994, Saewyc, *et al.* 2004). As a corollary, a disproportionately large number of young women who become pregnant during adolescence have been found to be victims of childhood sexual abuse (Boyer and Fine 1992, Stevens-Simon and McAnarney 1994, Nagy, *et al.* 1995). Furthermore, adolescent women who have been sexually abused are more likely not to use contraception, so their risk of unintended pregnancy will be increased (Boyer and Fine 1992, Nagy, *et al.* 1995, Esparza and Esperat 1996, Dietz, *et al.* 1999).

Boyer and Fine (1992) reported that two-thirds of a sample of 535 women from the state of Washington who had become pregnant as adolescents, had been sexually abused. They also found that these sexually victimised teenagers started intercourse a year earlier, were more likely to have used drugs and alcohol and were less likely to practise contraception. In addition, they were more likely to have been hit, slapped or beaten by a partner or to have exchanged sex for money, drugs or a place to stay. Furthermore, they were more likely to report that their own children had been abused or had been taken from them by the Child Protective Services.

Bayatpour, *et al.* (1992) analysed data from a sample of 352 pregnant adolescent women in California, whose average age was 15 years. They found that 82% of the women were of ethnic-minority descent, 23% had been sexually or physically abused, and all of them were receiving public assistance. When they compared adolescents who had been sexually or physically abused with those who had not, their results revealed significant differences with regard to marijuana and cocaine use, as well as self-destructive behaviours, such as suicidal thoughts and actions.

Labour and birth

Labour and birth can be frightening for any woman, but for those with a history of childhood sexual abuse the experience of childbirth may remind them of the times when they were attacked as children (Simpkins 2005). They may feel out of control; immobilisation on a bed, pain, and subjection to intrusive procedures such as vaginal examinations may make them feel objectified and depersonalised. The list of procedures that many women undergo in these days of institutionalised birth is lengthy and includes abdominal palpations, vaginal examinations during pregnancy and labour, ultrasound scanning, induction of labour by rupture of the amniotic membranes or by pharmacological methods, monitoring of uterine contractions and fetal heart rate, insertion of intravenous/urinary catheters, immobilisation in lithotomy stirrups, epidural or other pharmacological analgesia, episiotomy, forceps/ventouse and caesarean section delivery. Although these procedures may be of value for some women, they may make the woman who has been sexually abused as a child (or raped at any age) feel tied up and powerless. The use of lithotomy is something that many midwives and healthcare professionals take for granted, but it may induce particularly violent memories for women who have been sexually abused. Wet pads and sheets may bring flashbacks of ejaculated semen. Touching women in certain ways, such as helping to move their legs into the lithotomy poles or opening their legs in preparation for a vaginal examination or birth, may also bring back memories. Lee, *et al.* (2007) found that women in their small cross-sectional pilot study reported significantly more anticipated anxiety during breast, pelvic and rectal examinations when the clinician was male. Sensitive midwifery practice is required here to meet the needs of survivors of sexual abuse to avoid causing further trauma.

Kitzinger (1992) explored and compared the language used by women who were survivors of sexual violence with that of 345 women who had experienced traumatic births. She found that their descriptions were very similar. One woman said that the obstetrician 'hauled me around like a slab of meat', while others felt 'skewered, trussed up like an oven-ready turkey' or 'like a fish on a slab' or 'a carcass'. Both groups used the language of waste disposal, such as 'trash', 'rubbish', 'shit' and 'a bloody mess' (Kitzinger 1992: 74). It is important to note that the midwife or healthcare professional may not always realise what the woman perceives to be traumatic, especially if the outcome is a healthy baby.

As mentioned previously, one of the ways in which women survivors of sexual abuse may cope with the overwhelming feelings they encounter during labour and birth is to dissociate themselves from the experiences as a means of having some control over the situation. This means that there is a separation of body and mind as a survival technique. In order to cope with their experiences of sexual abuse, women may have repressed memories of the abuse, but the invasive methods described above can reproduce overwhelming flashbacks of that abuse (Smith 1998). Dissociation provided a way to gain some control for some participants in a study by Parratt (1994). Susan felt that her births were 'easy' and that dissociation helped:

> I think I always would have given birth fairly easily, but I think that being able to dissociate . . . and to have sort of accepted interference as a matter of course might have meant that in some ways it was less traumatic. (Parratt 1994: 33)

In a very informative article, Gutteridge (2001) relates her experiences of being a survivor of childhood sexual abuse to her experiences of being a midwife who has given birth in the current maternity services. She describes dissociation as a method that she has perfected throughout her life, and how she may slip into it when faced with problems. Those around her do not understand what is happening, and she is perceived as being impassive or submissive.

Midwives and healthcare professionals may congratulate a mother who has dissociated herself from her labour, and may tell her how brave she was because she was so quiet and good with her breathing. This happened to Margaret, who had a long labour:

> It was a long time and I just kept quiet and I just did my breathing. I just got on with what I had to do and I breathed away every contraction. And then when it came to the second stage, when I actually wasn't allowed to push but wanted to, I panted away like mad . . . I got it right. I do remember being told, 'Wow, you did well with your breathing!' (Smith 1993: 95)

Rhodes and Hutchinson (1994) describe retreating as taking the form of reliving the sexual abuse. During the course of labour, some women may become confused and disorientated with regard to place and time. Some assume a childlike voice and protective body postures, such as curling into a fetal position or hiding under the bedcovers. Rhodes and Hutchinson (1994) quote the recollection of one nurse-midwife about a 16–year-old survivor who was unresponsive to those around her:

> In active labour she assumed a childlike voice, threw her head up to the ceiling, clearly was not in the same room with the rest of us in her mind, and pleaded quietly but hysterically: 'Don't hurt me there. If you'll stop hurting me I'll be good. I promise I'll be good. I promise I won't tell anybody!'. (Rhodes and Hutchinson 1994: 218)

This reliving of sexual abuse is consistent with PTSD; the 16–year-old survivor re-experienced her abuse because the dynamics of her giving birth had similarities with her past trauma. Crompton (1996) considers PTSD and postulates that women may come to childbirth with or without a history of previous trauma. They may or may not be traumatised or further traumatised during the event. However, their experience of childbirth may on the one hand be a healing event (which allows them to integrate their past trauma), or it may cause them to develop PTSD. This is clearly food for thought for midwives and healthcare professionals. The key aims are to prevent women from feeling traumatised during childbirth, and to help women with a history of sexual abuse remain 'grounded' so that they do not dissociate or relive their past experiences. In this way, childbirth could be a healing experience for them.

Maintaining control is very important to survivors of childhood sexual abuse. Rhodes and Hutchinson (1994) quote the following words from a woman speaking of her feelings during childbirth:

> The birth terrified me. I thought I was going to die. I felt like that during the sexual abuse. When you get in a situation where you feel like you've been violated or you feel like your life is in danger, or someone has so much power over you they can do anything, you're out of control . . .. That's terrifying, and that's the feeling I remember when I was giving birth. I was going to die and there were no two ways about it. (Rhodes and Hutchinson 1994: 219)

For a woman to feel in control, it may be easier if she has as few midwives as possible during her pregnancy and birth, and this is best achieved through caseload practice or in a small team.

Language

Women tend to give birth in institutions that are hierarchical, paternalistic and scientific, and which have their own language that is foreign to most people. Such a power base may alienate women, and there is also a tendency to infantilise them. Below is a short list of phrases that the midwife and healthcare professional will have heard – and maybe used.

- Lie still dear, this won't hurt (it always does, and the woman knows it).
- Just open your legs a little bit wider. THAT'S GOOD! WELL DONE!
- Lift your bottom up for me. THAT'S GOOD! WELL DONE!
- Just popping a little finger inside.
- 'You'll feel me touching you, sweetie' (Bergstrom, *et al.* 1992: 10).
- Good girl, you're doing very well.

It is not difficult to see that survivors may find such language reminiscent of the way in which the abusers spoke to them during the abuse when they were children.

Language is power, and underlying this is the way in which midwives control and manipulate women in a hierarchical, institutionalised setting, according to policies and procedures that could be said to control midwives as well as other women. Although it is difficult in such a culture, it would be beneficial for midwives to take the time to listen carefully to every woman's story and then carefully and individually formulate responses (Tilley 2000, Simkin and Klaus 2004).

Unhappiness after birth

As was mentioned earlier in this chapter, a number of studies have highlighted the association between childhood sexual abuse and later adult mental health problems (Bifulco, et al. 1991, Yellowlees and Kaushik 1994). However, there is a paucity of research into the possible relationship between childhood sexual abuse and unhappiness after birth.

Buist and Barnett (1995) reviewed voluntary admissions to a mother-and-baby unit and found that 40% of mothers reported a history of sexual abuse, with the figure rising to 54% when a broader definition of abuse (to include physical and/or sexual abuse) was used. For all of these women this was their first psychiatric admission, and all of them displayed symptoms of high levels of anxiety and low levels of self-confidence, which were also related to their infant care. The researchers found an unusually low tolerance of frustration, which is of particular concern when survivors need to cope with the many and unpredictable demands and stresses of caring for babies and children. They may also be bringing up their children in families that are experiencing poverty, with alcohol and physical abuse prevalent as added stressors (Mullen, et al. 1993). Buist and Barnett (1995) postulated that a history of childhood sexual abuse may be a risk factor not only for the *occurrence* of postnatal depression, but also for its severity, duration and outcome. Clearly there are long-term issues to be addressed for these women not only with regard to their becoming mothers, but also with regard to maintaining relationships with their partners and raising their children.

Buist (1998) has reported the first stage of a three-year follow-up study of 56 women who were admitted with postpartum depressive disorders. They were assessed with regard to their well-being, relationships and infant interaction. In total, 28 women had a history of sexual abuse before the age of 16 years, 9 women had a history of physical/emotional abuse and 19 women had no history of abuse. It was found that the effects of childhood sexual abuse were indistinguishable from those of childhood physical and emotional abuse. These results support previous research findings, such as those of Mullen, et al. (1993). The most significant finding was a detrimental effect on the mother–infant relationship in those women who had a history of abuse. This finding has obvious long-term implications, and further research into this area is clearly required.

Breastfeeding

It is of interest that a the literature search undertaken for this chapter revealed very little about childhood sexual abuse and breastfeeding. Article after article finishes after the birth, yet the action of the baby suckling on the breast and the release of fluid (which may remind the woman of ejaculation) might be considered to be obvious areas of concern. Some survivors will have no difficulties with breastfeeding, while others will not even tolerate the thought of it; some may find it a healing experience and others will have neutral feelings about it and wish to breastfeed their babies because they want what is best for them.

Kendall-Tackett (1998) has written an extensive and useful article in which she describes what is known about the effects of childhood sexual abuse and how they might relate to breastfeeding. For example, she describes what she calls 'cognitive distortions', whereby a survivor who has felt so powerless and out of control in the past may feel the same as a mother and may underestimate her ability to protect and provide for her baby. She may also experience postnatal depression. If she experiences breastfeeding difficulties, she may feel that yet another part of her body is letting her down and that there is little she can do to remedy the situation.

Bowman (2007) published a review of the available literature on the mental health consequences of childhood sexual abuse that may influence the feeding decisions of adolescent mothers. She postulates that there is sufficient evidence to consider a possible link between childhood sexual abuse and the propensity of adolescent mothers to bottle feed their babies. She suggests that their abuse suffered as children predisposes them to emotional distance, emotional numbing and discomfort with intimacy.

Kendall-Tackett (1998) also provides some interesting practical information that may not otherwise be considered, and suggests that there are three key problem areas: night feeding, the early postpartum period, and playful older infants. She discusses the issue of night-time breastfeeding in relation to the fact that it may be a particularly stressful time for the survivor if her abuse used to occur at that time. She suggests that some survivors may prefer to express their breast milk and use a bottle or ask for someone else to take on the night feeds.

Simkin (1996) considers that some women have an aversion to breastfeeding because the breasts must be available to the baby 'on demand'. This implies a kind of ownership, and therefore a loss of control over her body by the mother. She has also described how breastfeeding can be a source of difficulty if the abuse was associated with the developing breasts (Simkin 1994). The midwife or healthcare professional who holds a survivor's breast in order to help her to suckle her baby needs to keep this possibility in mind; there are other ways of helping women to breastfeed their babies.

EFFECTS OF CHILDHOOD ABUSE ON CLINICIANS' PERSONAL AND PROFESSIONAL LIVES

A number of informative and courageous articles have been published about midwives and healthcare professionals who have been sexually abused (Rouf 1999, Tilley 2000, Gutteridge 2001, Copping 2005).

Denham (2003) published a descriptive study in the US to compare past and current abuse experiences in pregnant women and their healthcare workers. She found that assessment of pregnant women for abuse is important, but that it was unknown whether nurses and other healthcare workers could effectively assess for abuse if they had unresolved personal experiences involving abuse. Denham suggests that there should be improved methods to educate nurses about abuse assessment, and policies should be put in place to support pregnant women and their healthcarers.

Jackson and Nuttall (1997) investigated whether the experience of childhood abuse actually affected the clinical judgements of various clinicians. In their initial survey, they drew a random stratified sample of 1635 clinicians from the national directories of clinical social workers, paediatricians, psychiatrists and clinical psychologists (who all worked with children) in the US. These clinicians were then given 16 vignettes of case histories of sexual abuse and asked whether they believed the victim's story.

Importantly, their findings seem to demonstrate that interpretations of sexual abuse allegations can be highly subjective and that, despite the fact that all of the respondents were experienced in working with cases of child abuse, they took factors into account that were beyond the boundaries of clinical relevance. Clearly this is an area in need of further research involving healthcare professionals who work with women in childbirth.

CONCLUSION

Supporting survivors of childhood sexual abuse through their pregnancies, births and beyond is both challenging and rewarding for midwives and all those involved. It seems reasonable to consider that there are significant numbers of midwives and healthcare workers who have been sexually abused themselves, but it is unclear as to the effects that their own personal experiences might have on their practice. Urgent research is needed here. Midwives may of course be with women unaware that they have suffered sexual abuse during their childhood, or the survivor herself may occasionally be unaware of her past tragic history. Having a positive pregnancy and birth can be a powerful and healing experience for a survivor and may help her to come to terms with the pain and betrayal of the past. On the other hand, insensitive care during pregnancy or a traumatic birth may re-create the pain that the woman endured as a child, with devastating long-term effects. Midwives who listen and practise sensitively and with insight are in a key position to help the survivor in her transition to being a mother, and to help her achieve this with strength and confidence.

KEY POINTS

- ↪ Many women are survivors of sexual abuse, and some will not have disclosed their experiences.
- ↪ Many women who have haphazard pregnancies, self-destructive behaviour or miss antenatal appointments may well have a history of sexual abuse.
- ↪ Procedures and practices associated with birth have real potential to make survivors re-enact their experiences of childhood sexual abuse.
- ↪ Language is power, and the use of childlike phrases may make the survivor relive her childhood experiences.

- ↪ Childhood sexual abuse is a real problem, and society needs to acknowledge this in order to help to prevent it and enable a change in attitude to the survivors.

USEFUL ADDRESSES

Childline
Studd Street
London N1 0QW
Free telephone number for young people and children to ring in emergencies:
0800 1111
Tel: 0207 239 1000
Fax: 0207 239 1001

CISters (Childhood Incest Survivors)
PO Box 119
Eastleigh
Hampshire SO50 9ZF
Tel: 0238 033 8080
Email: admin@cisters.wanadoo.co.uk

Kidscape
2 Grosvenor Gardens
London SW1 0DH
Tel: 0207 730 3300
Fax: 0207 730 7081

National Association of People Abused as Children (NAPAC)
42 Curtain Road
London EC2A 3NH
Tel: 0800 085 3330
Website: www.napac.org.uk

National Children's Bureau
8 Wakeley Street
London EC1V 7QE
Tel: 0207 843 6000
Fax: 0207 278 9512

National Society for the Prevention of Cruelty to Children (NSPCC)
42 Curtain Road
London EC2A 3NH
Tel: 0207 825 2763
Fax: 0207 825 2763
Email: infounit@nspcc.org.uk

National Childbirth Trust
Alexandra House
Oldham Terrace
London W3 6NH
Tel: 0870 444 8707

The Association of Postnatal Illness
145 Dawes Road
London SW6 7EB
Telephone helpline: 0207 386 0868
Fax: 0207 386 8885
Email: info@APNI.org
Website: www.APNI.org

REFERENCES

Ahmad S. (2006) Adult psychosexual dysfunction as a sequela of child sexual abuse. *Sex Rel Therapy.* **21**(4): 405–18.

Al Mamun A, Alati R, O'Callaghan M, *et al.* (2007) Does childhood sexual abuse have an effect on young adults' nicotine disorder (dependence or withdrawal)? Evidence from a birth cohort study. *Addiction.* **102**(4): 647–54.

Araji S, Finkelhor D. (1986) Abusers: a review of the research. In: Finkelhor D, editor. *Sourcebook on Child Sexual Abuse.* London: Sage.

Bachman G, Moeller T, Bennet J. (1988) Childhood sexual abuse and the consequences in adult women. *Obstet Gynecol.* **71**: 631–41.

Bala M. (1994) Caring for adult survivors of child sexual abuse: issues for family physicians. *Can Fam Physician.* **40**: 924–31.

Bayatpour M, Wells RD, Holford S. (1992) Physical and sexual abuse as predictors of substance use and suicide among pregnant teenagers. *Soc Adolesc Med.* **13**: 128–33.

Bergstrom L, Roberts J, Skillman L, *et al.* (1992) 'You'll feel me touching you, sweetie': vaginal examinations during the second stage of labor. *Birth.* **19**: 10–18.

Bifulco A, Brown G, Adler Z. (1991) Early sexual abuse and clinical depression in adult life. *Br J Psychiatry.* **159**: 115–22.

Bohn DK, Holz KA. (1996) Sequelae of abuse: health effects of childhood sexual abuse, domestic battering and rape. *J Nurse Midwifery.* **41**: 442–56.

Bowman KG. (2007) When breastfeeding may be a threat to adolescent mothers. *Issues Ment Health Nurs.* **28**: 89–99.

Boyer D, Fine D. (1992) Sexual abuse as a factor in adolescent pregnancy and child maltreatment. *Fam Plann Perspect.* **24**: 4–19.

Buist A, Barnett B. (1995) Childhood sexual abuse: a risk factor for post-partum depression? *Aust NZ J Psychiatry.* **29**: 604–8.

Buist A. (1998) Childhood abuse, parenting and postpartum depression. *Aust NZ J Psychiatry.* **32**: 479–87.

Bunting L. (2005) *Females Who Sexually Offend Against Children: responses of the child protection and criminal justice systems.* London: National Society for the Prevention of Cruelty to Children.

Bunting L. (2007) Dealing with a problem that doesn't exist? Professional responses to female perpetrated child sexual abuse. *Child Abuse Review.* **16**: 252–67.

Burke Draucker C. (2000) *Counselling Survivors of Childhood Sexual Abuse.* 2nd ed. London: Sage.

Bushnell JA, Wells JE, Oakley-Browne MA. (1992) Long-term effects of intra-familial sexual abuse in childhood. *Acta Psychiatr Scand.* **85**: 136–42.

Cawson P. (2002) *Child Maltreatment in the Family: the experience of a national sample of young people.* London: National Society for the Prevention of Cruelty to Children.

Cawson P, Wattam C, Brooker S, *et al.* (2000) *Child Maltreatment in the United Kingdom: a study of the prevalence of child abuse and neglect.* London: National Society for the Prevention of Cruelty to Children.

Christensen M. (1992) Birth rape. *Midwifery Today.* **22**: 34.

Cohen T. (1995) Motherhood among incest survivors. *Child Abuse Negl.* **19**: 1423–9.

Copping C. (2005) Reawakened trauma. *Nurs Stand.* **20**(13): 32–3.

Courtois CA. (1993) Adult survivors of sexual abuse. *Prim Care.* **20**: 433–47.

Crompton J. (1996) Post-traumatic stress disorder and childbirth. *Br J Midwif.* **4**: 290–4.

Denham SA. (2003) Describing abuse of pregnant women and their healthcare workers in rural Appalachia. *Am J Matern Child Nurs.* **28**(4): 264–9.

Dietz PM, Spitz AM, Anda RF, *et al.* (1999) Unintended pregnancy among adult women exposed to abuse or household dysfunction during their childhood. *JAMA.* **282**: 1359–64.

Esparza DV, Esperat MCR. (1996) The effects of childhood sexual abuse on minority adolescent mothers. *J Obstet Gynecol Neonatal Nurs.* **25**: 321–8.

Feerick MM, Snow KL. (2005) The relationships between childhood sexual abuse, social anxiety, and symptoms of post-traumatic stress disorder in women. *J Family Violence.* **20**(6): 409–19.

Finkelhor D. (1990) Early and long-term effects of child sexual abuse: an update. *Prof Psychol Res Pract.* **21**: 325–30.

Finkelhor D. (1994) The international epidemiology of child sexual abuse. *Child Abuse Negl.* **18**: 409–17.

Finkelhor D. (1997) Child sexual abuse. In: Barnett OW, Miller-Perrin CL, Perrin RD, editors. *Family Violence Across the Lifespan.* Thousand Oaks, CA: Sage.

Fitzsimons P. (1999) Michel Foucault: regimes of punishment and the question of liberty. Revised extract. *Int J Sociol Law.* **27**: 379–99.

Fleming JM. (1997) Prevalence of childhood sexual abuse in a community sample of Australian women. *Med J Aust.* **166**(2): 65–8. Available at: www.mja.com.au/public/issues/jan20/fleming/fleming.html (accessed 2 Jan 2009).

Ghate D, Spencer L. (1995) T*he Prevalence of Child Sexual Abuse in Britain.* London: HMSO.

Gladstone GL, Parker GB, Mitchell PB, *et al.* (2004) The implications of childhood trauma for depressed women: an analysis of pathways from childhood sexual abuse to deliberate self-harm and revictimisation. *Am J Psychiatry.* **161**(8): 1417–25.

Griffing S, Fish Ragin D, Morrison SM, *et al.* (2005) Reasons for returning to abusive relationships: effects of prior victimisation. *J Family Violence.* **20**(5): 341–8.

Gutteridge KEA. (2001) Failing women: the impact of sexual abuse on childbirth. *Br J Midwif.* **9**: 312–15.

Hackett S, Uprichard E. (2007) *Animal Abuse and Child Maltreatment: a review of the literature and findings from a UK study.* London: National Society for the Prevention of Cruelty to Children.

Hallett C. (1995) Child abuse: an academic overview. In: Kingston P, Penhale B, editors. *Family Violence and the Caring Professions.* Basingstoke: Macmillan.

Hendricks-Matthews MK. (1993) Survivors of abuse: healthcare issues. *Prim Care.* **20**: 391–406.

Herman JL, Russell DEH, Trocki K. (1986) Long-term effects of incestuous abuse in childhood. *Am J Psychiatry.* **143**: 1293–6.

Hillis SD, Anda RF, Dube SR, *et al.* (2004) The association between adverse childhood experiences and adolescent pregnancy, long-term psychosocial consequences and fetal death. *Pediatrics.* **113**(2): 320–7.

Holz KA. (1994) A practical approach to clients who are survivors of childhood sexual abuse. *J Nurse Midwifery.* **39**: 13–18.

Home Office, Department of Health, Department of Education and Science and Welsh Office. (1991) *Working Together Under the Children Act 1989.* London: HMSO.

Home Office. (2008) *Saving Lives. Reducing Harm. Protecting the Public. An action plan for tackling Violence 2008–11.* London: The Stationery Office. Available at: www.homeoffice.gov.uk/documents/strategy_2008 (accessed 2 June 2008).

Horan DL, Hill LD, Schulkin J. (2000) Childhood sexual abuse and preterm labor in adulthood: an endocrinological hypothesis. *Women Health Issue.* **10**(1): 27–33.

Inter-departmental Ministerial Group on Sexual Offending. (2007) *Cross Government Action Plan on Sexual Violence and Abuse.* London: The Stationery Office.

Jackson H, Nuttall R. (1997) *Childhood Abuse: effects on clinicians' personal and professional lives.* London: Sage.

Jehu D. (1988) *Beyond Sexual Abuse: therapy with women who were childhood victims.* Chichester: John Wiley & Sons.

Johnson CF. (2001) Abuse and neglect of children. In: Behrman RE, Kliegman RM, Jenson HB, editors. *Nelson Textbook of Pediatrics.* Philadelphia, PA: WB Saunders Co.

Johnson RJ, Rew L, Sternglanz RW. (2006) The relationship between childhood sexual abuse and sexual health practices of homeless adolescents. *Adolescence.* 41(162): 221–34.

Kendall–Tackett K. (1998) Breastfeeding and the sexual abuse survivor. *J Hum Lactation.* 14: 127–30.

Kitzinger S. (1992) Birth and violence against women: generating hypotheses from women's accounts of unhappiness after childbirth. In: Roberts H, editor. *Women's Health Matters.* London: Routledge.

Koci A, Strickland O. (2006) Relationship of adolescent physical and sexual abuse to perimenstrual symptoms (PMS) in adulthood. *Issues Ment Health Nurs.* 28(1): 75–87.

Koss MP, Heslet L. (1992) Somatic consequences of violence against women. *Arch Fam Med.* 1: 53–9.

Lee SJ, Tolman RM. (2006) Childhood sexual abuse and adult work outcomes. *Soc Work Res.* 30(2): 83–92.

Lee TT, Westrup DA, Ruzek JI, *et al.* (2007) Impact of clinician gender on examination anxiety among female veterans with sexual trauma: a pilot study. *J Women Health.* 16(9): 1291–9.

Masho SW, Ahmed G. (2007) Age at sexual assault and post-traumatic stress disorder among women: prevalence, correlates and implications for prevention. *J Women Health.* 16(2): 262–71.

Miller DK. (2006) The effects of childhood physical abuse or childhood sexual abuse in battered women's coping mechanisms: obsessive-compulsive tendencies and severe depression. *J Family Violence.* 21(3): 185–95.

Mullen P, Martin J, Anderson J, *et al.* (1993) Childhood sexual abuse and mental health in adult life. *Br J Psychiatry.* 163: 721–32.

Nagy S, DiClemente R, Adcock A. (1995) Adverse factors associated with forced sex among southern adolescent girls. *Pediatrics.* 96: 944–6.

National Center on Child Abuse and Neglect. (1978) *Child Sexual Abuse: incest, assault and sexual exploitation: a special report.* Washington, DC: National Center on Child Abuse and Neglect.

Ompad DC, Ikeda RM, Shah N, *et al.* (2005) Childhood sexual abuse and age at initiation of injection drug use. *Am J Pub Health.* 95(4): 703–9.

Parratt J. (1994) The experience of childbirth for survivors of incest. *Midwifery.* 10: 26–39.

Petersen AC. (1993) *Understanding Child Abuse and Neglect.* Washington, DC: National Academy Press.

Polusny MA, Follette VM. (1995) Long-term correlates of child sexual abuse: theory and review of the empirical literature. *Appl Prev Psychol.* 4: 143–66.

Rahm GB, Renck B, Ringsberg KC. (2006) 'Disgust, disgust beyond description': shame cues to detect shame in disguise, in interviews with women who were sexually abused during childhood. *J Psychiatr Ment Health Nurs.* 13(1): 100–9.

Rayworth BB, Wise LA, Harlow BL. (2004) Childhood abuse and risk of eating disorders in women. *Epidemiology.* 15(3): 271–8.

Rhodes N, Hutchinson S. (1994) Labor experiences of childhood sexual abuse survivors. *Birth.* 21: 213–21.

Rouf K. (1999) Child sexual abuse and pregnancy: a personal account. *Pract Midwife.* 2: 29–31.

Saewyc EM, Magee LL, Petingell SE. (2004) Teenage pregnancy and associated risk behaviours among sexually abused adolescents. *Perspect Sex Reprod Health.* 36(3): 98–105.

Salmon P, Skaife K, Rhodes J. (2003) Abuse, dissociation, and somatisation in irritable bowel syndrome: towards an explanatory model. *J Behav Med.* 26(1): 1–18.

Sanci L, Coffey C, Olsson C, *et al.* (2008) Childhood sexual abuse and eating disorders in females:

findings from the Victorian adolescent health cohort study. *Arch Pediatr Adolesc Med.* **162**(3): 261–7.

Saradjian J. (1996) *Women Who Sexually Abuse Children: from research to clinical practice.* Chichester: John Wiley & Sons.

Scott A. (1996) *Real Events Revisited: fantasy, memory and psychoanalysis.* London: Virago.

Sedlack AJ, Broadhurst DD. (1996) *Third National Incidence Study of Child Abuse and Neglect.* Washington, DC: Department of Health and Human Services.

Seng J, Low LK, Sparbel K, *et al.* (2004) Abuse-related post-traumatic stress during the childbearing year. *J Adv Nurs.* **46**(6): 604–13.

Simkin P, Klaus P. (2004) *When Survivors Give Birth: understanding and healing the effects of early sexual abuse on childbearing women.* Seattle, WA: Classic Day Publishing.

Simkin P. (1994) Memories that really matter. *Childbirth Instructor Magazine.* **39**: 20–3.

Simkin P. (1996) Childbirth education and care for the childhood sexual abuse survivor. *Int J Childbirth Educ.* **11**: 31–3.

Simpkins R. (2005) The effects of sexual abuse on childbearing: antenatal care. *Br J Midwif.* **14**(3): 162–3.

Smith M. (1998) Childbirth in women with a history of sexual abuse. 1. *Pract Midwife.* **1**: 20–3.

Smith P. (1993) *Childhood Sexual Abuse, Sexuality, Pregnancy and Birthing: a life history study.* Palmerston North, New Zealand: Inside-Out Books.

Stevens-Simon C, Kaplan DW, McAnarney ER. (1993) Factors associated with preterm delivery among pregnant adolescents. *J Adolesc Health.* **14**: 340–2.

Stevens-Simon C, McAnarney ER. (1994) Childhood victimisation: relationship to adolescent pregnancy outcome. *Child Abuse Neglect.* **18**: 569–75.

Stevens-Simon C, Reichert S. (1994) Sexual abuse, adolescent pregnancy and child abuse: a developmental approach to an intergenerational cycle. *Arch Pediatr Adolesc Med.* **148**: 23–7.

Tilley J. (2000) Sexual assault and flashbacks on the labour ward. *Pract Midwife.* **3**: 18–20.

Treuer T, Koperdák M, Rózsa S, *et al.* (2005) The impact of physical and sexual abuse on body image in eating disorders. *Eur Eat Disord Rev.* **13**: 106–11.

Unikel C, Gomez-Peresmitre G, Gonzalez-Forteza C. (2006) Suicidal behaviour, risky eating behaviours and psychosocial correlates in Mexican female students. *Eur Eat Disord Rev.* **14**: 414–21.

Villano CL, Rosenblum A, Magura S, *et al.* (2007) Prevalence and correlates of post-traumatic stress disorder and chronic severe pain in psychiatric outpatients. *J Rehabil Res Dev.* **44**(2): 167–77.

Walker A, Kershaw C, Nicholas S. (2006) *Crime in England and Wales: 2005/6. Home Office Statistical Bulletin* (July 2006/December 2006). Available at: www.homeoffice.gov.uk/rds/pdfs06/hosb1206.pdf www.homeoffice.gov.uk/rds/index.htm (accessed 8 Jan 2009).

Wallace H. (1999) *Family Violence: legal, medical and social perspectives.* 2nd ed. London: Allyn and Bacon.

Wallace JD. (2007) Woman with incontinence and a history of childhood sexual abuse. *Urol Nurs.* **27**(1): 38–9.

Walling MK, Reiter RC, O'Hara MW, *et al.* (1994) Abuse history and chronic pain in women. 1. Prevalences of sexual abuse and physical abuse. *Obstet Gynecology.* **84**: 193–9.

Warm A, Murray C, Fox J. (2003) Why do people self-harm? *Psychol Health Med.* **8**(1): 72–9.

Warne T, McAndrew S. (2005) The shackles of abuse: unprepared to work at the edges of reason. *J Psychiatr Ment Health Nurs.* **12**(6): 679–86.

Yellowlees PM, Kaushik AV. (1994) A case-control study of the sequelae of childhood sexual assault in adult psychiatric patients. *Med J Aust.* **160**: 408–11.

Young L. (1992) Sexual abuse and the problem of embodiment. *Child Abuse Neglect.* **16**: 89–100.

CHAPTER 16

Assisted conception: threat or opportunity?

Marilyn Crawshaw

This chapter looks at the use of medically assisted conception treatments within a medical, legal and social framework. The author seeks to separate the facts from both the ways in which those facts have been interpreted and the ways in which professional practices in the field have developed.

Using this framework, certain areas of practice have been considered in more detail, namely access to treatments, and the treatments themselves. Statutory requirements with regard to 'the welfare of the child', counselling, the licensing of treatments, the inspection process, and preparation for parenthood are all discussed.

The author concludes that there is a potential for prejudicial professional practice and policies to develop; that critical awareness of the social context of developments in the new reproductive technologies is essential to counteract this; and that the separate influences of the medical, legal and social frameworks can be diluted or reinforced when they interweave with each other.

INTRODUCTION

People who enter the world of assisted conception treatments as patients may find themselves faced with medically, ethically and socially complex decisions and they do so within a context of intense media interest. The treatment decision that they face today may be the subject of a documentary or magazine article tomorrow. A decision to withdraw from treatment and 'move on' with their lives may be thrown into turmoil when the newspaper headline the following week claims an exciting new breakthrough.

As people move from the private world of 'trying for a baby' to the public world of seeking medical assistance with conception, they little know how extended their transition to parenthood may become, if indeed it ever culminates in parenthood. For those who achieve parenthood, their fertility impairment is rarely altered – only circumvented.

And it is not just people having difficulty conceiving who struggle to make sense of the world of reproductive technology. The confusion and ambivalence that many people experience will reflect their thoughts and feelings about the relationship between medicine, science and human reproduction. While they welcome some interventions as offering hope for people who find the route to parenthood blocked, uneasy visions of 'Frankenstein monsters' may lurk in the shadows. We use terms like 'designer' babies to express our revulsion at the notion of pre-selecting for 'social' characteristics in our offspring. Yet no equivalent value-laden term is accorded to the process of pre-implantation genetic diagnosis (PGD) or antenatal screening, reflecting our dual standards when the selection is designed to eliminate people with certain health conditions or impairments.

As a result of assisted conception techniques, new family forms are created for which our cultural, emotional and social understandings lag behind scientific understanding. Women have acted as surrogates for their daughters and given birth to their own grandchildren. Twins have been born years apart from frozen embryos. Men have fathered children after their death through posthumous conception. Reproductive tissue from young children undergoing treatment for cancer is stored for possible maturation and use in many years' time. New techniques offer the possibility of people being conceived using the gametes of two females alone and scientists claim that they are on the brink of cloning a human being. Babies can now be conceived who have up to 4 parents and 12 or more grandparents at birth – if the genetic mother donates her egg, the genetic father donates his sperm and the embryo that is created is donated to a couple in which the woman carries the fetus and gives birth to the baby for whom she and her partner will be the social parents (four parents). If each of the social parents has two genetic parents, each of whom is with a new partner, there is the potential for the baby to have four genetic grandparents (from their gamete donors) and eight social grandparents. Previously simple classroom tasks in which children are asked to draw their family tree may now present some unexpected challenges for the unsuspecting teacher!

Health- and social care professionals who are providing a service to women (and their partners if they have them) in the antenatal, delivery and postnatal periods following assisted conception treatment, have to manage their own feelings and views about the treatments in order to be emotionally and factually clear enough to provide an appropriate service. Some may have personal experiences either from their own lives or from their circle of family or friends. Others may hold strong views due to religious, moral or political standpoints. All of these may prove unexpectedly difficult to sustain when faced with the immediate pain (or joy) that an individual or couple bring to the professional encounter.

It is important to be aware of one's personal values and the way in which they interact with the professional task. Equally, it is important to be clear about one's factual knowledge base in order to keep the boundaries between fact and opinion clear. Finally, this needs to be encompassed by the development and maintenance of a rigorous and reflective critical awareness of the influence of the social context in which the new reproductive technologies have been, and continue to be, developed. A framework that may assist with this is outlined below.

A FRAMEWORK FOR UNDERSTANDING MEDICALLY ASSISTED CONCEPTION TREATMENT

The term 'the new reproductive technologies' is used to encompass new forms of intervention to do with human reproduction, including medically assisted conception treatment. They can be analysed within three main frameworks – medical, legal and social. By considering how far each of these frameworks, separately and in conjunction with each other, influences the way that we make meaning of these technologies, we can become clearer about their effects on the individuals who directly provide, use, and are affected by treatment services.

Medical framework

A medical framework seeks to understand difficulties in conceiving, primarily in terms of bodily malfunction, with a view to repairing or circumventing the malfunctioning parts. It fuels the drive to acquire new information about the functioning of the human reproductive system, with the body and body parts as the main site for technical exploration. It uses determinants of success, which have clear parameters, usually the achievement of a pregnancy, and more specifically, the birth of a single live baby free of any impairment and a birth mother who remains physically healthy. This approach also allows unsuccessful treatments to continue if they hold the promise of greater rewards. Thus, the (relatively) low success rates of in vitro fertilisation (IVF) when measured by live birth rates (see Human Fertilisation and Embryology Authority website www. hfea.gov.uk/en/1626.htm) are defended on the basis that improved knowledge about reproductive function might lead to lowered miscarriage rates, improved preventative work, and increased understanding of genetics. At its most reductionist, humans are seen as the sum of their body parts and determined in large part by their genetic make-up. This potentially allows an individual's function within the medical process to be given primacy over them as a whole person. For example, a sperm donor may be seen primarily as having a time-limited role through providing gametes for donation (biological function), obscuring the more complex and potentially longer-term social and emotional aspects of such a transaction.

Legal framework

A legal framework considers the way in which society regulates matters (primarily but not exclusively) in the public domain by administering and interpreting a codified set of rules that are determined in the first place by its legislature. Regulatory mechanisms to put those rules into operation may be proactive or reactive:

- **Proactive mechanisms** include inspection systems that are designed to ensure that rules and standards are maintained or promoted. Those relevant to reproductive technologies are invested in bodies such as the Human Fertilisation and Embryology Authority (HFEA), the regulators of professional conduct (e.g. the General Medical Council) and the Care Standards Commission and National Health Service (NHS) clinical governance frameworks.
- **Reactive mechanisms** include the courts of law, and ethics committees that are used when rules are breached or adjudication is required.

Interpretation of the law also takes place within policy making forums (e.g. health authorities), within individual professional practices and elsewhere.

The legal framework is premised on the belief that the common good can be determined in a civilised society by using rational analysis based on a set of rules.

Social framework

A social framework seeks to understand human actions at individual, group and societal levels, by considering the extent to which they are affected by the wider social context in which they occur. This is achieved through a variety of routes, including the following:

- ➡ data collection, which looks for trends or patterns associated with social characteristics such as age, gender, ethnicity, impairment and sexual orientation;
- ➡ research, discussion, and development of theoretical constructs on psychosocial issues.

A social framework thus considers where there may be causal links between experiences among those who share social characteristics and identities and prompts attention to the ways in which individual (patient, professional and lay) actions and experiences can be understood in psychosocial terms. An illustration of this is the way in which recent developments in the science of genetics have been accompanied by changes in the ways in which social relationships are described. For example, where one might previously have said 'X is Y's biological father' one may now say 'X is Y's genetic father'. A social framework approach considers the significance of such a change in discourse, particularly in relation to kinship (Franklin 1997) and encourages consideration of the interrelationship between scientific developments and the way we think about relationships, including those between prenatal genetic predisposition and postnatal socialisation.

USING THE FRAMEWORK TO AID PROFESSIONAL INTERVENTIONS

By separating factual information from interpretation within this framework and considering the reinforcing or diluting influence of each component on the other, professionals can better understand their own reactions in this complex area and, in turn, improve their potential to offer a more patient-centred approach to their service.

This can be illustrated by examining two key aspects of medically assisted conception services:

- ➡ Who gains access to treatments?
- ➡ What do the treatments involve and what happens when they end in pregnancy?

Who gains access to treatments?

What does the law say?

The relevant legal framework is to be found mainly in the Human Fertilisation and Embryology Act 1990 (HFE Act*) and the subsequent Code of Practice drawn up by the HFEA and regularly updated. The HFEA was established in 1991 with publicly appointed members, a Chairperson and a small paid staff under a Chief Executive in order to:

---

* Note that a new Human Fertilisation and Embryology Bill was going through Parliament at the time of writing and has since received Royal Assent (2008). This is the first major revision of the HFE Act..

- set standards and license and regulate clinics where licensed treatments are offered, where gametes are stored and/or where certain specified research is being undertaken;
- publish a Code of Practice;
- monitor new developments internationally and consult with both professional and patient groups and the general public to determine whether to license new treatments;
- publish information for patients;
- maintain the confidential Register of Information, the purpose of which is to enable people over the age of 18 (or 16 if contemplating marriage) to find out, after being offered 'appropriate counselling', whether they were born as a result of licensed fertility treatment, *and* whether they are related to someone whom they intend to marry. This latter clause was inserted in response to concerns about consanguinity although, surprisingly, was agreed as applicable to anyone below the age of 18 *only* if they were intending to marry and not if they were to enter a sexual relationship outside marriage, perhaps reflecting the social mores of the era in which the legislation was passed.

Under the new legislative proposals, the function of the HFEA remains substantially the same, though the conditions under which information relating to donor conception can be released are set to expand substantially. This is returned to later in the chapter.

There are three key gate-keeping points for entry into treatment, at each of which medical and social frameworks intermingle with the legal one:

- At the point of seeking referral – that is, *political practice*. Those seeking NHS-funded treatment have to meet the eligibility criteria drawn up by the health authority in whose area they reside *and* obtain funding from their local primary care trust. A major cause of controversy with regard to access to assisted conception treatments is the regional variation in NHS eligibility criteria and funding levels and the fact that, overall, the majority of assisted conception treatments are available in the private health sector rather than the NHS. This impacts most heavily on people from low-income groups who may thus be excluded from treatment if NHS routes are blocked to them. (Fuller information and discussion of these issues can be obtained from the National Infertility Awareness Campaign – see Useful Addresses section).
- At the point of referral, where individual referring doctors may operate their own (unpublished) criteria – that is, *professional practice*.
- At the point of entry into treatment, when some clinics have selection criteria (published or otherwise) – that is, *political or professional or commercial practice*.

The Act itself does not restrict treatments to any category of people. However the interpretation of it, most notably the section relating to the 'welfare of the child' (Section 13(5)), almost certainly has resulted in discrimination against lesbian couples and single women (no official figures are kept). It is noteworthy that the HFEA has never withdrawn a clinic's licence on the grounds that its selection criteria prohibit access to specific social groups. Despite the wording of the HFE Act, there does not appear to be any *obligation* for clinics to treat those referred. This is perhaps compounded by the dominance of private healthcare provision. However, fear that automatic refusal to treat certain patient groups may have been challenged under the Human Rights Act 1998, did appear to lead some clinics to modify their practice by removing overt reference to such exclusions from their patient information. No such legal challenges have yet been mounted.

In drawing up criteria for deciding which NHS patients may be eligible for referral for treatment, policy makers are required to interpret the HFE Act's stipulations. Here again the intertwining of the three frameworks is evident. As well as setting out the medical criteria, this requirement means that they, *as well as the professionals providing the treatment services*, are likely to take account of the welfare of any children potentially or actually involved and the emotional needs of those seeking treatment. The Act itself states that:

- ⇒ 'a woman shall not be provided with treatment services unless account has been taken of the welfare of any child who may be born as a result of the treatment (including the need of that child for a father), and of any child who may be affected by the birth' (Section13(5));
- ⇒ people must be given 'a suitable opportunity to receive proper counselling about the implications of taking the proposed steps' (Section 13(6); Schedule 3, paragraph 3(1)(a)).

This is the only area of law where such conditions apply in relation to either medical treatments or entry into parenthood, perhaps reflecting the unease with which this area of work was viewed in Parliament.

What does the 'welfare of the child' mean?

The HFEA Code of Practice (2007: Sections S.7.1 and G.3) provides the standards and guidance that need to be taken into account when conducting the assessment of prospective parents with regard to the 'welfare of the child/ren' who may be born or affected. Prior to the current Code of Practice, specific guidance was given as to what needed to be considered as part of this assessment, including additional criteria when it was proposed that donated gametes would be used. Following national consultations on the 'welfare of the child' procedures and on the Code of Practice itself, key changes were brought in (Human Fertilisation and Embryology Authority 2005). The Code of Practice now confines itself to publishing national standards to which clinics are expected to conform (and by which they are inspected) together with more limited guidance than previously to address procedure rather than content. The standards were drawn up in consultation with the relevant professional bodies and are identified clearly with the Act and accompanying Regulations.

The Code of Practice requires clinics to have procedures in place for conducting 'welfare of the child' assessments and for dealing with any issues arising prior to treatment commencing. It provides guidance on the situations in which assessments should be repeated and recommends that written records are kept in all cases. Following the 'welfare of the child' national consultation, it was agreed that a lighter-touch approach should be used in the majority of situations. Information from professionals and agencies outside of the licensed centre is now only sought (with the consent of those concerned) when there is 'cause for concern' as indicated by one or more of the following situations:

➡ information provided by those seeking treatment is lacking, inconsistent or suggests that serious harm may be caused to the child;
➡ there is evidence of deception;
➡ there are staff concerns.

Each clinic must have an ethics committee or access to a setting in which complex issues, such as those relating to the welfare of children, can be discussed. However, it is perhaps surprising that there is no statutory requirement for professional child welfare expertise to be included in such forums and their inclusion is not commonplace. Whatever the outcome of any risk assessment, the final decision always rests with the clinician responsible for administering the treatment. Where treatment is refused, however, clinics are now expected to provide their reasons to those affected, to explain any remaining options and to offer opportunities for counselling.

Guidelines from professional bodies rather than the Code of Practice thus now provide the reference point for 'good practice' in relation to the 'welfare of the child' assessments and, as such, are not enforceable by the HFEA. Indeed, current Code of Practice references to the implications of using donated gametes have been relocated to the guidance section on 'Providing proper information' (Section G5 2007) (though this is likely to change if more liberal conditions for seeking information proposed in the new Human Fertilisation and Embryology Bill are accepted, as seems likely – *see* below). The most relevant non-medical professional guidelines are published by the British Infertility Counselling Association (BICA) (BICA 2004, 2007, Section 5). In drawing these up, BICA has adopted a policy on the need for a clear separation to be made between assessing people's suitability to parent, and the need to give them an opportunity to receive professional help in thinking through their decisions and preparing for parenthood. While the former is not a counselling task, the latter is.

It remains too soon to know how far these changes are making a difference to practice on the ground. It was certainly the case in the past that assessments were not always made with sufficient transparency. There was ample opportunity for facts and opinion to become blurred and discrimination to occur. In some clinics, counsellors were involved in conducting assessments and their role as counsellors was compromised. The inclusion of child welfare experts and the use of a child welfare/protection evidence base in the assessment process was rare.

Within mainstream child protection work, full risk assessments in relation to an unborn child are among the most complex to undertake and are always done by a team of social workers and other professionals trained and skilled in such work. When a recommendation is made that prospective parents should be denied the opportunity to have care of their baby, the decision is taken at a multi-disciplinary, multi-agency Child Protection Case Conference and is open to the independent scrutiny of the courts. Even in the 'new world' of HFEA regulation, however, it remains the case that there is no statutory requirement for multi-disciplinary and multi-agency involvement in risk assessments in the assisted conception setting (i.e. before a pregnancy is achieved) and no route for independent scrutiny through the courts.

Now it could be argued that the two situations are very different, and at one level, they are. However, the current system in assisted conception clinics contains two areas where potential flaws can still arise:

➥ the 'facts' on which decisions are made might not hold up under scrutiny according to an accepted child welfare/protection evidence base;

➥ decisions will, in the main, be made by professionals who are not trained in child welfare/protection risk assessments.

The potential for prejudicial situations to arise remains of concern, especially given evidence from wider society that some groups may be particularly vulnerable to challenges to their parenting abilities. This includes those whose lifestyle (e.g. sex workers, drug users), physical attributes (e.g. wheelchair users, people who are HIV positive), learning difficulties or sexual orientation may be deemed unsuitable to equip them to be parents (Campion 1995, Saffron 2001, Olsen and Clarke 2003). Careful monitoring of the situation is called for.

The question of whether or not the use of donor–assisted conception treatment should merit any particular attention with regard to 'welfare of the child' assessments, is interesting. Child welfare issues that apply here are at least as controversial as those already discussed. In particular, some might argue that treatment should be refused on 'welfare of the child' grounds, to prospective parents who state their unwillingness to disclose the nature of their origins to any child conceived through donor–assisted treatment. I discuss this in more detail in a later section.

Finally, the debates on the Human Fertilisation and Embryology Bill 2008 gave scant attention to some of the child welfare aspects raised above. Instead they focused almost exclusively on the proposal to remove the 'need for a father' and whether or not this would be detrimental. A government amendment to change the requirement to become 'the need of child for supportive parenting' appears to have been sufficient to quieten the demand for the retention of the 1990 Act wording and looks likely to be enacted. In practice, the new wording is unlikely to bring about any substantial changes to existing assessment practices and hence will not address some of the concerns noted here. However, in one important area, the new Bill has strengthened the call for the law to reflect standards of 'good parental practice', namely in relation to the use of donated gametes. Not only does the original Bill include reference to the importance of openness between parent and child from early infancy, but it has been amended to make the provision of such information to prospective parents a legal requirement that will therefore be inspected against, giving more strength to the HFEA. Although it stopped short of linking this directly to 'welfare of the child' assessments and of including other more controversial clauses such as a requirement for birth certificates to include reference to donor conception, this is a significant step forward.

What are the requirements with regard to counselling?

Although the offer of counselling is a legal requirement, the way in which it is offered and provided is open to interpretation. The Code of Practice states that at least one of the counselling staff should hold a recognised qualification (HFEA 2007, Section G1: 4). In practice, this has proved difficult to verify, given the number of unregulated general counselling awards now available. (Readers who are interested in the long-standing discussions and developments about infertility counselling accreditation should refer to the BICA website: www.bica.net)

The following types of counselling should be made available:
- **implications counselling** – to enable the person concerned to understand the implications of the proposed course of action for themselves, their family and any children who are born as a result;
- **support counselling** – to offer emotional support at times of particular stress (e.g. failure to achieve a pregnancy);
- **therapeutic counselling** – to help people cope with the consequences of infertility and treatment and to help them resolve any problems that these may cause. It includes helping people to adjust their expectations and to accept their situation.

Only implications counselling *must* be offered: provision of the other types of counselling carries a lower mandate. Perhaps because it is usually offered at the same time as the patient is being considered for treatment, and uptake may be seen by some professionals and patients as an indication of poor coping or emotional instability, (even though the Code of Practice stresses it should not be seen in this light) the uptake of implications and other types of counselling remains low unless attendance is a condition of treatment (Boivin, *et al.* 1999). Moreover, many clinics only provide one free session and the financial pressure on couples, particularly those accessing private treatment, may preclude them from engaging in further contact. The HFEA Code of Practice stipulates that counselling should also be made available at all stages in the treatment process, including when it ends and at points in the future. However clinics are only required to assist people in *obtaining* counselling, but do not necessarily have to *provide* it, especially in the later stages of contact.

When one takes into account the growing body of evidence of the emotional and social strains associated with managing fertility difficulties and/or assisted conception treatment regimes, the low provision of psychosocial services is of concern (Burns and Covington 2006, Eugster and Vingerhoets 1999, Greil 1997, Throsby 2004, Verhaak, *et al.* 2005). This undoubtedly reflects in part the dominance of the medical framework approach and the resultant medicalisation of the 'problem' and its 'solution', which in turn encourages those affected to see their reactions as due primarily to emotional inadequacy.

How is the quality of services assured?

'Welfare of the child' assessments, provision of counselling, and all other requirements of the HFE Act and Code of Practice, must be carried out to the satisfaction of HFEA Inspectors. There have been some changes in recent years to the ways in which inspections are conducted, which have been largely welcomed and represent significant shifts in the inspection culture. Prior to 2005, annual inspections were conducted by a team drawn from appointed external Clinical, Scientific, and Social and Ethical Inspectors together with an internal HFEA Inspector, or by an HFEA Inspector working alone. The following changes are included.
- The bulk of inspections are now conducted by an in-house team of inspectors, who draw on a small group of expert external advisers only when they have concerns or feel that certain aspects of the inspection require this.
- Not all centres undergo full inspections each year though no more than three years can elapse between full inspections.

➥ Patients' views are sought as part of the information gathering process.
➥ Inspection reports are published on the HFEA website.

As before, inspection reports are prepared for the HFEA Licensing and Fees Committee where the final decision is made about renewal of licences and any imposition of conditions.

The inspection process and the system for appointing inspectors were not without controversy in the past, both from those opposed to it and from those who consider that it should have been more rigorous (Crawshaw 1999). For all areas *except counselling* that are required by law to be inspected (i.e. the medical and scientific aspects) 'external' inspectors with the relevant qualifications were appointed. External inspectors were used spasmodically, leading to concerns about their ability to maintain competence. Little or no effective training and updating was provided.

There continue to be concerns about the present arrangements, although the potential for greater consistency is apparent. Changes to the Code of Practice (cited above) have been largely welcomed, in particular the separation of 'Standards' from 'Guidance'. The inclusion of professional guidelines as the indicators of good practice have moved the process more into line with other statutory regulatory processes. However, psychosocial expertise is limited within the in-house inspection team and it appears that external advisers are being called on infrequently. The potential to lower the rigour with which psychosocial matters are inspected is apparent.

The difficulty for treatment providers and regulators alike remains that there is no public forum for debate on inspection regimes and little involvement of the courts in creating case law to guide future actions. Wide interpretations of practice in controversial areas such as 'welfare of the child' and counselling are therefore not surprising. For example, clinics where the provision of counselling is virtually non-existent or only available if paid for by patients, may be judged as being as acceptable as those where there is unlimited free counselling. Even in areas where there may be more so-called 'hard' evidence to draw on, for example, regarding the number of embryos to transfer to reduce the risk of multiple births, reaching a consensus has proved difficult.

What do the treatments involve and what happens when they end in pregnancy?

What is classed as a licensed treatment?

Treatments fell into two categories for their regulation under the HFE Act 1990:
➥ Licensed treatments included the following:
   — IVF including that with donor sperm, eggs or embryo
   — Intra-Cytoplasmic Sperm Injection (ICSI)
   — Donor Insemination (DI)
   — Pre-Implantation Genetic Diagnosis (PGD)
➥ Non-licensed treatments included the following:
   — Gamete Intra Fallopian Transfer (GIFT)
   — ovulation induction
   — Intrauterine Insemination with husband/partner's sperm (IUI).

Although this division was deemed controversial by many, alterations to what is licensable came not from a change in primary legislation but from one designed to ensure new quality and safety standards in scientific procedures. The European Union Tissues and Cells Directive (EUTCD) was implemented in 2007 with the result that all assisted conception treatments are now within the HFEA's regulatory framework.

Although not a medical treatment, surrogacy is also subject to regulation either through the surrogacy legislation alone where licensed treatment is not involved – in particular, the Surrogacy Arrangements Act 1995, Parental Orders (Human Fertilisation and Embryology) Regulations 1994, and Parental Orders (Human Fertilisation and Embryology)(Scotland) Regulations 1994 – or, where it is involved, through both these and the HFE Act.

What do the treatments entail?

There are many texts on the market to explain medical interventions from the perspective of those administering them (Balen and Jacobs 1997, Lockwood, *et al.* 2007, Winston 1996, 2008). There is also a growing number of publications that offer accounts from the perspective of people who have undergone the interventions (Barnby 1995, Benson and Robinson-Walsh 1998, Brian 1998, 2007, Gallup 2007, Lorbach 2003).

One of the key features of fertility treatments is that, regardless of whether or not the woman has any fertility impairment herself, she will be centrally involved in undergoing treatment. She will therefore be exposed to the associated risks from drug regimes, anaesthetics, surgical procedures as well as any emotional risk or consequences from having to take time off work. This is a not inconsiderable fact that has to be managed by the woman and her partner (if she has one) given that less than one-third of impairments are thought to be located in the female partner alone. This is one of the few areas where treatments are undergone by a non-impaired individual in order to 'overcome' the impairment of another person.

Why were some treatments licensed and others not?

Some interesting decisions were made by Parliament about which treatments were to be licensed. This led to the two-tier system referred to above whereby, until 2007, health facilities that only offered non-licensed treatments (e.g. GIFT, IUI and ovulatory treatments) were not required to be licensed or inspected by the HFEA. Where such treatments were offered alongside licensed treatments, *all* the treatments were inspected!

The yardsticks for determining which treatments to include were not apparently related to the complexity or innovatory nature of the treatments. Bennett and Harris (1999) have suggested that they may have been more to do with how closely the treatments mimic the natural process. Thus they argued that GIFT, IUI and ovulation induction remained unlicensed because fertilisation did not take place outside the body. However, this did not account for the inclusion of DI, perhaps the oldest (and previously unregulated) form of treatment, and surrogacy via other regulatory legislation. For these, one can only conclude that it was the presence of a genetic parent who did not become the social parent that led Parliament to favour external regulation.

Where similarly constituted families are formed *as a result of professional involvement* (e.g. adoption, fostering), there has also traditionally been a legal framework to regulate professional involvement and monitor the children's well-being. However, there are important differences from the HFE Act which may reflect the non-medical rather than the medical professional involvement and setting. In mainstream children's legislation

(Children Act 1989 which, interestingly, went through Parliament at almost the same time as the HFE Act 1990 under the same Government, and the more recent Adoption and Children Act 2002) and surrogacy arrangements:

•◦ the welfare of the child has paramountcy over that of all other interested parties;
•◦ children have the right, at the age of majority, to have access to their public agency records including identifying information about their genetic parents.

In the HFE Act, these principles did not apply even when, as is the case with the use of donated embryos, neither of the social parents had a genetic link to the child. Despite changes (through Regulations) in 2005 to the rights of donor-conceived adults to receive identifying information about the person who supplied half of their genetic material (i.e. the donor), there remains no legal requirement for parents to inform their children of their origins. Indeed the HFE Act made it legal for the non-genetic father to be named on the birth certificate. Unlike the situation with surrogacy or adoption, there is nothing on the birth certificate to alert the person to their genetic origins and therefore no independent route for them to find out. This brings up the curious situation whereby when surrogacy takes place in a licensed centre and involves the use of a donated egg, the offspring may gain access to their original birth certificate but this will *not* tell them that their birth mother was not their genetic mother. In the recent debates on the new HFE Bill, attempts to bring in changes to the way that birth certificates are notated for those conceived using donated gametes, were unsuccessful, although the Government did concede that it will keep the situation under review. For now, donor offspring can only find out if they were donor conceived if someone chooses to tell them this in either a planned or an unplanned way or through DNA testing.

Neither are there sanctions against clinics that do not insist on prospective parents discussing their strategies for dealing with the needs arising with regard to openness with their child and with family members (see above) as only the *offer* of implications counselling is mandatory.

This raises the question of why such differences were enacted in 1990 and have not been fully removed, even in the current HFE Bill. After many years of debate and consultation, the Government finally agreed to introduce Regulations to lift donor anonymity on the grounds that it was morally right to enable donor-conceived adults to be able to access information in full, which is stored on them in public records (i.e. the HFEA Register of Information). (For a fuller discussion of this, *see* Wincott and Crawshaw 2006.) The changes were effected prospectively in 2005. One might assume that good parental practice should therefore now be seen to include making children conceived using donated gametes aware of the nature of their genetic origins. Given this, it would be difficult to imagine how prospective parents could be assessed as being of low or no risk of causing their children 'serious psychological or medical harm' (Section G.3.4.5.) if they have a stated intention of secrecy. And yet this is the case. In perhaps the nearest equivalent professional setting where suitability is assessed in relation to parenting a child who is not genetically related (i.e. adoption) intended secrecy would constitute grounds for refusal.

A culture of preference towards secrecy undoubtedly still remains in some professionals' practice and among some prospective parents (though this is shifting, see Crawshaw 2008). Some procedural obstacles also remain:

•• Unlike earlier changes to the adoption law, the new Regulations to lift donor anonymity were not applied retrospectively. Thus the first opportunity for a donor offspring to gain access to identifying information may be as far away as 2024.

•• Under the new Regulations, existing donors can re-register as 'willing to be known' and parents can be given non-identifying information to assist them in bringing up their children. However there has been no national campaign to advise affected parties of these changes and clinic practices are likely to continue to vary in how proactive they are in promoting them or responding to approaches from 'old' donors.

•• The HFEA has still to determine the services and processes that it will provide to those donor offspring seeking non-identifying information from their Register of Information even though some are now eligible to do so.

•• There has been, and continues to be, considerable variation in the quantity and quality of information collected about, and from, donors. This is true for information collected at the point of donation and that offered by donors at a later stage. This may reflect varying views within the professional community about the wisdom or importance of recording such information. The outcome is that some of those seeking information about their donor will find there is little to receive.

•• Patients undergoing (licensed) treatment have to give their signed consent to disclose any information about their treatment to any health professional outside of the centre, enabling those inclined towards secrecy to refuse and thus remain unchallenged by professionals that they subsequently come into contact with, including midwives, health visitors, GPs and so on.

•• For those who were conceived *prior* to the enactment of the HFE Act, the government has funded a voluntary register, UK DonorLink, to facilitate information exchange and contact between those genetically related through donor conception. However, the limited funding available has severely restricted its promotion. Additionally, those seeking information have no legal right of access to any medical records surrounding their conception and there are no legal safeguards to prevent the destruction of such records. 'Matching' is therefore reliant on DNA testing with all the uncertainty that entails (Crawshaw and Marshall 2008).

It has been suggested that by not giving paramountcy to the welfare of children or the family unit to be formed, the welfare of the adults present at the time of decisionmaking unhelpfully takes precedence (Freeman 1996, Goodchild 2008, International Donor Offspring Alliance 2008, Speirs 1998). Indeed a recent policy statement from the medically dominated professional association, the British Fertility Society, has prioritised the demand from prospective parents for access to donated gametes over the social and emotional consequences of expanding the number of families that might be formed from a single donor (Hamilton, *et al.* 2008). Evidence from adult donor offspring coming forward and from parents who are committed to openness, is putting increasing pressure on this situation. It is clear that donor offspring (and their parents) may want to know the full details of their genetic origins and may want to restrict the numbers of families being formed. They argue that there is an important emotional, social and medical significance to the nature of their conception that some professionals and policy makers have hitherto minimised (Daniels 2004, Donor Conception Support Group 1997, Gollancz 2001, Kirkman 2004, Lorbach 2003, McWhinnie 2006, Morrissette 2006, Turner and Coyle 2000, Whipp 1998).

However, there have also been some measurable shifts in social understanding as well as in considerations of what kinship might mean to those affected, which look set to be reflected in the new HFE Bill, namely:

- the right for donor-conceived adults to be provided with information about the numbers, gender and year of birth of any donor half-siblings;
- the right for donors (though not their non-donor conceived offspring) to be given similar information about anyone conceived as a result of their donation;
- the rights of same sex couples in a civil partnership to have shared parental responsibility and legal parentage of any children born to them through assisted conception treatments.

Shifting the culture even further will only come as the issues are conceptualised and debated increasingly within legal and social frameworks rather than the medical one as hitherto. Prospective parents receive medical interventions for extended periods of time. Dangers remain from their transition to parenthood being framed as a medical event that requires a medical solution, rather than a social and emotional one that requires attention to their psychosocial needs as prospective parents. It is to this that I now turn.

What help do people get in preparing for parenthood?

Health professional involvement in the transition to parenthood is regularly provided through monitoring of the pregnancy and helping the prospective parents to prepare for the parenting tasks ahead. In the non-medical arena, this element of preparation is also maintained, for example in adoption preparation.

However, there is no requirement for assisted conception clinics to provide help with preparation for this particular form of parenthood, even in cases where donated gametes are used. Indeed the emphasis on 'welfare of the child' assessments may actually marginalise preparation needs. Patients who achieve a pregnancy are usually transferred to the care of antenatal services – who may or may not be aware of the particular circumstances of the conception. Although the Code of Practice states that clinics should be prepared for future contact from donors, parents, offspring or others affected by treatment, the approach to inspection outlined earlier makes this difficult to enforce or to prescribe minimum standards. The clinic's only further involvement may therefore be to notify the HFEA Register of Information when the woman informs them of the birth. (Note that when the woman gives birth, she is required to notify the Centre where she had the treatment so that they in turn can notify the HFEA Register of Information. There are no penalties attached to failure to notify and, until recently, no official system for tracking how often this actually happens.)

Parents, offspring and others are therefore left to manage the resulting personal and family dynamics unaided, with no publicly funded specialist service taking ongoing responsibility for them. This is of concern when one considers the potential vulnerabilities of these family members, including:

- evidence suggesting that some adults can continue to hold (and possibly repress) unresolved feelings about their use of donated gametes as a route to becoming parents (Daniels, *et al.* 1995, Hargreaves and Daniels 2007, Kirkman 2003, Snowden and Snowden 1998);
- evidence suggesting that parents who use donated gametes are more likely to downplay the influence of genetic inheritance (as part of their adjusting to treatment) than are parents with genetically related offspring, raising concerns that they may find such views difficult to sustain in the longer term (Grace and Daniels 2007, van den Akker 2000, Waterman 2003);
- the lack of biographical and identifying information available to parents who choose to be open in order to help their child integrate the facts of his or her identity into the process of growing up;
- the potential medical disadvantages of not having full access to information about, or even awareness of, genetic heritage (Simpson 1998);
- the dangers associated with accidental disclosure as apparent from adoption research (Hill and Shaw 1998, Howe and Feast 2000, Keefer and Schooler 2000, Triseliotis, *et al.* 2005) as well as from research involving donor offspring themselves (McWhinnie 2006, Morrissette 2006, Turner and Coyle 2000, Whipp 1998);
- the socially isolating effect of the culture of secrecy that can lead to family members having reduced access to formal and/or informal support systems;
- the psychological effect of managing any stigma that is felt by coming to parenthood through medically assisted conception.

If indeed it is the medicalisation of the process – along with the social stigma (especially where the process involves the use of donated gametes) – that has silenced or at least delayed the debate about parenthood, then dilution of its influence is imperative.

CONCLUSION

This chapter has considered the use of medically assisted conception treatments and sought to identify the medical, legal and social frameworks within which they are practised. It has suggested that professionals who are working with women and couples in the antenatal, delivery and postnatal periods need to be vigilant about the potential for their personal values and experiences to affect professional tasks. It has argued that the development of a clear factual base means separating fact from opinion. This needs to be encompassed with a rigorous and reflective critical awareness of the influence of the social context in which new developments arise. Awareness of the diluting or reinforcing effect of the interweaving of medical, legal and social strands can better enable the professional to maintain a patient–centred approach to their work, where the uniqueness of the patient's situation is viewed against this backdrop.

Specific aspects of the new reproductive technologies (access to treatments and their regulation, counselling and 'welfare of the child' requirements) have been considered in order to illustrate both their complexities and their potential for social manipulation. In particular, the position of people who are conceived by the use of donated gametes has been highlighted. The media tend to express opposition to the new reproductive technologies too simplistically, arising *either* from a religious standpoint *or* from an inadequate understanding of these technologies. This brief examination makes it clear that it is infinitely more complex to try and answer the question of whether the new reproductive technologies represent a threat or opportunity.

KEY POINTS

- ⮞ Personal values and experience can prejudice the performance of professional tasks.
- ⮞ Critical awareness of the social context of developments in the new reproductive technologies is essential.
- ⮞ The separate influences of medical, legal and social frameworks can be diluted or reinforced when they interweave with each other.

USEFUL ADDRESSES
Patient organisations
ACeBabes
www.acebabes.co.uk

DC Network
PO Box 7471
Nottingham NG3 6ZR
Information line: 0208 245 4369
www.donor-conception-network.org

Infertility Network UK (INUK)
(including National Infertility Awareness Campaign (NIAC)
and More to Life)
Charter House
43 St Leonards Road
Bexhill on Sea
East Sussex TN40 1JA
Tel: 0800 008 7464
www.infertilitynetworkuk.com

Pink Parents
Box 55
Green Leaf Bookshop
82 Colston St
Bristol BS1 5BB
Tel: 0117 377 5794/904 4500
www.pinkparents.org.uk

Surrogacy UK
PO Box 24
Newent
Gloucestershire GL18 1YS
Tel: 0153 182 1889/0169 829 3744
www.surrogacyuk.org

Other organisations

British Infertility Counselling Association
111 Harley St
London W1G 6AW
www.bica.net

Human Fertilisation and Embryology Authority
21 Bloomsbury St
London WC1B 3HF
Tel: 020 7291 8201
www.hfea.gov.uk

National Gamete Donation Trust
helpline: 0845 226 9193
www.ngdt.co.uk

UK DonorLink
31 Moor Rd
Headingley
Leeds LS6 4BG
Tel: 0113 278 3217
www.ukdonorlink.org.uk

REFERENCES

Balen A, Jacobs HS. (1997) *Infertility in Practice.* London: Churchill Livingstone.

Barnby K. (1995) *Labours of Eve: women's experiences of infertility.* London: Boxtree Ltd.

Bennett R, Harris J. (1999) Restoring natural function: access to infertility treatments using donated gametes. *Hum Fertil.* 2(1): 18–21.

Benson J, Robinson–Walsh D. (1998) *Infertility and IVF: facts and feelings from patients' perspectives.* London: Scarlet Press.

Blyth E, Crawshaw M, Speirs J, editors. (1998) *Truth and the Child 10 Years On: information exchange in donor assisted conception.* Birmingham: BASW Publications.

Boivin J, Scanlan LC, Walker SM. (1999) Why are infertile patients not using psychosocial counselling? *Hum Reprod.* 14(5): 1384–91.

Brian K. (1998) *In Pursuit of Parenthood: real-life experiences of IVF.* London: Bloomsbury Publishers Ltd.

Brian K. (2007) *The Complete Guide to Female Infertility.* London: Piatkus Books.

British Infertility Counselling Association. (2004) *Implications Counselling for People Considering Donor-assisted Conception.* London: BICA Publications.

British Infertility Counselling Association. (2007) *Guidelines for Good Practice in Infertility Counselling.* 2nd ed. London: BICA Publications.

Burns LH, Covington SN. (2006) *Infertility Counselling: a comprehensive handbook for clinicians.* 2nd ed. Carnforth: Parthenon.

Campion MJ. (1995) *Who's Fit to be a Parent?* London: Routledge.

Crawshaw M, Marshall L. (2008) Practice experiences of running UK DonorLink, a voluntary information exchange register for adults related through donor conception. *Hum Fertil.* 11(4): 231–7.

Crawshaw M. (2008) Prospective parents' intentions regarding disclosure following the removal of donor anonymity. *Hum Fertil.* 11(2): 95–100.

Crawshaw MA. (1999) What do BICA licensed centre counsellors think should be covered as part of a good quality HFEA inspection of counselling services? *J Fertil Counsel.* 6(3): 21–4.

Daniels KR, Lewis GM, Gillett W. (1995) Telling donor insemination offspring about their conception: the nature of couples' decision making. *Soc Sci Med.* 40(9): 1213–20.

Daniels KR. (2004) *Building a Family with the Assistance of Donor Insemination.* Palmerston North, New Zealand: Dunmore Press.

Donor Conception Support Group of Australia. (1997) *Let the Offspring Speak: discussions on donor conception.* Georges Hall, NSW, Australia: Donor Conception Support Group.

Eugster A, Vingerhoets AJJM. (1999) Psychological aspects of in vitro fertilisation: a review. *Soc Sci Med.* 48: 575–89.

Franklin S. (1997) *Embodied Progress: a cultural account of assisted conception.* London: Routledge.

Freeman M. (1996) The new birth right: identity and the child of the reproduction revolution. *Int J Child Rights.* 4(3): 273–97.

Gallup C. (2007) *Making Babies the Hard Way: living with infertility and treatment.* London: Jessica Kingsley Publishers.

Gollancz D. (2001) Donor insemination: a question of rights. *Hum Fertil.* 4: 164–7.

Goodchild S. (2008) *Donor children demand to be told parents' ID.* London: Evening Standard; 31 March 2008. Available at: www.highbeam.com/doc/1P2-15596327.html (accessed 3 Jan 2009).

Grace VM, Daniels KR. (2007) The (ir)relevance of genetics: engendering parallel worlds of procreation and reproduction. *Sociol Health Illn.* 29(5): 692–710.

Greil AL. (1997) Infertility and psychological distress: a critical review of the literature. *Soc Sci Med.* 45(11): 1679–704.

Hamilton M, Pacey A, Tomlinson M, *et al.* (2008). Working party report on sperm donation services in the UK: report and recommendations. *Hum Fertil.* 11(3): 147–58.

Hargreaves K, Daniels KR. (2007) Parents dilemmas in sharing donor insemination conception stories with their children. *Children Soc.* 21(6): 420–31.

Hill M, Shaw M, editors. (1998) *Signposts in Adoption: policy, practice and research issues.* London: British Association for Adoption and Fostering (BAAF).

Howe D, Feast J. (2000) *Adoption, Search and Reunion.* London: The Children's Society.

Human Fertilisation and Embryology Authority. (2005) *Tomorrow's Children: report of the policy review of welfare of the child assessments in licensed assisted conception clinics.* London: HFEA. Available at: www.hfea.gov.uk/docs/TomorrowsChildren.pdf (accessed 3 Jan 2009).

Human Fertilisation and Embryology Authority. (2007) *The HFEA Code of Practice.* London: HFEA. Available at: http://cop.hfea.gov.uk/cop/ (accessed 3 Jan 2009).

International Donor Offspring Alliance. (2008) *Human Fertilisation and Embryology Bill: Birth Certificates: the case for reform – briefing for members of the House of Commons.* Available at: http://web.jaguarpaw.co.uk/~tom/idoa-briefing-latest.pdf (accessed 3 Jan 2009).

Keefer B, Schooler JE. (2000) *Telling the Truth to Your Adopted or Foster Child.* Westport, CT: Bergin and Garvey.

Kirkman M. (2003) Parents' contributions to the narrative identity of offspring of donor-assisted conception. *Soc Sci Med.* 57: 2229–42.

Kirkman M. (2004) Genetic connection and relationships in narratives of donor-assisted conception. *Aust J Emerg Technol Soc.* 2(1): 1–20.

Lockwood G, Anthony-Ackery J, Meyers-Thompson J, *et al.* (2007) *Fertility and Infertility for Dummies.* London: John Wiley and Sons.

Lorbach C. (2003) *Experiences of Donor Conception.* London: Jessica Kingsley Publications.

McWhinnie A. (2006) *Who Am I? Experiences of donor conception.* Leamington Spa: Idreos Education Trust.

Morrissette M, editor. (2006) *Behind Closed Doors: moving beyond secrecy and shame.* Minneapolis, MN: Be-Mondo Publishing.

Olsen R, Clarke H. (2003) *Parenting and Disability: disabled people's experiences of raising children.* Bristol: The Policy Press.

Saffron L. (2001) Decision making among lesbians wishing to get pregnant. *J Fertil Counsel.* 8(2): 31–6.

Simpson SA. (1998) Truth and the child: a genetic perspective. In: Blyth E, Crawshaw M, Speirs J, editors. *Truth and the Child 10 Years On: information exchange in donor assisted conception.* Birmingham: BASW Publications.

Snowden R, Snowden E. (1998) Families created through donor insemination. In: Daniels KR, Haimes E, editors. *Donor Insemination: international social science perspectives.* Cambridge: Cambridge University Press.

Speirs J. (1998) Children's rights or adult's rights. In: Blyth E, Crawshaw M, Speirs J, editors. *Truth and the Child 10 Years On: information exchange in donor assisted conception.* Birmingham: BASW Publications.

Throsby K. (2004) *When IVF Fails: feminism, infertility and the negotiation of normality.* Basingstoke: Palgrave Macmillan.

Triseliotis J, Feast J, Kyle F. (2005) *The Adoption Triangle Revisited: a study of adoption, search and reunion experiences.* London: British Association for Adoption and Fostering (BAAF).

Turner AJ, Coyle A. (2000) What does it mean to be a donor offspring? The identity experience of adults conceived by donor insemination and the implications for counselling and therapy. *Hum Reprod.* 15(9): 2041–51.

Van den Akker O. (2000) The importance of a genetic link in mothers commissioning a surrogate baby in the UK. *Hum Reprod.* 15(8): 1849–55.

Verhaak CM, Smeenk JMJ, van Minnen A, *et al.* (2005) A longitudinal, prospective study on emotional adjustment before, during and after consecutive fertility treatment cycles. *Hum Reprod.* 20(8): 2253–60.

Waterman B. (2003) *The Birth of an Adoptive, Foster or Stepmother: beyond biological mothering attachments.* London: Jessica Kingsley Publishers.

Whipp C. (1998) The legacy of deceit: a donor offspring's perspective on secrecy in assisted conception. In: Blyth E, Crawshaw M, Speirs J, editors. *Truth and the Child 10 Years On: information exchange in donor assisted conception.* Birmingham: BASW Publications.

Wincott E, Crawshaw MA. (2006) From a social issue to policy: social work's advocacy for the rights of donor-conceived people to genetic origins information in the UK. *Soc Work Health Care.* 43(2/3): 53–72.

Winston RML. (1996) *Infertility: a sympathetic approach.* London: Optima.

Winston RML. (2008) *A Child Against All Odds.* London: Bantam Books.

CHAPTER 17

Fetal surveillance

Christine Grabowska

This chapter will challenge accepted opinion on fetal screening and ask the reader to explore the wider, covert issues related to the production of human beings. Eugenics and politics will be discussed in attempting to highlight some of the reasons for the availability and eventual outcomes of screening. This chapter will consider the acceptance of tests on the fetus using the ideas mainly of Foucault and Parsons, for sociological interpretation. An explanation of the social influences upon the individual and the organisation will lead the reader to the possibilities for the future. These theories are applied to practice.

The chapter asks the practitioner to explore why screening is adhered to routinely. It asks who is in control of the process – the woman or the doctor and what is the actual purpose of screening, is it to create a uniformity of acceptable human beings or to reduce suffering? It briefly considers the moral questions of whether the fetus is always entitled to life or is society at liberty to choose a suitable commodity in the form of a child? It demonstrates that women, though at the centre of the screening process, have little say on screening and even less say on the outcomes.

INTRODUCTION

The fetus is the 'ideal' subject for the perfect system of surveillance, which is one that observes the silent body of the non-consenting fetus, the body that cannot object or eagerly participate. Its mother, who is obeying social norms, or accepted practice, sees the surveillance as 'normal'. The question of normality is explored and concludes that it is a social convention. It has no meaning other than it is what is happening to the majority of people. Normality knows no boundaries and society can push its meaning in any direction. It is only morality that puts a stop to the proceedings.

WHAT IS SURVEILLANCE?

Surveillance, simply defined, means nothing more than 'keeping a close eye on', or according to Collins dictionary (1998), 'to keep watch'. The word may conjure up images of Closed Circuit Television (CCTV) within shops and other public places. The idea of 'Big Brother is watching you' has less impact today than when Aldous Huxley published *Brave New World* in 1932 or when George Orwell's *Nineteen Eighty Four* was published in 1949. We live in an age of technology, machinery and gadgets; people have been subsumed into the mechanistic era and have integrated 'Big Brother' as part of their existence. Surveillance has become 'normal' and is no longer seen or acknowledged as untoward. The maternity contract between hospital providers and users may be said to have the same implicit message.

The benefits of fetal surveillance may be considered overrated; it would be negligent and untrue to suggest that we have the technology to prevent fetal 'abnormalities' yet somehow the public are led to believe this is possible and they have the expectation that it will be the result of fetal surveillance. If the system fails them, litigation or revenge is often the next step. Is the current system of fetal surveillance desirable? Should society be free of so-called 'abnormalities'? The control over applied genetics rests with the scientists, doctors, insurance companies, medical suppliers and the Government.

WHAT ARE THE CONSEQUENCES OF FETAL SURVEILLANCE?

Fetal surveillance has enhanced the personal blame culture of the materialist world. In other words, the individual is directly responsible within a world where monetary profit is a priority. Because 'abnormalities' can be destroyed it is up to the individual to take the responsibility to do so. The popular culture is one where facilities and resources to care for the 'disabled' are reducing and there is a social stigma and stereotype that exists around disability. The fetus can thus become a commodity like anything else that can be purchased and it depends on surveillance to be accepted or rejected. Parenting for a child becomes conditional until the quality of the child is approved through technology. People, which include mothers and practitioners, are now secondary in the process.

THE EMERGENCE OF SURVEILLANCE

Foucault (1973) considers that medicine has moved away from listening and seeing to a three-dimensional examination involving the physical, technical and laboratory. Classically, doctors would listen to the patient and base their diagnosis on the 'story'. Treatment was based on the traditional fifteenth century diagnosis of 'humours', which included 'blood', 'black/green bile' or 'mucus'. Finally, with the introduction of the post-mortem into medical school curricula, doctors could discover the body away from the patient. Post-mortems moved life, disease and death to a technical arena (Eribon 1992). The doctor learned about non-living tissue; tissue that could not tell its 'story' and tissue that was abstracted from life (Armstrong, *et al.* 2007). This is the place that doctors often start their careers today.

The three-dimensional examination takes on objectivity, as the doctor does not have to be influenced by the patient. It becomes truly objective when a specimen can be removed from the patient, tested in the laboratory, and a diagnosis made without the patient ever being present. Compare this with the fetus under the ultrasound scan, the fetus being the specimen observed, and having no choice and no say. The diagnosis on this 'specimen' may result in having to make one of two choices, one of life and the other of death.

Foucault (1974) would liken fetal surveillance to the Panopticon – the perfect system of surveillance. He takes his thoughts from the model of a prison that Jeremy Bentham described in 1786 (Boyne 2000). This is an eight-sided building with two windows to each cell. The prison warder is able to view each prisoner from a central area. The light from the window meant that the warder could view each prisoner, but the prisoner could not see the warder. The warder could stand in one place and view those all around. Foucault called this 'the gaze', where everyone could be viewed from a vantage point. He observed that hospitals and schools, as well as prisons, have been built to incorporate 'the gaze' and he called this institutional surveillance. The nurse, in the hospital, could view everyone from the middle of a nightingale ward; the teacher, in schools, could gaze upon the pupils in their rows from the podium. The patients or pupils, though, did not have the same vantage point as the nurse or teacher in that they could not gaze upon each other in totality.

The ultimate purpose of 'the gaze' is to reduce deviancy, through self-conformity. Consider a prisoner planning an escape but not knowing when he is being gazed upon. Foucault calls this mechanism that produces conformity through observation, the 'Disciplinary Power'. 'What is being punished is non-conformity which the exercise of disciplinary power seeks to correct' (Smart 2002: 86).

Koskela (2003: 301) notes that 'the Panopticon operates to maintain normality' in society and certainly, with the use of CCTV, laser scanning in shops and paying with credit cards, everyone is being surveyed and gazed upon and they believe this to be 'normal' (Koskela 2003). 'A gaze which each individual under its weight will end by interiorising to the point that he is his own overseer, each individual thus exercising this surveillance over, and against himself' (Foucault 1972: 155). Thus the perfect 'disciplinary power' is instituted and becomes part of the culture. The individual is automatically partaking and accepting 'the gaze' with little awareness of their own involvement. Routine ultrasound in pregnancy provides the milieu for panopticon-like surveillance. The woman brings her fetus to be viewed and yet the fetus has no choice. Foucault's (1977: 204) 'laboratory of power' is applicable in this setting where fetuses are labelled and either accepted or rejected. The woman's responsibility for the pregnancy and its natural course is being impeded by the ultrasonic panopticon and the fetus has 'no possibility to "respond" or "oppose" the gaze' (Koskela 2003: 298).

The gaze is thus turned in on the person herself and this results in self-discipline or conformity. Surveillance has made it possible for medicine to change from being involved with sickness alone, to having the potential to discover abnormality and to blame the victim, in this instance, the mother (Petersen and Bunton 1997).

The message of health promotion is that health impairment is avoidable by making the right choices; in this case responsibility for choosing is given to the mother. Katz Rothman (1986: 14) suggests that choice is an illusion because the mother ends up 'taking the least awful choice'. She is 'trapped, caught . . . in a nightmare' (1986: 189). The 'forced choice' (1986: 180) is of whether she will devote her life to caring for a handicapped child, in the midst of social disapproval, or whether she will destroy the life.

WHO IS MAKING CHOICES?

The gaze is extended into all areas of life, for instance, the male gaze upon the female body. Males have culturally developed an 'appetite' for certain bodily characteristics by gazing at models. Females are complicit in the process; on seeing the same media propaganda they aspire to copy the body image so that they too will be gazed upon. The rise in cosmetic surgery supports the notion that people are aiming to be similar (King 1999). The gaze is so strong that society is trying to improve its so-called health by trying to look similar to an established norm. This appears to boost the ego. The way to achieve it is often said to be through 'healthy' living, including working out, dieting, lipo-suction and so on (Baron 2007).

The gaze will produce uniformity (thus conformity) of looks and expectations. 'Because most people don't want to become delinquent, they accept normative values that are supposed to make them "good" citizens' (Danaher, *et al.* 2000: 60). However, this leads to self-punishment, when the gaze is turned in upon the self (Koskela 2000) and at the extreme, it produces eating disorders, excruciating work-outs and subjecting the body to cosmetic surgery. In a similar way, women will tolerate pain (via an amniocentesis or vaginal ultrasound scan, for instance) in order to gaze upon the fetus. Screening is seen as demanded by women themselves. The choices women make are therefore socially created as well as socially constrained. When the gaze is applied to the fetus it will be possible to not only reject the sex of the child but also their height, weight, and eye, hair and skin colour (Koskela 2003). Again, this will achieve uniformity. If this appears abhorrent, consider this: the orthodox church in Cyprus, prior to marriage, asks couples to produce their thalassaemia carrier status. The church will marry couples who are both carriers, only on the premise that they will use prenatal diagnosis and abortion. The church does not condone abortion for other reasons (Richards 1993: 573, Statham, *et al.* 2000). The point is this: thoughts originate in culture (Foucault 1974: 50) and can then become normalised.

The pregnant woman conforms by taking the fetus to be gazed upon. The woman knows that the fetus is being surveyed, but does not know everything that is seen. The technician who has this information therefore wields power. Merquior (1985: 236) tells us that power is associated with repression. Power allows people to exploit others for their own gain (Brewis 2001). Cousins and Hussain (1984: 210) suggest that power is not always isolated to an individual but can originate from the needs of capitalism, so people express this in the power exerted. It is the Marxist notion that women will reproduce according to the capitalist needs; therefore the woman will be alienated from the end product, just like the car assembly worker who has only a small part to play in the car's production (Koch 2005). She is the commodity that serves political and economic needs.

> The biological traits of a population become relevant factors for economic management and it becomes necessary to organise around them an apparatus which will ensure not only their subjection but the constant increase of their utility. (Foucault 1972: 172)

Materialism is promoted by capitalism. Machinery manufacturers, for instance continuously create even more 'precise' equipment such as with ultrasound, which is welcomed by the maternity system.

It can be seen that the technology, which is established to further the capitalist economy, holds a powerful footing. The problem with power is that it can be belittled or removed and therefore to prevent this from happening it becomes important to subordinate women, and create a continuous struggle to develop 'secret' knowledge (which is expressed through the manipulation of machinery, technology and gadgets). Nola (1998) tells us that Foucault recognised that knowledge creates and results in domination. Subordination is evident not just in hospitals, but in every area of society where power is to be maintained and this includes even the micro-structure of the family (Lindahl, *et al.* 2004). Generally, what is observed during an ultrasound scan examination is a subordinate woman lying, often silently, looking at the screen, hoping to have the pleasure of seeing a 'normal' baby.

Foucault (1972: 119) acknowledges that the ultrasound scan will produce knowledge which in turn 'produces discourse'. The discourse, or discussion, is usually amongst professionals and it is this discourse that increases the body of knowledge (Vailly 2006). The doctor's gaze relates symptoms and signs, and the description of the dis-ease is then formulated (Cousins and Hussain 1984: 159). Foucault (1974: 87) simply says that language is the basis of knowledge. Language 'is a necessary medium for any scientific knowledge that wishes to be expressed in discourse' (1974: 296). It is the medically formulated language of the uncertain, or previously unknown, that is transmitted as knowledge (Cousins and Hussain 1984: 161).

Without language the dis-ease could not be labelled and therefore could not be treated or obliterated. Therefore, the label given allows the doctor to reason and create what is acceptable or not. Merquior (1985: 146) suggests that 'reason itself is a technology of power, science and an instrument of domination'. Thus, if women questioned the dis-ease they would be driven into subordination by the act of reasoning. The reasoning will validate surveillance, which will have included machinery, technology or gadgets (which are venerated with the truth) (Kuhn and Kramer 2000).

The creation of knowledge, which often is an agreed opinion, gives power and status, not to the specimen that was gazed upon, but to those that created the label to describe what was gazed upon (Vailly 2006). Smart (2002) tells us that knowledge creates power and advances in knowledge are an expression of that power. Nola (1998) goes one step further in suggesting that the subjects of truth, knowledge and what is considered right are all creating power. It is power that creates what is then accepted as truth (Kuhn and Kramer 2000).

The human genome project creates the perfect objective gaze because in order to know the truth of a pathological fact the doctor must abstract the patient (Foucault 1973). Danaher, *et al.* (2000: 50) inform us that 'one of discipline's concerns is with producing docile healthy bodies'. Ultimately, the production of designer children will be possible if this trend is continued, thus creating children that conform to ethnocentric ideas of normality and desirability (Pinker 2003).

Foucault (1973) explains that at the end of the eighteenth century the life/death continuum started to change from being normal to abnormal. The only abnormal death prior to this time resulted from murder/war. Birth and death now happen mainly in hospital. The hospital depicts Max Weber's 'ideal type' of institution (Sung 2007) that is a rational, hierarchical, bureaucratic structure, whereby everyone performs a unique function/skill for a minimum cost to the organisation. To ensure efficiency everyone is overseen and thus will be subordinated to some part of the hierarchy – 'The hierarchy established to provide a progression towards the more complex and the less exact' (Foucault 1974: 246). It can be seen from this that allowing birth/death to happen naturally can overturn the 'ideal type'; therefore both ends of the continuum are manipulated with the help of machinery, technology and gadgets. This change is seen as normal (Kuhn and Kramer 2000).

Normality is therefore socially constructed (O'Donnell, *et al.* 2005). Look at the statistical norm and its place in the histogram (or bell shaped curve), the majority are the social creation of normal. It appears as follows in figure 17.1.

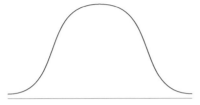

FIGURE 17.1 A normally spread histogram

The norm is a line drawn in the middle to represent the greatest number of the population. Therefore, if this is a representation of pregnant women undergoing ultrasound scans, in this country, the majority will actually have a scan and the bell will be very narrow (as shown in Figure 17.2).

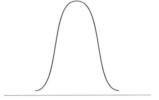

FIGURE 17.2 A narrow histogram

It can thereby be concluded that it is normal for women to have ultrasound scans during pregnancy (Whittle 2000). This is very different from natural.

Consider the difference between a natural and a normal birth. What is now conceived as normal cannot be termed natural (Royal College of Midwives 2007). Most 'normal births' will have occurred as a result of the use of machinery, technology and gadgets as opposed to natural births, which will not have made use of these (Kennedy and Shannon 2004). Equally, death that has occurred with the use of technology involving drugs cannot be conceived as natural (Howitt Wilson 2000). This is easier to see in the fetus than in the adult. For instance, injecting potassium chloride into the fetal heart with the intention of committing fetocide, some might argue, is no different to the morphine that is offered as 'pain relief' to the terminally ill adult.

The changing social view of normality may originate in the scientific or technocratic community. Doctors define a 'normal' or 'abnormal' baby today (Vailly 2006). A technological diagnosis is made through chromosome analysis, for instance, and if the result is 'abnormal' the doctor offers death of the fetus to the parents. This is termed a 'therapeutic abortion', but for whom is it therapeutic? A similar option would not be given to parents if a doctor deemed the baby to be 'normal'. Consider the possibility of parents wanting a baby who has an abnormality as a preference in order to replicate their own genes, would this be supported by doctors (Atkinson 2008)? Foucault (1972: 177) considers 'the hospital is more the seat of death for the cities where it is sited than a therapeutic agent for the population as a whole'. Informed choice includes looking at all the options and yet the options appear limited when that of termination of the pregnancy dominates the conversation. This may be argued to be the present day form of eugenics.

EUGENICS

Historically, eugenics might have been said to originate to prevent the higher social classes being burdened by 'social problems' (Koch 2004). Marie Stopes, one of the original eugenicists, in 1919, wrote that she developed contraception to produce 'more children from the fit, less from the unfit' (Cantwell and Enyeart 2007). But it was Francis Galton, a statistician, who founded the Eugenics Society (Eugenics Society 1982) and in 1883 first used the term 'eugenics' (Wikler 1999) originating from the Greek 'eugenes' meaning 'good stock'. Thus Galton developed an interest in obtaining 'good human stock'. He noted that farmers and horticulturists could obtain an improved variety of animal or plant and saw a normal development of applying this to human beings. Thus developed the Eugenics Society, which included members such as Charles Darwin's nephew, Leonard Darwin, who in 1926, suggested ways of getting rid of the inferior by 'the lethal chamber, murder, segregation by imprisonment, confinement and supervision, sterilisation and family limitation by contraception or abstinence' (1926: 114).

Publishing one's thoughts was considered 'normal' in the 1920s and the notion of 'political correctness' certainly did not prevail. It is easy to see how Adolf Hitler's ideas of producing the Aryan race did not cause a public outcry. Following a historical eugenicist example will enlighten as to where current day practices may lead.

The state of Indiana passed the first eugenic sterilisation Act in the USA in 1907. The Sheppard-Towner Act introduced Indiana's Division of Infant and Child Hygiene in 1920 (Stern 2002). The 'better baby contest' was introduced into the state at this time. It excluded entries from African American children. These 'better baby contests' began to be included in state fairs across the USA. State fairs traditionally exhibited livestock and agricultural produce and thus many eugenic organisations originated from agricultural breeders' associations whose aim was to improve animal breeds and plant types (Pernick 2002). Eugenics and 'racial hygiene' were introduced into the medical school curricula, in Germany by 1933. It could be argued that Nazi racial policy originated thus from the scientific community (Annas and Grodin 1992). Galton introduced pedigrees into England prior to this time (Galton.org 2008) but Nazi Germany introduced them under the race laws. On 14 July 1937 the sterilisation law was passed for the prevention of genetically diseased offspring and hundreds of thousands of people were sterilised under these laws. Euthanasia was introduced legally for the mentally ill, handicapped and infirm, which meant that homes and hospitals could be closed down because in-patient numbers were declining. The war years brought mass extermination of human beings to prevent their reproduction. This potted history misses much but allows consideration of the 'slippery slope'.

The majority now saw eugenics, post war, as abhorrent (Koch 2004). The word 'eugenics' was interpreted as racism in the USA (Wasserman and Asch 2006). The eugenicist publications were changing their name to genetics in the title and interestingly the first genetic advisory clinic in Britain was commenced in 1946. It used pedigrees in the history-taking process, as do genetic counsellors of today.

Fetal surveillance took on a different meaning in 1967 since it was the first time that abortion could be offered legally. Even though amniocentesis was a technique familiar to the medical profession prior to 1967, it did not become available to pregnant women until 1967, when a fetus deemed to be 'abnormal' could be terminated, a procedure termed, as already mentioned, 'therapeutic abortion'. Is this therapeutic for the fetus or society?

The human genome project could be said to be the continuation of eugenics. It identifies all the material in the 23 pairs of chromosomes giving information about a person that until now was unknown and unseen. It was Watson and Crick, in 1953, who discovered the double helix structure of DNA and ultimately initiated the Human Genome Project. It is now known that there are three billion base pairs of human genetic make up (Conrad and Gabe 1999). The question remains as to what will be done with all this information. It will be expensive to buy the information on one individual. It is thought that some employers would be willing to pay the price in order to avoid a 'bad' risk. Equally, insurance companies may choose to do the same (Nuffield Council on Bioethics 2002). This could work to their advantage or disadvantage. The companies may not insure 'bad' risks, but then people with 'good' health may decide they do not need the insurance. The premiums thus would increase dramatically so that people requiring insurance could not afford them (Kaufert 2000). Bunton and Petersen (2005) review the increase in inequality from surveillance and wonder if regulation would intensify the danger because of the self-interests of the body that would make up the scrutiny committee.

The human genome project is funded jointly by the United States Department of Energy and National Institutes of Health, other Government agencies worldwide, and by private biotechnology companies. Blood samples are obtained for testing/experimentation from the poorer peoples of the world. Whilst these people may receive a small sum of money for their participation, there do not appear to be any plans for a return or direct benefit to the people who contributed to the discovery of the genome (Alliance for Human Research Protection 2002).

ETHICAL CONSIDERATIONS

Jackson (2000) tells us that the fetus has no rights as a person in the law and therefore cannot have full moral status (Gillam 1999). Doctors have been performing abortions for unwanted babies despite the potential healthy status of the baby and these abortions may be considered 'non-healing' (Wasserman and Asch 2006: 53). Wasserman and Asch (2006) suggest that abortion does not follow other health measures. The mother increases her risks by having an abortion (NHS Direct 2008), and thus if the fetus has no rights in law, the doctor's duty is to cause no harm to the mother. Today, with the 1990 Human Fertilisation and Embryology Act (House of Commons 1990), termination of pregnancy can be carried out at any gestation if there is a serious fetal handicap.

Kuhse and Singer (1999) pose the question – is abortion for fetal abnormality any different to paediatric euthanasia? Currently, this *is not* a 'normal' or legal procedure, whilst fetal euthanasia *is* an acceptable and legal practice. Ethically, Kuhse and Singer cannot quantify a difference. Gillam (1999) suggests that selective abortion is equivalent to non-voluntary euthanasia. However, the challenge is to question the moral outrage this can engender (until the time when it becomes 'normal'). Since January 1995 the Chinese Government has forbidden couples with a serious genetic disease from having children, and this is enforced through abortion. The GMTV poll on 15 February 1995 asked the public whether doctors should kill 'abnormal' babies and the majority of respondents agreed with this action. The social conventionist view is that it is humans that determine normality, not nature (Watson 2008). Fetal deformity has been interpreted as a burden to society and women have been accused of child abuse for choosing to pass on 'abnormalities'. The language used is in relation to fetal rights to 'health' as opposed to fetal rights to life, but the definition of health is socially produced; the individual's understanding of health will be determined by their own opinion of 'normality'.

Destruction of life for 'abnormalities' can be traced back to the classics. Aristotle suggested that the ideal legislation, in his politics, was to destroy deformed infants. Plato, not only agrees with Aristotle, in 'The Republic', but adds that the destruction of babies who are the result of 'unfit' parents, or produced by parents past the ideal childbearing age, would also be beneficial (Tooley 1983).

Analysing the reasons for fetal surveillance poses two questions: is its purpose to remove genetic defects or to produce individuals with more desirable qualities? Given that fetuses have been killed because they have cleft lips or are female, for instance, it may be the latter. From an ethical viewpoint it could be argued that removing pain and suffering from the potentially disabled child through prevention of their life is beneficence, based on the belief that no harm is caused. Equally, a child born disabled could sue her/his parents for a tort of wrongful life. None of this, though, can be enforced on moral grounds (Clarkeburn 2000). Is it the parents who are making the decision of what is genetically worthy, or is it the doctor, on behalf of society, who acts as the detective in the technical screening process and then acts within the eugenic principles of enforcing abortion through social control? Mendonca (2000) suggests that leadership, as in the case of the doctor, can only be ethical when it is based on altruism and not egotism.

The Abortion Act (House of Commons 1967), however, reiterates the doctor's choice (as two doctors have to sign it – not the woman). If women's autonomy is to be respected then medicine cannot be paternalistic. Autonomy is a person's ability to make her/his own decisions and act upon them. In order to be able to fulfil the individual requirement of autonomy, informed consent is essential before submission to any medical procedure. Women therefore, who 'choose' the option of abortion, freely, are also willing to accept responsibility for this decision, which would include the possibility of sterility (Gargaro.com 2008).

The technology behind surveillance cannot be neutral. There is an argument that would suggest that the technology is:

➥ sexist, from a feminist point of view
➥ ableist, from a disabled rights point of view
➥ racist, from a race relations point of view.

1 Some feminists see technology as abusing women and their bodies (McElroy 2008). Women tend to accept the procedural norms of the maternity system, often not

questioning, nor receiving sufficient information (Klein, *et al.* 2006). Information has to be given to avoid litigation, but enough can be withheld to ensure compliance. Women are coerced (by the doctor, their family, the genetic counsellor or the midwife) to have an abortion for fetal abnormality, whilst believing that they have made the choice themselves (Epstein 2003). The technology can be seen as a form of harassment, which is formulated by the male gendered medical profession against women (Brewis 2001, McElroy 2008).

2   Disabled Rights organisations acknowledge that due to the increase in abortion, there are dwindling resources to support disability in society, and with a gradual removal of disabled rights there is less likelihood of trying to find a cure (Jackson 2000). This is probably the result of cause and effect. Prenatal diagnosis and abortion are cheaper in most cases than financially supporting an 'abnormal' person. Disability is seen as undesirable, whilst able people are seen as desirable, therefore by implication, people who already exist with a disability are also undesirable (Snyder and Mitchell 2006). However, prenatal diagnosis and selective abortion are juxtaposed with an increasing number of people surviving with 'abnormalities' such as diabetes or cardiac disease (Williams 2006). They would otherwise have not been conceived, been miscarried, been a stillbirth or died in life. These people now exist because of the efforts of technology. It is also incongruent when able-bodied people are being sent to wars to be killed or maimed and thus become disabled.

3   Racism arises from the issue of trying to narrow the gene pool or promote a certain genetic stock – in principle suggesting that every other resulting human being is unworthy of human status (Nuffield Council on Bioethics 2002). Caplan, *et al.* (1999) argue that eugenics is producing a desirable phenotype or genotype that is different from what parents would choose (thus overriding individual choice). This is racist. What does this say about a society that will not tolerate differences and is there not a duty to let all humans live (Persson 1999)?

WHO HAS THE POWER?

Parsons (1951), a structural functionalist, was clear that power was with the doctor. He recognised that the pregnant woman had an obligation to obey the doctor. Parsons considered the doctor to have social influence and this alone would ensure that patients would carry out their duties and obligations. The mother is seen to have a duty to subordinate her own interest of having a child to that of the greater interest of the society in the creation of 'normality' (Klein, *et al.* 2006).

Parsons thought the woman would not be able, or competent, to make a technical decision. In fact he alludes to her subjectivity and thus irresponsibility. It is important to view this in context. Consider the 1950s, in the USA, and the role of women. The social expectation was that women would be mothers and housewives. Value was placed on the capitalist ethic of economic productivity, as today; hence women who were unpaid for their work derived low status and were often disempowered. However, Parsons saw the doctors gaining the empowerment and economic reward and it is from this social context that Parsons was able to write:

> Birth and the rearing of a child constitutes a 'cost' to the society, through pregnancy, childcare, socialisation, formal training and many other channels. Premature death,

before the individual has had the opportunity to play out his full quota of social roles, means that only a partial 'return' for this cost has been received. (Parsons 1951: 430)

Parsons, it could be argued, was a linear reductionist in that he was able to 'box everything' simply or put it in its place. All human beings were shown to have social roles, which defined their existence. He literally was able to discuss one set of human activities and show how it would go on to affect another set of human activities. However, he dealt only with the external environmental role (or how the individual interacted in society) and did not explore internal issues (Berezin 2003). Parsons, before Foucault, considered the sick role as one of a disciplinary process – 'The sick role allowed exemption from normal responsibilities but (the individual had) an obligation to seek medical help' (Frank 1991: 207). Again, like Foucault, he recognised that there is a choice between obeying procedural norms or an alternative of punishment. Choice is not available when carrying out an obligation.

Parsons sees handicap as dysfunctional. It cannot fit into the scheme of society. Handicap is being labelled as 'useless' to society and therefore has to be obliterated (Johnson 2001). The human activity associated with handicap is not seen as productive to the society from a capitalist perspective, and therefore it would not set off the linear set of human activity associated with capitalism. One way of obliterating handicap is through socialising women into accepting fetal surveillance. On entering the hospital and the maternity system, it is, for the majority of women, an unspoken contract to obey procedural norms, and for Parsons, women should have no say (Sethuraman 2006).

The hospital is an institution of social control (Silverman 2003). Medicine can label our dis-eases and make them real. Disability is thus seen as the problem rather than prejudiced attitudes; as Wasserman and Asch (2006: 54) point out, the attitude is similar to 'being African American or female in America'.

The technology originated, not as a result of public demand, but as a response to demand from doctors, scientists and big multinational pharmaceutical and machinery companies (Parsons and Atkinson 1993, Vailly 2006) thus promoting the capitalist ethos. Talcott Parsons might say that the institutionalisation and therefore normalisation of fetal surveillance means that women will find the procedure comforting and thus worthwhile. Women want confirmation of normality (Press and Browner 1997, Kowalcek 2007). But if the sick role is to become the health role then the domination of the doctors will take on less importance whilst there will be an engendering of self-interest and responsibility by the woman (Frank 1991: 209).

PREVENTION

The majority of 'abnormalities', after all, result from the environment not from the gene pool (Brent 2004). Genetic disorders account for 3–5% of handicap and 2% are born with a congenital abnormality (Statham and Green 1993: 126). Consider also the possibility that technology is increasing genetic 'abnormalities'. Reproductive technology outcomes, for instance, show higher rates of babies born with a congenital 'abnormality' as opposed to those conceived naturally (Bowdin, *et al.* 2007, Rugg-Gunn, *et al.* 2007). More babies are now born with serious medical conditions because their mothers were assisted in maintaining their pregnancies (Williams 2006, Office of National Statistics

2008). Perhaps, in an effort to prevent 'abnormality', attention needs to be directed towards the prevention of war, poverty, environmental hazards/pollutants, accidents and disease (Wertz 1997, Brent 2004). The capitalist economy exists whereby big multi-national companies may consider profit before health and thus handicap will result from food pollution, chemical contamination, nuclear power, the effects of acid rain on fish and so on. Policies to change employment, state benefit, housing and taxation are some areas that need to be addressed to prevent 'abnormality' in order to gain the long-term benefit in the production of healthy children.

The prevention of poverty and deprivation would be costly and have less effect on the development of careers and personal interests. Fetal surveillance is given prefer-ence because it is cheaper than social welfare. Nutrition, for instance, affects our cell production; social pressure can affect our immune response. Social policy to better our nutritional status, housing and economic support can be ignored if the origins of 'abnor-mality' are cast back on the individual as is happening in this victim-blaming society.

The victim-blaming perspective could be used to provide an elitist model, which would make use of a person's genetic profile to determine her/his 'worthiness' for dif-ferent jobs, insurance risks, reproductive mates and material wealth. Clearly, this is a huge political issue, which, if tackled, would need to change the ethos in society from the 'I'm all right Jack' culture to develop the sense of community, which has been lost in many major cities of the world. Wasserman and Asch (2006) see that social, legal and institutional change is the answer to potentially changing individual attitudes to 'abnormality' and in fact that change would re-define the social meaning of the word and eradicate the present day perception of 'normality'.

CONCLUSION

Surveillance has become normalised through the ritual of maternity care. Merquior (1985: 94) notes that where rituals contain within them observation and supervision then the 'right to punish [is] deeply entwined'. How many women 'give in' to the ritual for fear of being reprimanded? Will the 'slippery slope' develop the continuum of what is genetically worthy based on the scientific community's opinion? Is it possible that, on the other hand, the nature of society will change from the competitive, materialist world to acceptance of diversity and improvement of the environment, which will enhance the lives of all human beings?

KEY POINTS

- ꙅ Fetal normality is defined within the scientific community.
- ꙅ Eugenics originated within the scientific community.
- ꙅ Technology originates from the needs of capitalism.
- ꙅ Technology can be viewed as sexist, ableist and racist.
- ꙅ Fetal surveillance is a process designed to select desirable individuals.

REFERENCES

Alliance for Human Research Protection. (2002) *Chinese Farmers Not Well-Informed About Genetic Probe.* Available at: www.hartford-hwp.com/archives/55/203.html (accessed 4 Jan 2008).

Annas GJ, Grodin MA, editors. (1992) *The Nazi Doctors and the Nuremberg Code.* New York: Oxford University Press.

Armstrong D, Lilford R, Ogden J, *et al.* (2007) Health-related quality of life and the transformation of symptoms. *Sociol Health Illn.* **29**(4): 570–83.

Atkinson R. (2008) *When disability becomes illegal: we can screen abnormalities out before birth, but should we?* London: BBC; 31 March. Available at: www.bbc.co.uk/ouch/features/when_disability_becomes_illegal_we_can_screen_abnormalities_out_before_birth_but_should_we.shtml (accessed 4 Jan 2009).

Baron J. (2007) *Against Bioethics.* Cambridge, MA: The MIT Press.

Berezin M. (2003) *Emotions and the Economy.* CSES Working Paper Series No 12. Available at: www.economyandsociety.org/publications/wp12_berezin_03.pdf (accessed 4 Jan 2009).

Bowdin S, Allen C, Kirby G, *et al.* (2007) A survey of assisted reproductive technology births and imprinting disorders. *Hum Reprod.* **22**(12): 3237–40.

Boyne R. (2000) Post-Panopticism. *Econ Soc.* **29**(2): 285–307.

Brent RL. (2004) Environmental causes of human congenital malformations: the pediatrician's role in dealing with these complex clinical problems caused by a multiplicity of environmental and genetic factors. *Pediatrics.* **113**(4 Suppl.): 957–68.

Brewis J. (2001) Foucault, politics and organizations: (re)-constructing sexual harassment. *Gend Work Organ.* **8**(1): 37–60.

Bunton R, Petersen A, editors. (2005) *Genetic Governance: health, risk and ethics in the biotech age.* London: Routledge.

Cantwell RJ, Enyeart KA. (2007) *Women & Eugenics.* Available at: http://wiki.dickinson.edu/index.php?title=Group_1:_Women_and_Eugenics (accessed 4 Jan 2009).

Caplan AL, McGee G, Magnus D. (1999) What is immoral about eugenics? *BMJ.* **319**(7220): 1284–5.

Clarkeburn H. (2000) Parental duties and untreatable genetic conditions. *J Med Ethics.* **26**(5): 400–3.

Collins English Dictionary & Thesaurus. 5th ed. (1998) Glasgow: Harper Collins.

Conrad P, Gabe J. (1999) Sociological perspectives on the new genetics: an overview. *Sociol Health Illn.* **21**(5): 505–16.

Cousins M, Hussain A. (1984) *Michel Foucault.* Houndmills: MacMillan Education Ltd.

Danaher G, Schirato T, Webb J. (2000) *Understanding Foucault.* St Leonard's: Allen & Unwin.

Darwin L. (1926) *The Need for Eugenic Reform.* London: John Murray.

Epstein CJ. (2003) Is modern genetics the new eugenics? *Genet Med.* **5**(6): 469–75.

Eribon D. (1992) *Michel Foucault.* Boston: Harvard University Press.

Eugenics Society. (1982) *Sir Francis Galton 1822–1911.* London: The Eugenics Society.

Foucault M. (1972). *Archaeology of Knowledge.* New York: Pantheon.

Foucault M. (1973) *The Birth of the Clinic: an archaeology of medical perception.* London: Tavistock.

Foucault M. (1974) *The Order of Things: an archaeology of the human sciences.* London: Tavistock.

Foucault M. (1977) *Discipline and Punish: the birth of the prison.* London: Allen Lane.

Frank AW. (1991) From sick role to health role: deconstructing Parsons. In: Robertson R, Turner BS, editors. *Talcott Parsons: theorist of modernity.* London: Sage.

Galton.org (2008) *Francis Galton and composite portraiture.* Available at: http://galton.org/composite.htm (accessed 4 Jan 2009).

Gargaro.com (2008) *Abortion Related Medical Complication: sterility.* Available at: www.gargaro.com/healthproblems.html (accessed 4 Jan 2009).

Gillam L. (1999) Prenatal diagnosis and discrimination against the disabled. *J Med Ethics.* **25**: 163–71.

Green J, Statham H. (1993) Testing for fetal abnormality in routine antenatal care. *Midwifery.* **9**(3): 124–35.

House of Commons. (1967) *The Abortion Act*. London: HMSO.

House of Commons. (1990) *The Human Fertilisation and Embryology Act*. London: HMSO.

Howitt Wilson MB. (2000) *Killing Me Softly: should doctors decide whether a life is worth living?* Available at: http://www2.netdoctor.co.uk/editors_voice/index.asp?mode=showentry&entryId=35 (accessed 4 Jan 2009).

Huxley A. (1932) *Brave New World*. Harmondsworth: Penguin.

Jackson E. (2000) Abortion, autonomy and prenatal diagnosis. *Soc Leg Stud.* **9**(4): 467–94.

Johnson M. (2001) *Airing the 'disability perspective' but getting few converts*. Available at: www.ragged-edge-mag.com/0101/0101bkrev1.htm (accessed 4 Jan 2009).

Katz-Rothman B. (1986) *The Tentative Pregnancy*. London: Pandora.

Kaufert PA. (2000) Health policy and the new genetics. *Soc Sci Med.* **51**(6): 821–9.

Kennedy HP, Shannon MT. (2004) Keeping birth normal: research findings on midwifery care during childbirth. *J Obst Gynecol Neonatal Nurs.* **33**(5): 554–60.

King DS. (1999) Preimplantation genetic diagnosis and the 'new' eugenics. *J Med Ethics.* **25**(2): 176–82.

Klein MC, Sakala C, Simkin P, *et al.* (2006) Why do women go along with this stuff? *Birth.* **33**(3): 245–50.

Koch AM. (2005) *Romance and Reason: ontological and social sources of alienation in the writings of Max Weber*. Lanham, MD: Lexington Books.

Koch L. (2004) The meaning of eugenics: reflections on the government of genetic knowledge in the past and present. *Sci Context.* **17**: 315–31.

Koskela H. (2000) 'The gaze without eyes': video surveillance and the changing nature of urban space. *Prog Hum Geogr.* **24**(2): 243–65.

Koskela H. (2003) 'Cam Era': the contemporary urban Panopticon. *Surveill Soc.* **1**(3): 292–313.

Kowalcek I. (2007) Stress and anxiety associated with prenatal diagnosis. *Best Pract Res Clin Obstet Gynecol.* **21**(2): 221–8.

Kuhn RL, Kramer J. (2000) *Technology and Society*. London: Hay House Audio Books (Closer to Truth Series).

Kuhse H, Singer P, editors. (1999) *Bioethics: an anthology*. Oxford: Blackwell.

Kuhse H, Singer P. (1985*) Should the Baby Live? The problem of handicapped infants*. Oxford: Oxford University Press.

Lindahl KM, Malik NM, Kaczynski K, *et al.* (2004) Couple power dynamics, systemic family functioning and child adjustment: a test of a mediational model in a multiethnic sample. *Dev Psychopathol.* **16**(3): 609–30.

McElroy W. (2008) *Feminists Against Women: the new reproductive technologies*. Available at: www.wendymcelroy.com/e107_plugins/content/content.php?content.111 (accessed 4 Jan 2009).

Mendonca M. (2000) Personal mastery in ethical leadership. *Med Law.* **19**(4): 855–62.

Merquior JG. (1985) *Foucault*. London: Fontana Press.

National Health Service (NHS) Direct. (2008) *Abortion Risks*. Available at: www.nhs.uk/Conditions/Abortion/Pages/Risks.aspx?url=Pages/what-is-ait.aspx (accessed 4 Jan 2009).

Nola R. (1998) *Foucault*. London: Frank Cass.

Nuffield Council on Bioethics. (2002) *Genetics and Human Behaviour: the ethical context*. London: Nuffield Council on Bioethics.

O'Donnell JJ, Brown A. White TD, *et al.* (2005) *The Nature of Normal Human Variety*. Available at: www.edge.org/3rd_culture/leroi05/leroi05_index.html (accessed 4 Jan 2009).

Office of National Statistics. (2008) *Congenital Abnormalities*. Available at: www.statistics.gov.uk (accessed 7 Mar 2009).

Orwell G. (1949) *Nineteen Eighty Four*. New York: Penguin.

Parsons E, Atkinson P. (1993) Genetic risk and reproduction. *Sociol Rev.* **41**(4): 679–706.

Parsons T. (1951) *The Social System*. London: Routledge, Kegan & Paul.

Pernick MS. (2002) Taking better baby contests seriously. *Am Pub Health Assoc.* **92**(5): 707–8.

Persson I. (1999) Equality and selection for existence. *J Med Ethics.* **25**: 130–6.

Petersen A, Bunton R. (1997) *Foucault, Health and Medicine.* London: Routledge.

Pinker S. (2003) *The designer baby myth.* Manchester: Guardian; 5 June. Available at: http://education. guardian.co.uk/higher/research/story/0,970359,00.html (accessed 4 Jan 2009).

Press N, Browner CH. (1997) Why women say yes to prenatal diagnosis. *Soc Sci Med.* 45(7): 979–89.

Richards MPM. (1993) The new genetics: some issues for social scientists. *Sociol Health Illn.* 15(5): 567–86.

Royal College of Midwives, National Childbirth Trust, Royal College of Obstetricians. (2007) *Making Normal Birth a Reality.* London: Royal College of Midwives.

Rugg-Gunn PJ, Ferguson-Smith AC, Pedersen RA. (2007) Status of genomic imprinting in human embryonic stem cells as revealed by a large cohort of independently derived and maintained lives. *Hum Mol Genet.* 16(R2): R243–51.

Sethuraman KR. (2006) Professionalism in medicine. *Regional Health Forum.* 10(1): 1–10. Available at: www.searo.who.int/LinkFiles/Regional_Health_Forum_Volume_10_No_1_01-Professionalism_ in_Medicine.pdf (accessed 4 Jan 2009).

Silverman WA. (2003) Vital decisions. *Paediatr Perinat Epidemiol.* 17(1): 1–2.

Singer P, Wells D. (1984) *The Reproductive Revolution.* Oxford: Oxford University Press.

Smart B. (2002) *Michel Foucault.* London: Routledge.

Snyder SL, Mitchell DT. (2006) *Cultural Locations of Disability.* Chicago: University of Chicago Press.

Statham H, Green J. (1993) Serum screening for Down's syndrome: some women's experiences. *BMJ.* 307(6897): 174–6.

Statham H, Solomou W, Chitty L. (2000) Prenatal diagnosis of fetal abnormality: psychological effects on women in low-risk pregnancies. *Baillieres Best Pract Res Clin Obstet Gynaecol.* 14(4): 731–47.

Stern AM. (2002) Making better babies: public health and race betterment in Indiana 1920–1935. *Am J Public Health.* 92(5): 742–52.

Sung Ho Kim. (2007) Max Weber. In: *Stanford Encyclopedia of Philosophy.* Stanford, CA: Stanford University. Available at: www.seop.leeds.ac.uk/entries/weber/ (accessed 4 Jan 2009).

Tooley M. (1983) *Abortion and Infanticide.* Oxford: Oxford University Press.

Vailly J. (2006) Genetic screening as a technique of government: the case of neonatal screening for cystic fibrosis in France. *Soc Sci Med.* 63(12): 3092–101.

Wasserman D, Asch A. (2006) The uncertain rationale for prenatal disability screening. *Virtual Mentor.* 8(1): 53–6.

Watson I. (2008) *The common triggers of synesthesia are social conventions* [online]. Available at: www. ianwatson.org/common_triggers.pdf (accessed 4 Jan 2009).

Wertz DC. (1997) Society and the not-so-new genetics: what are we afraid of? Some future predictions from a social scientist. *J Contemp Health Law Policy.* 13: 299–346.

Whittle MJ. (2000) *Ultrasound Screening.* London: Royal College of Obstetricians and Gynaecologists. Available at: www.rcog.org.uk/index.asp?PageID=1185 (accessed 4 Jan 2009).

Wikler D. (1999) Can we learn from eugenics? *J Med Ethics.* 25: 183–94.

Williams C. (2006) Dilemmas in fetal medicine: premature application of technology or responding to women's choice? *Sociol Health Illn.* 28(1): 1–20.

CHAPTER 18

Breastfeeding: a natural phenomenon or a cultural construct?

Cathryn Britton

There can be no dispute that breastfeeding can enhance the health of babies and their mothers. Yet despite the evidence of its health-enhancing properties, women in the UK often either choose not to breastfeed or curtail the activity after a relatively short time. Traditionally, health professionals have considered health promotion to be an important aspect of encouraging more women to breastfeed. There is an assumption that imparting knowledge may change attitudes and beliefs. However, it is naïve to assume that if women are simply given more information about breastfeeding, the rates of breastfeeding will increase. The majority of women in the UK are not ignorant of the health benefits of breastfeeding. However, a variety of influences affect their infant feeding decisions. The main focus of this chapter will be on the social and cultural influences that exist within the UK that might help or hinder breastfeeding.

INTRODUCTION

It is generally accepted that most women, after giving birth, are physiologically able to lactate. The biology of lactation has been well described elsewhere (e.g. Rankin 2005, Riordan 2005). Women, like all female mammals, have breasts in order to suckle their young. There is an implied natural law and naturalness with regard to breastfeeding. Lactation occurs without question – women expect their breasts to produce milk. In many societies in the world breastfeeding is performed not only by the infant's mother, but is shared by other members of the kin group (Hrdy 2000). This type of 'wet-nursing' has an important function in strengthening kin ties. It might be considered that breast milk will transmit important qualities to the infant (Parkes 2004). In societies where breastfeeding of the infant is not confined to the infant's mother, milk kinship might be formed with the other women who feed the infant (Ensel 2002, Parkes 2004, Parkes

2005). The breastfeeding woman might not be biologically related to the infant, but through a milk tie, a powerful bond is created between the child, woman and wider kin group (Lambert 2001, MacClancy 2003).

Around the world women breastfeed without question. There is a natural assumption that the breast will be offered to the newborn infant and that breast milk will nourish the infant until weaning. In many societies there is little discourse on the health benefits of breastfeeding, because the latter is fundamental to child survival. There is one exception to this, namely the ingestion of colostrum. Ergenekon-Ozetci, *et al.* (2006) and McLachlan and Forster (2006) provide examples of negative health beliefs associated with colostrum and their effect on the initiation of breastfeeding. Commonly quoted views are that colostrum is 'dirty', 'bad for the baby' and 'old and stale'. It is difficult to explain why these beliefs about colostrum exist.

However, in the UK, the dominant discourse of breastfeeding focuses on promoting the activity by emphasising its health benefits.

HEALTH BENEFITS

There are many health benefits to be gained by a mother breastfeeding her baby. Many research studies have demonstrated a positive correlation between breastfeeding and subsequent health in childhood. These include studies showing a reduction in gastrointestinal infections (Kramer, *et al.* 2003), respiratory infections (Quigley, *et al.* 2007, Bachrach, *et al.* 2003), ear infections (Ip, *et al.* 2007), allergic diseases (Rothenbacher, *et al.* 2005) and insulin-dependent diabetes mellitus (Sadauskaite-Kuehne, *et al.* 2004). There is also evidence that infant–parent co-sleeping and breastfeeding may reduce the risk of sudden infant death syndrome (McVea, *et al.* 2000, Ip, *et al.* 2007). Other studies have demonstrated that breastfed children achieve higher scores in standardised tests of mental development than do children who have been fed artificial formula milk (Kramer, *et al.* 2008, Caspi, *et al.* 2007).

Although breastfeeding is usually promoted as an infant health issue, there is little doubt that there are health benefits for women too (Labbok 2001). For women who have a history of breastfeeding, scientific studies have demonstrated a lower incidence of premenopausal breast cancer (Ip, *et al.* 2007), ovarian cancer (Ip, *et al.* 2007), and an improvement in bone density, which could reduce the incidence of hip fractures in later life (Paton, *et al.* 2003).

Despite the evidence that breastfeeding is a health–enhancing activity, the breastfeeding rates in the UK are disappointing. In the recent *Infant Feeding Survey 2005* the incidence of breastfeeding at birth increased (Bolling, *et al.* 2007). However the prevalence of breastfeeding at one week after birth was 63%, which fell to 48% by six weeks and 25% by the time the baby was four months old (Bolling, *et al.* 2007).

So the question that needs to be asked is this. If breastfeeding is so good for the infant and the mother, why do more women not do it?

If it is accepted that most women are able to lactate and understand the health benefits of breastfeeding, it is essential to look at those forces that affect the everyday life of breastfeeding women in the UK and consider what makes them decide to breastfeed initially and what makes them give up or continue breastfeeding. However, before considering the contemporary life of women in the UK, it is useful to discuss the historical context of infant feeding, which has affected modern practices.

HISTORICAL INFLUENCES

It is useful to consider breastfeeding within a historical context in order to understand the prevailing attitudes towards infant feeding. Giving an infant nourishment other than their mother's milk is not a new phenomenon. Throughout world history there are accounts of infants being given breast milk from other women (wet-nursing) or milk from animals (Fildes 1986, 1988). Between 1500 and 1900 the use of wet-nurses in England was commonplace, especially. among the wealthy. Although it later became uncommon in England, some industrialised nations (e.g. Austria, Italy and the USA) were using wet-nursing as an alternative to maternal breastfeeding until at least the 1940s (Fildes 1988). Historical records suggest that infants were commonly given food-stuffs such as bread and broth as a complement to or substitute for breast milk (Fildes 1986, Apple 1987). Artificially formulated milk from animals became widely available in Europe, Australia and the Americas during the late 1800s, when the scientific community became interested in the subject of infant nutrition (Apple 1987, Latteier 1998). During the Second World War, national dried milk was introduced to encourage women into the workplace, and following the war the infant formula industry became very competitive, with intense marketing strategies equating bottle-feeding with affluence and consumerism. The marketing of artificial formula milk has received considerable attention as a major cause of the global decline in breastfeeding (World Health Organization [WHO]/UNICEF 2007, Palmer 2009). Human lactation as an unreliable body function became a cultural truth that has persisted to the present day (Wolf 2000).

The 'bottle-feeding culture' became a part of the medicalisation of infant feeding, where scientists and doctors became 'the experts'; various practices were introduced to control and regulate infant feeding, whereby predictability and measuring the baby's intake became important (Murphy 2003). As women were encouraged to approach the management of breastfeeding from a scientific paradigm, this caused a lack of confidence in their ability to nourish their babies, and this lack of confidence in breastfeeding persists in the UK today (Scott and Mostyn 2003, Dykes 2006). Despite the known health benefits of breastfeeding, prejudicial attitudes against breastfeeding in the UK still remain. Many of the people with whom a woman comes into contact during her reproductive life have been exposed to the 'norm' of bottle-feeding, and it is clear that the social milieu is a major influence on women's willingness to breastfeed.

THE SOCIAL EXPERIENCE OF BREASTFEEDING

The breastfeeding experience is not an isolated event but one that exists in a social context. Not only does a woman have to choose whether she will initially breastfeed her infant, but she may also need to consider the length of time for which she will breastfeed, how she will incorporate breastfeeding into her everyday life, where she will breastfeed, in whose company she feels comfortable breastfeeding, whether she will breastfeed during the weaning process and whose advice and opinions will guide her (e.g. family, friends and/or health professionals). These decisions are likely to be shaped by political, economic, social and cultural influences.

The WHO recommends that whenever possible infants should be fed exclusively on breast milk until six months of age (World Health Organization 2003). In the UK the public health message is that 'breast is best' and Government guidelines support the WHO recommendation (Scientific Advisory Committee on Nutrition 2008). Economic pressures to work during the breastfeeding period, might raise issues about access to a breastfeeding child in the workplace and the acceptability of breastfeeding or expressing the breasts during work time (Gatrell 2007). Social and cultural factors will determine the norms of behaviour with regard to breastfeeding – that is, what is tolerated, what is not, and how behaviour might be regulated.

In many societies in the world, breastfeeding is commonly continued into toddlerhood (Dettwyler 1995a). This does not mean that these women are exclusively breastfeeding two- or three-year-old children, but they continue to provide breast contact in some form along with other foodstuffs. This practice is not confined to 'other' societies – it also occurs in the UK (Britton 2000). It is difficult to determine the extent of long-term breastfeeding in the UK because national infant feeding statistics are not collected after the infant reaches nine months of age. Breastfeeding a toddler is not generally a publicly visible activity, as most women choose to confine the activity to the home (Britton 2000). In babyhood, breastfeeding is promoted as being the best form of nutrition for an infant, but as the child grows older, breastfeeding might become problematic in social situations. The mother might find herself having to defend her breastfeeding activity if others comment on the appropriateness of breastfeeding an older child. A range of opinions might be vocalised about when is too old to breastfeed a child. For some people there is a notion of what can be expected of a child at certain ages; a child who is still breastfeeding once they are wearing shoes, can articulate what they want, or have 'a mouthful of teeth', might be deemed too old to breastfeed (Britton 2000).

The public health message produced by the UK Government and reinforced by health professionals is that breastfeeding is right and proper until six months of age, after which the child should be encouraged to take supplementary foodstuffs and be 'weaned' (Department of Health 2008). The most recent Infant Feeding Survey (Bolling, *et al.* 2007) confirms that by six months of age very few infants receive any breast milk. Yet this is at odds with the WHO recommendation, which suggests that infants should be breastfed and given appropriate and nutritionally adequate complementary foodstuffs until the age of two years or beyond (World Health Organization 2003). Although the WHO has publicly supported the continuation of breastfeeding for at least the first two years of an infant's life, this has been ignored in the public health discourse on breastfeeding.

THE CONCEPT OF 'SUCCESS' IN BREASTFEEDING

Although the policy discourse encourages the notion that 'successful breastfeeding' equates to following the guidelines, it is important to gauge what constitutes success from the woman's perspective. The term *successful breastfeeding* is a value-laden term, as one person's view about successful breastfeeding may not be shared by another. For example, if a woman breastfed an infant for over a year, her concept of success might be to suckle subsequent children for at least one year. However, another woman might feel successful if she has breastfed her infant for a few weeks prior to returning to work. Health professionals also have their own ideas about optimal breastfeeding and might assume that a woman who starts to breastfeed is committed to do so for as long as possible. Therefore care needs to be taken to ensure that assumptions are not made.

WHY (NOT) BREASTFEED?

The reasons why some women either do not breastfeed or else breastfeed for only a limited period of time are multiple and complex. Breastfeeding is socially constructed and exists within a woman's social world. It is not an isolated event that can be readily assigned to scientific reasoning alone. Other issues that affect women's lives and have received little attention in the medical approach to breastfeeding are societal and cultural influences that will influence a woman's choice with regard to initiating and sustaining breastfeeding. A woman may experience conflicting roles as mother, wife and wage earner. Her infant feeding decisions might be influenced by her partner's views (Okon 2004) and women who feel unsupported by their partners with regard to their breastfeeding decision are less likely to be successful in breastfeeding (Swanson and Power 2005, Kong and Lee 2004). In the UK, many women return to work after the birth of their baby. For some, the return to the workplace makes breastfeeding problematic, as promotion of breastfeeding in the workplace is not seen as a priority for employers. The absence of breastfeeding facilities during the working day, limited or no access to the infant, and difficulties in expressing and storing breast milk all contribute to the early cessation of breastfeeding for many working women (Gatrell 2007). Many women believe that if they do not continue to express their breasts during the day their milk supply will cease. In the policy discourse, the promotion of breastfeeding is focused on the early weeks of the activity, not on long-term breastfeeding. The promotion of breastfeeding is targeted at the infant's first six months, and little attention is given to promoting the continuation of breastfeeding activities beyond the time when supplementary foods are expected to be introduced.

Research has been conducted to investigate why women choose not to breastfeed at all or else give up early (Earle 2000, Bailey, *et al.* 2004, Bolling, *et al.* 2007). A key focus of the studies has been to investigate the link between socio-demographic variables and the decline in breastfeeding. The outcomes of these studies demonstrate that women who are in the higher social classes, who have remained in full-time education until 18 years of age, and who live in southeast England, are all more likely to breastfeed. Although statistical analyses can be useful for detecting associations between socio-demographic factors and infant feeding choices, they are unable to explain the choices that are made by individual women. Differences in breastfeeding uptake cannot be explained by socio-demographic variables alone. Social and cultural factors may be important, but they have received little attention.

SOCIAL AND CULTURAL INFLUENCES

Women are exposed to a variety of social and cultural factors that influence their chosen feeding method (Kong and Lee 2004, Lavender, *et al.* 2006, McFadden and Toole 2006). The attitudes and opinions of family members, friends, and health professionals are likely to affect the uptake and continuation of breastfeeding (Lavender, *et al.* 2006, McInnes and Chambers 2008). Health professionals have traditionally encouraged women to breastfeed their babies, by giving information about its benefits. However, there may be other social and cultural values that affect the breastfeeding event, such as the dominant societal and media representations of breastfeeding, and feeling able to breastfeed in public.

These issues are influenced and underpinned by the way in which others regulate the body of an individual. Within each society an individual learns the cultural norms with regard to their body in everyday life (e.g. bodily adornment, private and public parts of the body, interpretation of bodily functions). The way in which the body is managed in everyday life and the impact that it has on others must also be considered (Schmied and Lupton 2001). For example, both emotional and physical control of the body will gain meaning from and be interpreted within cultural norms.

Religious beliefs, race and ethnicity may also impact on the reproductive life of some women. There are several instances where control of women's bodies has been driven by religious ideology. For example, the Catholic Church does not support contraception and abortion. The everyday life of women may be controlled by religious teachings such as the seclusion of women from public view (e.g. purdah in many Islamic societies).

In recent years the reproductive body has been a focus of attention in the disciplines of anthropology and sociology. The medicalisation of childbirth has been widely debated (e.g. Davis-Floyd 2001, Devries, *et al.* 2001, van Teijlingen 2005, Henley-Einion 2009), where childbirth has been defined as a 'problem' that needs to be controlled by experts and monitored by technology. Turner (1992) suggests that medicine, law and religion are preoccupied by the regulation of the body. In the UK there has been debate about protecting breastfeeding practices by law. Scotland is the only country in the UK to pass a law allowing women the right to breastfeed in public (Scottish Parliament 2005). In the USA there have been legal cases involving breastfeeding, such as the effect of breastfeeding on custody and visitation rights, the right to breastfeed at work and breastfeeding in public places. Consequently, breastfeeding legislation in many states of the USA has been developed in order to promote and encourage breastfeeding (Vance 2005).

In UK society, individuals learn from an early age that the body needs to be managed and disciplined (Shilling 1993). Drawing on the work of Elias (1982), the body has been subjected to the 'civilising process'. During the course of socialisation most natural functions have been classified as offensive and distasteful. Body fluids fit into this category very well – the sight or smell of body fluids such as urine, faeces or menstrual blood may be seen as 'matter out of place' (Douglas 1984). People expect to be in charge of their bodies, so if the body goes out of control it can be viewed as problematic – not only for others, but by the self as well (Isaksen 2002). Women have been socialised to control their body fluids and render them invisible (Britton 1996, Bramwell 2001). For example, during breastfeeding the leaking milk is contained by the use of breast pads. The control of decency may also be an issue when the breasts become 'public' during breastfeeding. However, concern about the public display of the breast during breastfeeding seems to be in direct contradiction to the media representation of the breasts in the popular press.

SOCIETAL NOTIONS OF THE BREAST AND BREASTFEEDING

Societal notions of the breast and breastfeeding in the UK are embedded in a cultural context that shapes people's opinions about the breast and attitudes towards breastfeeding activities. The visual and print media in any culture depict the 'desirable' female body in terms of the appropriate shape and size of the breast (Wykes and Gunter 2005). Women who are dissatisfied with their breasts seek assistance from surgeons with regard to reconstructive surgery to enable them to achieve the desired shape and size of breast.

The breast may also be perceived as an erotic body part, to be represented both in pornography and in the media as an essential feature for attracting heterosexual men.

Cross-cultural accounts provide evidence of societies, such as the UK and North America, where there is a strong association of the breast with sex (Dettwyler 1995b, Rodriguez-Garcia and Frazier 1995). The sexual nature of the breast in the UK means that breastfeeding is ultimately linked with female sexuality, and this might be an important factor influencing a woman's success in breastfeeding. At the other end of the spectrum there are societies, such as Mali, where the breast is not considered to be sexually arousing during sexual intercourse (Latteier 1998). There are also societies in which the breast is regarded as both sexual and maternal, which enables a breastfeeding culture to exist within a society that sexualises the breast (Latteier 1998).

The media have the ability to influence public opinion. Breastfeeding women are acutely aware of the media's interest in aspects of breastfeeding (Britton 2000). The sexualisation of the breast through media images has become commonplace in UK society, with various newspapers, magazines and television programmes portraying the female breast as sexual. In the UK there is a strong cultural preference for sexualised breasts. When women breastfeed they may be seen as transgressing the boundary between motherhood and sexuality (Young 1998). The media can also influence attitudes to breastfeeding (Henderson, *et al.* 2000). The media's interest in breastfeeding often focuses on problems associated with breastfeeding in the social world. For years there have been regular reports in popular magazines and newspapers encouraging public debate of topics, such as whether women should breastfeed in public or the merits of breastfeeding older children.

BREASTFEEDING IN EVERYDAY LIFE: THE PUBLIC DIMENSION

In everyday life a breastfeeding woman will breastfeed on someone's territory, whether it be a public place or in her own domestic space. In many societies breastfeeding in public is not an issue – the breastfeeding act is incorporated into everyday life without question. In the UK, breastfeeding in public has become a topic of debate. In recent years there has been plethora of newspaper and media articles questioning its appropriateness (*see* Figure 18.1). The very fact that it has become an issue for public debate indicates that it is a problematic activity for society in general. Many women in the UK find it difficult to breastfeed in public places (Britton 2000, Bolling, *et al.* 2007), and their concerns are reinforced when the media highlight their plight.

If women feel concerned about incorporating breastfeeding into their social life, they will give up breastfeeding in public or quickly develop an awareness of appropriate facilities, such as mother-and-baby rooms, which are regarded as areas of 'safe refuge'. Mother-and-baby facilities can offer women a place that is frequented by other women with children, which provides privacy away from the public gaze, and where their mothering capabilities are not on public display. However, the environment within such mother-and-baby rooms is not always ideal. Often the space is cramped, and chairs for breastfeeding may be placed next to nappy bins. If mother-and-baby facilities are not available, then women might find other 'safe' areas in which to breastfeed, such as restaurants and cafes, or they might negotiate an area with shop assistants. However, they may go to some length to create a safe space within these settings by placing themselves away from others in order to avoid the public gaze. When seeking a safe, private area in

---

Costa Coffee apologises to young mum for throwing her out for breastfeeding

Daily Mirror 21 April 2008

Mother told that customers had complained that her breastfeeding made them 'uncomfortable' and she was asked to leave the premises.

A parking ticket . . . for breastfeeding

Daily Express 22 June 2007

A new mum was given a parking ticket – while she was breastfeeding her baby in her car.

Mamaflaging, a decorous way to breastfeed

The Times 31 January 2008

The launch of a garment – Mamaflage – that conceals breastfeeding in public.

FIGURE 18.1 Examples of newspaper articles encouraging debate of breastfeeding in public

which to breastfeed their baby, a public toilet might be the only readily available place, which women loathe, as they equate breastfeeding with nourishment rather that with excretion (Britton 2000). Although 'safe refuges' are welcomed by most women, their presence can reinforce the social concerns about breastfeeding in public by reducing it to a clandestine activity.

In the early weeks of motherhood, women may express anxiety about going away from the home, because they will have to manage and regulate their baby in a social setting among strangers. First-time mothers in particular are conscious of their new role and have differing degrees of confidence in handling and managing a young baby. For some women, the public display of mothering is an anxious time if they believe that others might monitor their skills. The act of breastfeeding might be regarded as a public demonstration of how the woman copes with her baby and attends to its needs appropriately.

BREASTFEEDING IN EVERYDAY LIFE: THE DOMESTIC DIMENSION

The home is usually regarded as a safe, private place in which breastfeeding can take place. However, the presence of others within this space may impose a reordering of the place to breastfeed. Those women who would normally breastfeed in a 'day' area, such as a living-room, may retreat to a more private area, such as a bedroom, rather than breastfeed in the view of others in their domestic space.

In the domestic setting, public and private demarcations of space may change according to whether the woman is breastfeeding in front of friends and family. She may manage breastfeeding on her own, with her partner present, or in front of friends and family in different ways, depending on how comfortable she feels breastfeeding in front of these individuals. The domestic space may usually be regarded as private space in which a breastfeeding woman can choose where to feed her child. However, this may become disrupted when the domestic arena becomes public (e.g. when guests are invited into the home). A demarcation of public and private space might occur, with the woman removing herself to a private space should breastfeeding be necessary. What is interesting here is that for some breastfeeding women their domestic space has different meanings depending on who is present. Factors that influence the woman's choice of feeding venue include her relationship to the guest, the sex of the guest, and her partner's view on breastfeeding in front of 'others'. The woman's personal preferences also have to be considered, as well as those of the individuals who were invited into the home, and consequently a re-evaluation of the use of private and public domestic space may occur.

CONCLUSION

Scientific research can improve our understanding of the biological benefits of breast-feeding and influence the development of strategies to increase the number of women who initiate breastfeeding. However, the social context of breastfeeding must be considered in order to gain an improved understanding of the conflicts and dominant forces that shape breastfeeding for many women.

The reasons why some women do not breastfeed at all, or only breastfeed for a limited time, are multiple and complex. The dominant societal and cultural influences will affect a woman's decision about whether to initiate and sustain breastfeeding. By examining these forces, health professionals can identify how they may better support women who choose to breastfeed and appreciate the constraints to breastfeeding that women might encounter.

In the UK, the medical/scientific approach to breastfeeding in policy discourse is dominant, and little attention is given to the social and cultural values that underlie a woman's reasons for breastfeeding. Nevertheless, there is evidence that without an understanding of cultural attitudes the medical message is often unable to permeate to the wider audience. Despite women's knowledge that breastfeeding can be health enhancing, some women choose not to breastfeed. In order to promote breastfeeding, health professionals have used the dominant discourse of medicine to encourage an increase in the number of women who breastfeed. The strategies that they use are the provision of information about the health benefits and the use of scientific research to underpin advice about appropriate management of breastfeeding concerns. However, this is not enough – it is essential to acknowledge the cultural and social influences that might help or hinder the act of breastfeeding.

KEY POINTS

- ∞ Lactation is universal, but the act of breastfeeding is socially constructed.
- ∞ Breastfeeding does not take place as an isolated event, but is influenced by the social world of the woman.
- ∞ Political, economic, social and cultural influences may shape breastfeeding decisions.

USEFUL ADDRESSES

The Breastfeeding Network
PO Box 11126
Paisley PA2 8YB
Supporter line: 0844 412 4664
www.breastfeedingnetwork.org.uk

La Leche League (GB)
PO Box 29
West Bridgeford
Nottingham NG27NP
Tel: 0845 456 1855
www.laleche.org.uk

National Childbirth Trust
Alexandra House
Oldham Terrace
Acton
London W3 6NH
Tel: 0300 330 0770
www.nct.org.uk/home

Baby Milk Action
34 Trumpington Street
Cambridge CB2 1QY
Tel: 0122 346 4420
www.babymilkaction.org/

UNICEF UK Baby Friendly Initiative
Africa House
64–78 Kingsway
London WC2B 6NB
Tel: 0207 405 5592
www.babyfriendly.org.uk

Fatherhood Institute
9 Nevill Street
Abergavenny NP7 5AA
Tel: 0845 634 1328
www.fatherhoodinstitute.org/

REFERENCES

Apple R. (1987). *Mothers and Medicine: a social history of infant feeding, 1890–1950*. Madison, WI: University of Wisconsin Press.

Bachrach VR, Schwarz E, Bachrach LR. (2003) Breastfeeding and the risk of hospitalisation for respiratory disease in infancy: a meta-analysis. *Arch Pediatr Adolesc Med*. **157**: 237–43.

Bailey C, Pain R, Aarvold J. (2004) A 'give it a go' breastfeeding culture and early cessation among low-income mothers. *Midwifery*. **20**(3): 240–50.

Bolling K, Grant C, Hamlyn B, *et al.* (2007) *Infant Feeding Survey 2005*. The Health and Social Care Information Centre [online]. Available at: www.ic.nhs.uk/pubs/ifs2005 (accessed 5 Jan 2009).

Bramwell R. (2001) Blood and milk: constructions of female bodily fluids in Western society. *Women Health*. **34**(4): 85–96.

Britton C. (1996) Learning about 'the curse': an anthropological perspective on experiences of menstruation. *Women's Stud Int Forum*. **19**: 645–53.

Britton C. (2000) *Women's Experiences of Early and Long-term Breastfeeding in the UK*. [unpublished PhD thesis]. Durham: University of Durham.

Caspi A, Williams B, Kim-Cohen J, *et al.* (2007) Moderation of breastfeeding effects on the IQ by genetic variation in fatty acid metabolism. *Proc Natl Acad Sci U S A*. **104**(47): 18860–5. Available at: www.pnas.org/content/104/47/18860.full (accessed 5 Jan 2009).

Davis-Floyd R. (2001) The technocratic, humanistic, and holistic paradigms of childbirth. *Int J Gynecol Obstet*. **75**: S5–23.

Department of Health. (2008) *Weaning Leaflet* [online]. London: Department of Health. Available at: www.dh.gov.uk/en/Publicationsandstatistics/Publications/PublicationsPolicyAndGuidance/DH_4117080 (accessed 5 Jan 2009).

Dettwyler K. (1995a) A time to wean: the hominid blueprint for the natural age of weaning in modern human populations. In: Stuart-Macadam P, Dettwyler K, editors. *Breastfeeding: biocultural perspectives*. New York: Aldine de Gruyter.

Dettwyler K. (l995b) Beauty and the breast: the cultural context of breastfeeding in the United States. In: Stuart-Macadam P, Dettwyler K, editors. *Breastfeeding: biocultural perspectives*. New York: Aldine de Gruyter.

Devries R, Benoit C, van Teijlingen ER, *et al.*, editors. (2001) *Birth by Design: pregnancy, maternity care and midwifery in North America and Europe*. London: Routledge.

Douglas M. (1984) *Purity and Danger: an analysis of the concepts of pollution and taboo*. London: Ark Paperbacks.

Dykes F. (2006) *Breastfeeding in Hospital: mothers, midwives and the production line*. London: Routledge.

Earle S. (2000) Why some women do not breastfeed: bottle feeding and fathers' role. *Midwifery*. **16**(4): 323–30.

Elias N. (1982) *The Civilising Process*. Oxford: Basil Blackwell.

Ensel R. (2002) Colactation and fictive kinship as rites of incorporation and reversal in Morocco. *J N Afri Stud*. **7**(4): 83–96.

Ergenekon-Ozelci P, Elmaci N, Ertem M, *et al.* (2006) Breastfeeding beliefs and practices among migrant mothers in slums of Diyarbakir, Turkey, 2001. *Eur J Public Health*. **16**(2): 143–8.

Fildes V. (1986) *Breasts, Bottles and Babies: a history of infant feeding*. Edinburgh: Edinburgh University Press.

Fildes V. (1988) *Wet Nursing: a history from antiquity to the present*. Oxford: Basil Blackwell.

Gatrell C. (2007) Secrets and lies: breastfeeding and professional paid work. *Soc Sci Med.* **65**(2): 393–404.

Henderson L, Kitzinger J, Green J. (2000) Representing infant feeding: content analysis of British media portrayals of bottle feeding and breastfeeding. *BMJ.* **321**: 1196–8.

Henley-Einion A. (2009) The medicalisation of childbirth. In: Squire C, editor. *The Social Context of Birth.* 2nd ed. Oxford: Radcliffe Publishing.

Hrdy SB. (2000) *Mother Nature.* London: Vintage.

Ip S, Chung M, Raman G, *et al.* (2007) *Breastfeeding and Maternal and Infant Health Outcomes in Developed Countries* [structured abstract]. Rockville, MD: Agency for Healthcare Research and Quality. Available at: www.ahrq.gov/clinic/tp/brfouttp.htm (accessed 5 Jan 2009).

Isaksen LW. (2002) Toward a sociology of (gendered) disgust: images of bodily decay and the social organisation of care work. *J Fam Issues.* **23**(7): 791–811.

Kong S, Lee D. (2004) Factors influencing decision to breastfeed. *J Adv Nurs.* **46**(4): 369–79.

Kramer MS, Aboud F, Mironova E, *et al.* (2008) Breastfeeding and child cognitive development: new evidence from a large randomised trial. *Arch Gen Psychiatry.* **65**(5): 578–84. Available at: http:// archpsyc.ama-assn.org/cgi/content/short/65/5/578 (accessed 5 Jan 2009).

Kramer MS, Guo T, Platt RW, *et al.* (2003) Infant growth and health outcomes associated with 3 compared with 6 months of exclusive breastfeeding. *Am J Clin Nutr.* **78**(2): 291–5.

Labbok MH. (2001) Effects of breastfeeding on the mother. *Pediatr Clin North Am.* **48**(1): 143–58.

Lambert H. (2001) Village bodies? Reflections on locality, constitution and affect in Rajasthani kinship. In: Böck M, Rao A, editors. *Culture, Creation and Procreation: concept of kinship in South Asian practice.* Oxford: Berghahn Books.

Latteier C. (1998) *Breasts: the women's perspective on an American obsession.* New York: Harrington Park Press.

Lavender T, McFadden C, Baker L. (2006) Breastfeeding and family life. *Matern Child Nutr.* **2**(3): 145–55.

MacClancy J. (2003) The milk tie. *Anthropology of Food.* Available at: http://aof.revues.org/ document339.html (accessed 5 Jan 2009).

McFadden A, Toole G. (2006) Exploring women's views of breastfeeding: a focus group study within an area with high levels of socio–economic deprivation. *Matern Child Nutr.* **2**(3): 156–68.

McInnes R, Chambers J. (2008) Supporting breastfeeding mothers: qualitative synthesis. *J Adv Nurs.* **62**(4): 407–27.

McLachlan HL, Forster DA. (2006) Initial breastfeeding attitudes and practices of women born in Turkey, Vietnam and Australia after giving birth in Australia. *Int Breastfeed J.* **1**: 1–7. Available at: www.internationalbreastfeedingjournal.com/content/1/1/7 (accessed 7 Jan 2009).

McVea KL, Turner PD, Peppler DK. (2000) The role of breastfeeding in sudden infant death syndrome. *J Hum Lact.* **16**: 13–20.

Murphy E. (2003) Expertise and forms of knowledge in the government of families. *Sociol Rev.* **51**(4): 433–62.

Okon M. (2004) Health promotion: partners' perceptions of breastfeeding. *Br J Midwif.* **12**(6): 387–93.

Palmer G. (2009) *The Politics of Breastfeeding: when breasts are bad for business.* London: Pinter and Martin.

Parkes P. (2004) Milk kinship in southeast Europe: alternative social structures and foster relations in the Caucasus and the Balkans. *Soc Anthropol.* **12**: 341–58.

Parkes P. (2005) Milk kinship in Islam: substance, structure, history. *Soc Anthropol.* **13**: 307–29.

Paton LM, Alexander JL, Nowson CA, *et al.* (2003) Pregnancy and lactation have no long-term deleterious effect on measures of bone mineral in healthy women: a twin study. *Am J Clin Nutrition.* **77**(3): 707–14. Available at: www.ajcn.org/cgi/content/full/77/3/707 (accessed 5 Jan 2009).

Quigley MA, Kelly YJ, Sacker A. (2007) Breastfeeding and hospitalisation for diarrheal and respiratory infection in the United Kingdom millennium cohort study. *Pediatrics.* **119**(4): e837–42. Available at: www.pediatrics.org/cgi/content/full/119/4/e837 (accessed 5 Jan 2009).

Rankin J. (2005) The breasts and lactation. In: Stables D, Rankin J, editors. *Physiology in Childbearing.* 2nd ed. Edinburgh: Elsevier.

Riordan J. (2005) *Breastfeeding and Human Lactation.* 3rd ed. Sudbury, MA: Jones and Bartlett.

Rodriguez-Garcia R, Frazier L. (1995) Cultural paradoxes relating to sexuality and breastfeeding. *J Hum Lactation.* **11**: 111–5.

Rothenbacher D, Weyermann M, Beermann C, *et al.* (2005) Breastfeeding, soluble CD14 concentration in breast milk and risk of atopic dermatitis and asthma in early childhood: birth cohort study. *Clin Exp Allergy.* **35**(8): 1014–21.

Sadauskaite-Kuehne V, Ludvigsson J, Padaiga Z, *et al.* (2004). Longer breastfeeding is an independent protective factor against development of type 1 diabetes mellitus in childhood. *Diabetes Metab Res Rev.* **20**(2): 150–7.

Schmied V, Lupton D. (2001) Blurring the boundaries: breastfeeding and maternal subjectivity. *Sociol Health Illn.* **23**(2): 234–50.

Scientific Advisory Committee on Nutrition (SACN) (2008) *Infant Feeding Survey 2005: a commentary on infant feeding practices in the UK. A position statement.* London: The Stationery Office.

Scott JA, Mostyn T. (2003) Women's experiences of breastfeeding in a bottle-feeding culture. *J Hum Lactation.* **19**(3): 270–7.

Scottish Parliament. (2005) *Breastfeeding etc.* (Scotland) Act 2005. Available at: www.opsi.gov.uk/legislation/scotland/acts2005/asp_20050001_en_1 (accessed 5 Jan 2008).

Shilling C. (1993) *The Body and Social Theory.* London: Sage.

Swanson V, Power KG. (2005) Initiation and continuation of breastfeeding: theory of planned behaviour. *J Adv Nurs.* **50**(3): 272–82.

Turner B. (1992) *Regulating Bodies: essays in medical sociology.* London: Routledge.

van Teijlingen E. (2005) A critical analysis of the medical model as used in the study of pregnancy and childbirth. *Sociol Res Online.* **10**(2). Available at: www.socresonline.org.uk/10/2/teijlingen.html (accessed 10 Jul 2008).

Vance M. (2005) Breastfeeding legislation in the United States: a general overview and implications for helping mothers. *Leaven.* **41**(3): 51–4. Available at: www.llli.org/llleaderweb/LV/LVJunJul05p51.html (accessed 5 Jan 2009).

Wolf J. (2000) The social and medical construction of lactation pathology. *Women Health.* **30**: 93–110.

World Health Organization. (2003) *Global Strategy for Infant and Young Child Feeding.* Geneva: World Health Organization.

World Health Organization/UNICEF. (2007) *WHO and UNICEF call for renewed commitment to breastfeeding.* Press Release. Geneva: World Health Organization/UNICEF; 20 June. Available at: www.who.int/nutrition/topics/Breastfeeding_pressrelease.pdf (accessed 5 Jan 2009).

Wykes M, Gunter B. (2005) *The Media and Body Image.* London: Sage.

Young I. (1998) Breasted experience: the look and the feeling. In: Weitz R, editor. *The Politics of Women's Bodies: sexuality, appearance and behaviour.* New York: Oxford University Press.

CHAPTER 19

Experiencing disability

Harriet Clarke

Disabled people can experience significant barriers to accessing community services and universal and specialist services including health and social care. Attitudes to disabled people as parents can be discouraging to those anticipating parenthood and can mean that social and impairment-related support needs are either not acknowledged or appropriately provided. Midwives working with disabled women and with women who have disabled partners need to have an understanding of the social context of disabled people's lives; for parents, maternity services can be a key part of this social context. This chapter focuses on disability awareness and effective communication as fundamental in the delivery of care and support, in the context of legislative and organisational developments, which together seek to ensure equal access to services for all parents.

INTRODUCTION

In order to deliver supportive, high quality maternity services designed around women's and their babies' needs (Department for Education and Skills/Department of Health 2004), disabled women's experiences need to be made visible and included within mainstream planning and delivery of care. This chapter examines the issues relevant to disabled women in anticipating and becoming mothers, and the key messages for midwives and other professionals involved in their care. Issues of relevance to supporting families in which there is a disabled father are also included here. The material provided in this chapter should be considered alongside the wider material presented in this text, as disabled mothers are as diverse as non-disabled women in their social and personal circumstances.

UNDERSTANDING DISABILITY AND IMPAIRMENT

The language used to talk about the personal experiences of disability and impairment can differ within and between professional groups and academic disciplines. It is important that all professionals working with disabled people have knowledge of these differences, and the perspectives on disability that they represent. Understanding different perspectives and the contribution of disabled people to professional under-standings will support communication between health and social care workers, and between staff and disabled people. An overview is provided here before moving on to define the way in which 'disabled parents' as a term is used to refer to many parents and parents-to-be within this chapter.

Until recently the dominant way of understanding disability has focused on the individual experience of impairment. This has been the traditional medical approach to disabled people; the 'disability' is regarded as occurring within the individual, usu-ally as a result of an accident or illness. Indeed the term 'disability' has often been used to refer to an *impairment* (e.g. 'her disability is epilepsy', 'his disability is multiple sclerosis') and so terms such as '*people with disabilities*' has meant people who have an impairment. Disability can also be used within medical fields to refer to 'loss of func-tion', the restricted ability to carry out physical or personal and emotional tasks that have often been presented as inextricably the result of impairment. Such approaches are frequently termed *individual model* or *medical model* approaches, and arguably reflect the ways in which health professionals often focus on the bodily and functional experience of disabled people, usually within clinical rather than social settings.

A contrasting approach has been developed in the UK by disabled people, argu-ing that disability is located in social organisation and interpersonal interactions. The research field of Disability Studies in the UK has built on and debated the nuances of this approach, however it is very useful to begin with a clear definition, which has underpinned the *Social Model of Disability*.

> *Impairment* is the functional limitation within the individual caused by physical, mental or sensory impairment. *Disability* is the loss or limitation of opportunities to take part in the normal life of the community on an equal level with others due to physical and social barriers. (Barnes 1991: 2)

In other words, the *social context of disabled people's lives* is the source of many of the barriers to the fulfilment of desired roles and independent living, barriers that had previ-ously been regarded by professionals as the result of impairment. Physical barriers could include steps into health centres, shops and schools, lack of accessible transport, lack of accessible working environments, and so on. Social barriers can refer to social and economic features that can discriminate against some disabled people (such as restricted educational opportunities, disabling practice in the workplace). Crucially, social barriers can also occur at the *interpersonal level*, where discriminatory attitudes restrict a disabled person's power, choice and control within an interaction, role or relationship.

The Royal College of Nursing (RCN) stresses the importance of midwives and nurses having an understanding of the social model of disability:

> . . . understanding how society, rather than the individual, is the cause of disability will help avoid asking inappropriate questions rather than applying the medical model (which results in disabled people being asked about their impairment rather than the barriers they face in accessing services such as stairs, equipment, intercoms and voice-only telephones, poorly lit rooms, staff behind screens, or barriers in accessing information because of inappropriate formats). (RCN 2007: 7)

This is not to suggest that understanding disabled women's needs, fears, concerns or difficulties in relation to impairment is unimportant: however, professionals can distinguish between support requirements emanating from impairment-related issues, and those that should be understood in terms of ensuring equal access to mothering and parenting activities and challenging disability (barriers) where they occur. In order to understand the importance of this, the personal experience of barriers that mothers and mothers-to-be encounter need to be heard, acknowledged and responded to, most effectively through working in partnership with disabled women themselves. As Thomas (1997) highlights, this approach helps us to identify where change needs to happen.

Within this chapter we are focusing on the experience of disabled women as mothers and mothers-to-be. Each individual person carries with them their own understanding of impairment and experience of disability, and may use 'medical model' or 'social model' language to express this, or indeed draw on their own and others' 'everyday' language to express the meaning and nature of their experience. The language used in this chapter is based on the distinction between impairment and disability mentioned above. Further, disability is presented here as barriers experienced by disabled people in the context of their relationships: an important consequence of this is being aware that the family members of a disabled person may also experience 'disability' as a result of the barriers their child, partner, or parent experiences; relationships – both personal and professional – can also be a source of disability, particularly where women experience control of the mothering role being 'hijacked' by others. More positively, relationships with family members and with professionals are also a powerful conduit through which people can challenge disability.

DEFINING DISABLED PARENTS

Up until the 1990s disabled parents were largely invisible in accounts of human experience, research and practice. Such studies of disabled parents that were conducted, were often quite clinical or individual in focus, with interests in specific impairment 'groups' of disabled people. Such impairment-based definitions of disabled parents (with multiple sclerosis, learning difficulties, and so on) often looked for deficits in parenting and/or difficulties experienced by children, and neglected the social context in which disabled parents and their families were seeking to live their lives (*see* Olsen and Clarke 2003 for a review).

In this chapter, disabled parents are not identified in relation to a specific group of impairment experiences. Disabled parents are parents with additional support needs; they may face disabling barriers (attitudinal, material, structural) in areas of their lives, including parenting, and have difficulty obtaining support that prioritises parental choice and control in family life.

Throughout this chapter 'disabled parents' will be used to refer to parents experiencing social barriers, as the result of having one or more of a diverse range of impairments:
- parents with physical impairments
- parents with sensory impairments
- parents with learning difficulties
- parents with mental health support needs

- parents who identify as Deaf (i.e. part of the Deaf Community, linguistically and culturally)
- parents with long-term health conditions (including HIV and AIDS)
- parents living with substance misuse problems (alcohol, other drugs).

This definition reflects the inclusive approach of *Disabled Parents Network* and of Morris and Wates (2006, 2007) in their work for the Social Care Institute of Excellence, which looked at the ways in which social care services deliver care (and can improve that delivery) to disabled parents and their families.

Disabled parents are diverse not only in relation to the impairment experience, but also in relation to socio-economic position, ethnicity, gender, sexuality, and their own life histories. Women using maternity services may or may not self-identify as a 'disabled person', and may or may not see impairment and disability as central influences in their lives. What is important is that professionals can communicate effectively to support women to identify their own personal, emotional, social and physical support requirements and are able to understand their own role alongside those of others in responding to women in the provision of care and parenting support.

DISABILITY AND PARENTING IN SOCIAL CONTEXT
Disabling ideologies: then and now

For much of the twentieth century disabled people were positioned as dependants (rather than caregivers), and this led to practices such as institutionalisation rather than provision of support to enable them to live their lives in community (or family) settings. The most extreme disablist ideologies led to eugenic practices, particularly in parts of Europe and in many states in the USA, which removed the reproductive rights of many disabled people. In the UK eugenic programmes were not formalised, but some disabled people found that their sexuality, relationships and reproduction were controlled, for example through institutionalisation. It has been argued that there remains a 'long shadow' of eugenics that still has relevance for disabled people, particularly disabled women in relation to their reproductive rights (Sayce and Perkins 2004):

> It is worth asking why, in the aftermath of the horrors of World War II, a complete break was not made with the ideology of eugenics. Change did occur . . . The forced sterilisation law was repealed in . . . some . . . American States in the 1980s, Sweden's in 1976. However, just as people were to some extent freed from the view that their genes meant they should not breed, they were confronted by the view that they could not make good enough parents . . . In the UK, [mental health service users] are frequently actively encouraged to have abortions. If they do bear a child they often lose parental rights at, or even before, birth. (Sayce and Perkins 2004: 10).

We are currently living in a period of significant change in relation to disability rights and in challenging and seeking to end discrimination. Disabled women, including women who are mental health service users and women with learning difficulties, can (but do not always) receive appropriate support that recognises their positive mothering role. Sayce and Perkins (2004) remind us to question the extent of change, particularly where disabling attitudes inform professional interactions with parents. Olsen and Clarke (2003), speaking to disabled parents in the late 1990s, found that social care and other professionals sometimes expressed very negative attitudes to disabled women as mothers and to their aspirations for motherhood. For example, one mother related that she was told by a social worker that '. . . disabled people shouldn't have children if they cannot look after them'; similarly, a mother experiencing mental health difficulties said 'I've had social workers tell me not to have them (children)'. It has been argued that parents with mental health difficulties often receive a specific message that they:

> . . . have a moral responsibility not to have children in the interests of preventing further unnecessary suffering. (Beresford and Wilson 2002: 547).

All health and social care professionals should be aware of their own and others' attitudes to people using their services, and to disabled mothers and fathers; attitudes may be directly stated, or may be implied through behaviours, communication, or indeed a lack of communication. Those who reported receiving negative attitudes in Olsen and Clarke's study (2003) did become parents: however, the long-term impact for some mothers could be continued lack of trust in professionals. Others felt confident and strong in their own achievement in parenting and family life, whilst still feeling disappointment where the negative attitudes of others had been part of their experience. Wates (2003) highlights how disabled people are exposed to messages of concern and disbelief about parenting, through interpersonal interactions and the media, and stresses that understanding the impact of negative assumptions and countering them is an important way to stop antagonism developing within the professional-parent relationship.

(In)visibility of disabled parents

Until recently disabled parents were relatively invisible in research, policy and practice. Where disabled parents *were* of interest was often where specific 'problems' were identified as being the result of *impairment*, rather than a result of *disability*: that is, where disabled parents have been 'visible', it has been often in terms of identifying problems or 'pathology', rather than examining their experiences, choices and support requirements in relation to parenting. It has been suggested that the invisibility of disabled parents, in part, is the result of a disabling belief that disabled people are 'asexual', or, conversely, should have their sexuality controlled (for example to 'protect' them or their potential children from a presumed distress) (*see* Kallianes and Rubenfeld 1997). Such understandings are clearly linked to the 'othering' of disabled people, which has happened historically, as we noted briefly above.

Families that include disabled parents gained greater recognition in the UK during the 1990s, through the development of research work that explored the caring responsibilities of children and young people living with a disabled relative. Young people providing care, including to disabled parents, became known as 'young carers'. This area of work highlighted that many parents were receiving insufficient support; but the focus was largely on needs of children providing 'care', rather than on how to support parents to ensure they are not placed in a position of having to accept inappropriate support from their children. As the focus of 'young carers' research was children, it couldn't tell us in depth about parents-to-be or parents' perspectives and strategies around becoming and being a parent.

Moving beyond the shadow

There is increasing research knowledge around disabled people's experiences of services, including disabled mothers' experiences of healthcare and aspirations about becoming a parent. Positive experiences of disabled people as parents provide important messages to disabled and non-disabled people alike, challenging ideas that problematise disabled parents and their families. Increased visibility itself is an important consideration in health services and health information; it can help to ensure that support for disabled women in maternity services is not seen as 'special' but is provided as a result of good communication and organisation, which seeks to respond to the needs of (and ensure equal opportunities for) *all* parents, whatever their experience of illness, impairment and disability. The services women receive and their experiences of health professional work *is itself* an important aspect of the social context for disability and parenting.

ENABLING AND DISABLING PRACTICE

Pregnant disabled women's needs are fundamentally the same as all mothers and mothers-to-be. In order for healthcare needs to be met appropriately, midwives and healthcare professionals need to be aware of the ways in which discriminatory practice can occur, and their impact, and ensure that good practice is delivered to all mothers in their care.

Earlier we identified two main approaches to understanding disability. One approach, the 'medical model', has been primarily focused on impairment; such an approach if used uncritically and without a concern for social context can lead to a professional focus on 'risk' (to the mother; to family members) instead of a focus on supporting the mother's functional control within their pregnancy and birth situation, and a lack of concern for equal opportunities for choice and control in maternity care. The social model approach instead enables a focus on listening to and fully hearing disabled women, supporting choice and control, and removing barriers to equal opportunities in healthcare provision.

Ending disability discrimination and upholding rights has been a key focus of recent legislation. The Human Rights Act (1998) upholds the right to respect for private and family life (article 8) and the right to marry and found a family (article 12). The Disability Discrimination Act (2005, amending the 1995 Act) makes it unlawful for service providers to deliver a lower standard of service to disabled people: public authorities, including health and care providers, need to promote equality in the design and delivery of services.

Attitudinal barriers

Attitudinal barriers to receiving satisfactory (and good) care are arguably often the most significant: without positive attitudes to enabling good experiences for all women, including disabled women, other barriers to service delivery may not be sufficiently challenged; where other barriers are addressed, disabling attitudes will make a trust relationship between healthcare practitioner and mother difficult to build or sustain.

The Royal College of Nursing (2007) highlights the way in which negative terminology has previously been used to label disabled people, and how such negative terminology is discriminatory. This includes describing and objectifying people with reference to their impairment (e.g. 'epileptic', 'schizophrenic') rather than seeing the *person* first. People who have epilepsy, or have a diagnosis of schizophrenia, are much more than such labelling conveys. Such labelling suggests that the person using the label may be objectifying (making objects of) the people they are working with.

Disability awareness, including the important role of midwives and nurses in ensuring equality of access to services for disabled people, is an important issue for practitioners in their training and subsequent professional development (Rotherham and McKay-Moffat 2007). This is not only desirable to improve women's experience, but crucial, given that staff prejudices can impact on outcomes for mothers and children, as has been suggested in an enquiry into maternal deaths (Lewis and Drife 2004). Knowledge, understanding and working in partnership with disabled women are important elements of challenging discriminatory attitudes and practices, and equality training in disability issues has been identified as *one* element in supporting this cultural change process:

> Health providers have a responsibility to address explicitly the existence of discrimination and its implications for care. Disability equality training should be provided for all levels of staff, including non-medical personnel, e.g. domestic staff, and should be facilitated by disabled people themselves. Midwives with limited experience in caring for disabled women should seek advice and guidance from better informed services, professionals and colleagues and from women themselves, who are often the best source of information. (Royal College of Midwives 2000)

The involvement of disabled women, in the development of both personal plans and in policy, and the involvement of women in staff training and development, are clearly areas that require commitment from managers as well as active engagement by workers.

Communication

Communication barriers can impact on women's access to information before, during and after pregnancy, and during birth itself; all information should be available in accessible formats (Wates 2003). This can be a particular issue in relation to antenatal care, for example when parents can find that antenatal classes are not accessible, and this may be a particular concern for parents with sensory impairments (Morris 2003, Wates 2003).

Communication skills are vital for midwives with all women, in order to collate information from and provide information to them appropriately: where communication needs are not identified and addressed clearly, disabled mothers will face a significant barrier to receiving care centred on their needs and choices. Disabled Parents Network (DPN) highlighted this in their evidence to the House of Commons Health Committee in 2002–3:

> Disabled women are not always given the same choices as other parents, for example, decisions about the type of birth or anaesthesia and mode of delivery are taken by professionals without adequate discussion with the woman or her partner. Informed choice is often not an option for disabled women due to assumptions and decisions made by professionals. (House of Commons Health Committee 2003: 20)

McKay-Moffat (2007) highlights that communication that ensures good care happens in many formats between midwife and mother, and between midwife and other key professionals. For example, communication is both two-way (between the communicators) and across two broad channels (verbal/non-verbal or linguistic/non-linguistic). As Morris (2003) states, disabled women can find that communication barriers restrict the possibility of a trusting relationship developing, and this may be particularly so for Deaf parents (i.e. who identify as part of the Deaf community) deaf parents (who have hearing impairments and who may or may not use British Sign Language), and women with learning difficulties. Where a health worker is uncomfortable around meeting the needs of, or negative about, a disabled mother, this may be carried through into inappropriate bodily or verbal communication (e.g. speaking to the mother's partner rather than to the mother herself). Where a midwife is uncertain about a disabled woman's requirements or choices in terms of communication, this will again provide a barrier. When working with a D/deaf or disabled woman, it is important for the woman to identify her preferences (which she may feel are different in different circumstances – e.g. in consultations, and when delivering her child). McKay-Moffat (2007) also stresses the importance of pictures and models, and clearly expressed information resources, as well as translator services where appropriate. The complexity of all day-to-day communication, and even more so in relation to the journey of pregnancy, birth and early childcare, point to the importance of midwives gaining as much information as possible ahead of the first antenatal appointment (RCN 2007), so that women do not experience immediate barriers to forming a relationship with their healthcare providers at the first hurdle.

LIVED EXPERIENCE
Disabled women's experiences of pregnancy and early childcare

All women may have concerns and questions about how their pregnancy and birth experiences might impact on their well-being, whether short- or long-term. In relation to impairment related concerns, these will need to be considered by the woman within her own support and information networks, and with health practitioners. Disabled women should be supported by midwives in accessing information in appropriate formats relevant to their circumstances (e.g. for women with sensory impairments or learning difficulties).

Disabled parents may have been born with their impairments, acquired an impairment prior to becoming a parent, or after starting a family. Not all congenital or later-onset impairments are hereditary, but women with hereditary impairments may have specific feelings or questions about this issue. During early pregnancy women face a series of decisions around testing. This experience may be difficult for many women, but for disabled women – particularly those living with a congenital impairment – the issue may have particular resonance. As Crow (2003) recounts from her experience:

> Back in the early stages of pregnancy, the subject of screening was raised at every antenatal appointment, although it was stated clearly on my notes that I did not want any testing. As a disabled woman, I have thought harder than most about impairment and its realities. Screening is a judgement on me and my friends and all the people who never made it and every time testing was raised I felt a visceral reaction . . . When tests are carried out and people are supported in deciding on a course of action, or

> inaction, nothing in that process is neutral – the very language is steeped in bias: 'abnormalities', 'anomalies', 'defects' – every aspect is culturally constructed. (Crow 2003: 5–6)

This personal account reveals the extent to which medical intervention in pregnancy, including testing, has a political and social context; different women will have different responses and concerns about testing for impairment, but it is crucial that practitioners are informed about disability and impairment, and do not denigrate disabled people explicitly or implicitly in their practice. The Royal College of Midwives (2000) has stressed the importance of sensitive practice in antenatal screening (and that assumptions are not made about what is a 'desirable' outcome); it also highlights that antenatal and postnatal groups should be accessible and appropriately conducted, particularly where discussions about fetal 'abnormality' are undertaken.

Testing is clearly one subject in which a 'risk discourse' has particular connotations for disabled women. Thomas (1997) found that disabled women she interviewed experienced professionals as well as family members focusing on hereditary risk and risks to their own health (e.g. around use of medications during pregnancy, or on implications of pregnancy for impairment). Many women did not necessarily question these concerns, and would themselves make choices about whether or not to have more children based on risk assessments that they made for themselves, in the context of the wider discourse. Thomas highlights that whilst some disabled women may discuss reproductive risk issues with their practitioners, this does not mean that the conversation is not influenced by disabling ideas (for example, that disability is a 'tragedy' to be avoided, or that disabled women 'should not' have children):

> . . . [I]n 'disability rights' terms, the powerful medical (and wider) discourse on reproductive risk acts as a social barrier in the sense that it plays an important part in 'restricting activity'; in its light, decisions are made not to have a child/another child, or to be sterilised, or to terminate a pregnancy. (Thomas 1997: 633)

Women's experience of support in obtaining early childcare, in hospital settings, and at home, should ensure that their own control and confidence is supported. Thomas (1997) reports that the women she interviewed had a range of positive and negative experiences here. The barriers that people faced were feelings of being left out of decisions and activities about how care would be provided to their baby, with one woman reporting that midwives bathed her baby rather than providing appropriate assistance to enable her to do that herself. This taking away of the mothering role was also reported in relation to breastfeeding, where one woman reported that too much attempted intervention by others meant that she went to bottle feeding, where she felt she had more control and less fuss from others about her ability to feed her child. Information, appropriate aids, and space for women to find their own solutions are key ways in which women can be supported.

Disabled men's involvement in birth and early childcare

In much of the research into disabled parents' experiences, the focus has been (implicitly or explicitly) on mothers. Fathers can have a significant involvement in their partner's experience of the birth, and in early childcare. Both disabled fathers and non-disabled partners of pregnant women should have their own needs and questions considered when involved in their partner's care. With respect to 'woman-centred care' the Department of Health (2003) has highlighted in its vision for maternity services that there can be a central role for the father in achieving positive outcomes for mother and child:

> . . . [T]he priority is to ensure that maternity services are sensitive to each woman's needs . . . Services also need to focus on how best to involve the father in the process of supporting his partner and his child. (Department of Health 2003: 20)

In relation to disabled parents, the RCN (2007) has stressed the importance of involving fathers in all aspects of care to the degree that their partners want them to be; disabled fathers' support requirements should be responded to in the same way as mothers, so that access, information and communication needs are addressed. Where the mother herself has an impairment, it is important that workers do not look to a non-disabled partner to speak on behalf of the mother as this itself would be discriminatory and reduce the feelings of power and control that women should experience within a trusting relationship with their professional carers.

MIDWIFERY AND HEALTH PROFESSIONAL RESPONSIBILITIES

We are currently in a state of learning about disabled women's experiences of maternity and childcare services: however, there is growing evidence about what women find positive or negative in their use of maternity services.

McKay-Moffat and Cunningham (2006) report that in their interviews with five mothers who had physical impairments, there were specific concerns about midwives' lack of knowledge concerning impairment, disability awareness and attitudes, and communication (reflected through women's experiences as reported above). Interviews with eight midwives highlighted similar issues, as well as difficulties in working with multiple professionals and making appropriate referrals to specialists to support the woman during pregnancy, birth and into the early years of the child's life.

KEY ISSUES IN DELIVERING MIDWIFERY CARE TO DISABLED WOMEN

The following guidance is a summary of many of the key practice points from the RCN (2007).

Antenatal care
- Identify disabled clients early (from GP letter or at first visit).
- Identify any communication requirements or preferences at first booking visit.
- Offer home visits or clinic-based appointments – each as a positive choice.
- Agree time and frequency of visits.
- Ensure assessment of needs is from the woman's point of view: acknowledge her expertise.

- Use the social model – challenge barriers, identify strengths.
- Network to ensure appropriate multi-agency support.
- Prepare a plan of care with the parents, encompassing pregnancy, birth and postnatal care, and communicate this across the care team.
- Consider parents' ideas about bringing equipment or aids into hospital where this can be done safely.

Birth care
- Home birth may not pose increased risk for many disabled women and may be a positive choice.
- Partners may need somewhere to sleep in hospital during a hospital admission.
- Relevant equipment, aids and information should be sourced in advance.

Parenting
- Value of positive role models for parents – some disabled parents may want to access parenting support organisations including disabled parents groups.
- Access to mainstream services for parents of young children should be assessed and addressed.
- Support needs beyond disability (e.g. socio-economic factors that may impact on health) should also be considered.
- Midwifery care can continue as long as necessary following birth, and discharge plans should be made when and as appropriate.

The midwife can help disabled women to access social care services to support them in their everyday lives, including in their parenting role. Where professionals have concerns about the welfare of parents, referral (with consent of the parent) to adult social care services may be considered, or if women wish to consider self-referral, they can be provided with information, either at that time or in the future. Access to adult social care is determined by eligibility criteria, and parents with low-level and moderate support requirements can find it difficult to access services (this differs by locality). Local disability support organisations may be able to provide parents with further information and give support in accessing services; midwives and childcare professionals (including health visitors) may also be able to help parents identify local groups, organisations and services that support parents with young children.

Olsen and Tyers (2004) highlight the importance of responding appropriately to identified social support requirements, and understanding the value of support for parents in their own right. This particularly means recognising that parents' own support needs should be met before parents' are made to feel 'judged' in terms of their parenting. If child welfare concerns have arisen, practitioners should consider the parents' requirements and whether they are being supported in their parenting role:

> . . . [W]hen disabled parents come into contact with social services and other agencies, child welfare and/or child protection concerns can come unnecessarily to the fore. It is important that practitioners work to challenge this, (a) by acknowledging that such concerns may be the product of a failure of statutory agencies adequately to support

parents in the past, and (b) by separating abusive or neglectful behaviour on the part of parents from impairments and the need for assistance that may be associated with them. (Olsen and Tyers 2004: 78)

In relation to concerns about parent and child well-being, parents with learning difficulties or with severe enduring mental health difficulties are most at risk of having their needs as a parent viewed primarily through a 'risk' rather than a 'support' lens (RCN 2007). Midwives potentially have a key role in ensuring that parents receive early support, information and advice about adult social care and other areas of possible support (e.g. housing; benefits). Parents may face barriers in accessing the range of services that families find valuable, and midwives can help to minimise them by providing information and instilling confidence that services are focused on supporting them as parents.

CONCLUSION

There is clearly an identified need to keep building practitioner confidence and knowledge, and to ensure that professional networks (within healthcare and across health and social care) are supported through resources and clear lines of referral and responsibility. It is important to ensure that midwives have training and continuing professional development in impairment-specific needs, that they have an understanding of the social context of disabled women's lives and that they understand the fundamental importance of combating disability at structural and interpersonal levels.

KEY POINTS

- ↷ Disabled women's support requirements in relation to maternity are increasingly being recognised.
- ↷ The social model of disability is an important tool to support professional understanding of women's lives in the social context.
- ↷ Attitudinal barriers are often the major hurdle faced by disabled women seeking to be and becoming mothers.
- ↷ The midwife's role is fundamental in supporting access to woman-focused care, and communication is vital to this.
- ↷ Health professionals need to work in partnership with disabled women, and also, where appropriate, with other professionals and agencies to enable access to the range of supports for parents and families.

USEFUL ADDRESSES

Deaf Parenting UK (DPUK)
National Centre for Disabled Parents
DPUK is a registered charity providing information and support for deaf parents and parents-to-be who use British Sign Language, and to professionals.
Unit F9, 89–93 Fonthill Road
London N4 3JH
Tel: 020 7263 3088
Tel: 0800 018 4730 (information service)
Textphone: 0800 018 9949
Email: info@dppi.org.uk (enquiries)
Web: www.deafparent.org.uk

Disabled Parents Network
DPN is an organisation run by and for disabled parents (and for disabled people thinking about becoming a parent). As well as conducting consultation and training activities, it provides information, a helpline, and on-line discussions.
81 Melton Road
West Bridgford
Nottingham NG2 8EN
Email: information@DisabledParentsNetwork.org.uk
Tel: 0870 241 0450 (helpline and information)
Web: www.DisabledParentsNetwork.org.uk

Disability, Pregnancy and Parenthood international (DPPi)
National Centre for Disabled Parents
DPPi provides information to disabled parents and to professionals. It has a wide range of resources available, including a Journal (*see* website/contact DPPi for details).
Unit F9, 89–93 Fonthill Road
London N4 3JH
Telephone, textphone and email contacts for DPPi are listed above, under DPUK
Web: www.dppi.org.uk

Parental Mental Health and Child Welfare Network
Social Care Institute for Excellence (SCIE)
This network promotes and supports joint working between adult mental health and care services.
Goldings House
2 Hay's Lane
London SE1 2HB
Email: mhnetwork@scie.org.uk
Tel: +44 (0)207 089 6840
Web: www.scie.org.uk/mhnetwork/index.asp

REFERENCES

Barnes C. (1991) *Disabled People in Britain and Discrimination*. London: Hurst and Co.

Beresford P, Wilson A. (2002) Genes spell danger: mental health service users/survivors, bioethics and control. *Disabil Soc.* **17**(5): 541–53.

Crow L. (2003) *Invisible and Centre Stage: a disabled woman's perspective on maternity services*. Paper presented at the Department of Health Open Forum Event of the Children's National Service Framework (Maternity). Available at: www.leeds.ac.uk/disability-studies/archiveuk/Crow/Invisible%20and%20centre%20stage.0302.pdf (accessed 6 Jan 2009).

Deparment for Education and Skills and Department of Health. (2004) *National Service Framework for Children, Young People and Maternity Services*. London: Department of Health.

Department of Health. (2003) *Getting the Right Start: The National Service Framework for Children, Young People and Maternity Services – emerging findings*. London: Department of Health.

House of Commons Health Committee. (2003) *Choice in Maternity Services Ninth Report of Session 2002–3 Vol 1*. London: The Stationery Office.

Kallianes V, Rubenfeld P. (1997) Disabled women and reproductive rights. *Disabil Soc.* **12**(2): 203–21.

Lewis G, Drife J, editors. (2004) *Why Mothers Die: 2000–2002*. The Sixth Report on Confidential Enquiries into Maternal Deaths in the United Kingdom. CEMACH. London: RCOG Press.

McKay-Moffat S, Cunningham S. (2006) Services for women with disabilities: mothers' and midwives' experiences. *Br J Midwif.* **14**(8): 472–7.

McKay-Moffat S. (2007) Midwives' skills, knowledge and attitudes: how they can affect maternity services. In: McKay-Moffat S, editor. *Disability in Pregnancy and Childbirth*. Edinburgh: Churchill Livingstone/Elsevier.

Morris J, Wates M. (2006) *Supporting Disabled Parents and Parents with Additional Support Needs*. Adults' Services Knowledge Review 11. London: Social Care Institute for Excellence.

Morris J, Wates M. (2007) *Working Together to Support Disabled Parents*. Adults' Services Resource Guide 9. London: Social Care Institute for Excellence.

Morris J. (2003) *The Right Support: report of the task force on supporting disabled parents in their parenting role*. York: Joseph Rowntree Foundation.

Olsen R, Clarke H. (2003) *Parenting and Disability: disabled parents' experiences of raising children*. Bristol: Policy Press.

Olsen R, Tyers H. (2004) *Think Parent: supporting disabled adults as parents*. London: National Family and Parenting Institute.

Rotherham J, McKay-Moffat S. (2007) Maternity services and women's experiences. In: McKay-Moffat S, editor. *Disability in Pregnancy and Childbirth*. Edinburgh: Churchill Livingstone/Elsevier.

Royal College of Midwives. (2000) *Maternity Care for Women with Disabilities*. Position Paper 11a (Reviewed 2005). London: The Royal College of Midwives. Available at: www.rcm.org.uk/EasySiteWeb/GatewayLink.aspx?alId=12780 (accessed 6 Jan 2009).

Royal College of Nursing. (2007) *Pregnancy and Disability: RCN guidance for midwives and nurses*. London: Royal Collge of Nursing. Available at: www.rcn.org.uk/__data/assets/pdf_file/0010/78733/003113.pdf (accessed 6 Jan 2009).

Sayce L, Perkins R. (2004) 'They should not breed': feminism, disability and reproductive rights. *Women's Global Network for Reproductive Rights – Newsletter.* **81**: 9–12.

Thomas C. (1997) The baby and the bath water: disabled women and motherhood in social context. *Sociol Health Illn.* **19**(5): 622–43.

Wates M. (1997) *Disabled Parents: dispelling the myths*. Cambridge: National Childbirth Trust.

Wates M. (2003) *It Shouldn't be Down to Luck*. London: Disabled Parents Network.

Index